ALZHEIMER'S DISEASE IN THE MIDDLE-AGED

ALZHEIMER'S DISEASE IN THE MIDDLE-AGED

HYUN SIL JEONG
EDITOR

Nova Science Publishers, Inc.
New York

LIBRARY OF CONGRESS CATALOGING-IN-PUBLICATION DATA

Alzheimer's disease in the middle-aged / Hyun Sil Jeong (editor).
     p. ;cm.
Includes bibliographical references and index.
ISBN 978-1-60456-480-8(hardcover)
1. Alzheimer's disease—Age factors. 2. Middle-aged persons—Mental health. I. Jeong,Hyun Sil
[DLMN:1. Alzhemier Disease.2.Middle Aged. WT 155 A47882 2008]
RC523.A3973 2008
616.8'31—dc22   2008005120

Published by Nova Science Publishers, Inc. ✦ *New York*

CONTENTS

PREFACE

Dementia is a brain disorder that seriously affects a person's ability to carry out daily activities. The most common form of dementia among older people is Alzheimer's disease (AD), which involves the parts of the brain that control thought, memory, and language. Age is the most important known risk factor for AD. The number of people with the disease doubles every 5 years beyond age 65. AD is a slow disease, starting with mild memory problems and ending with severe brain damage. The course the disease takes and how fast changes occur vary from person to person. On average, AD patients live from 8 to 10 years after they are diagnosed though the disease can last for as many as 20 years. Current research is aimed at understanding why AD occurs and who is at greatest risk of developing it, improving the accuracy of diagnosis and the ability to identify those at risk, discovering, developing, and testing new treatments, and discovering treatments for behavioral problems in patients with AD. This new book gathers state-of-the-art research from leading scientists throughout the world which offers important information on understanding the underlying causes and discovering the most effective treatments for Alzheimer's Disease.

Chapter 1 – There is significant research suggesting that Alzheimer's disease (AD) initially begins as a stage of cognitive decline that is referred to as mild cognitive impairment (MCI). Individuals with MCI demonstrate cognitive deficits that are in excess of normal aging, but that are not yet sufficient for the diagnosis of AD. This chapter presents a comprehensive overview of the epidemiology and current clinical criteria for MCI, how it differs from normal aging and dementia, the subtypes of MCI, and some of the recent theories about its neuropathological underpinnings. To aid in the early detection of MCI, clinicians and researchers are increasingly relying on neuropsychological assessment, genetic testing, and the use of neuroimaging. The latter includes region-of-interest (ROI) approaches on MRI, FDG-PET imaging to measure neuronal loss and neuropathological hallmarks, and FDDNP-PET imaging of amyloid and tau. This chapter also discusses the efficacy of MCI treatment and the most appropriate methods for clinical intervention. This includes discussing the current research on pharmacological, healthy lifestyle, and cognitive interventions. Because of the risk that those with MCI will progress to AD, this review may be particularly important for detecting, diagnosing, and treating cognitive difficulties in the growing number of aging individuals experiencing MCI.

In our current neuropsychiatric climate, there no longer exists a discrete dichotomy between dementia and non-dementia among older adults, but rather many shades of gray representing differing levels of memory and cognitive impairments. In response to this, there has been a relatively recent surge in geriatric research towards gaining further understanding about the early stages of dementia and the clinical phenomenon that exist prior to onset. Increased attention has been particularly devoted to a pre-diagnostic stage referred to as mild cognitive impairment (MCI), with the most recent focus on early detection, lifestyle modifications, and both pharmacological and non-pharmacological interventions for MCI. Given the growing older adult population and the rising interest in longevity, it will be critical for clinicians to be familiar with this emergent area of science. This chapter will review the most current literature on diagnostic issues in MCI, early detection of MCI via neuropsychological and biological markers, and potential biological and cognitive treatment interventions for MCI.

Chapter 2 – There is a large body of evidence which has established the neural network supporting working memory (WM). Several functional imaging studies have identified functional changes within this network in the course of physiological brain ageing. Behavioural studies have also shown that in the course of pathological cognitive decline, for example that due to Alzheimer's disease (AD), WM deficits are detectable very early and appear different from those of normal ageing. In normal ageing, WM decline may be due to slower processing, a reduced capacity for inhibition or a less highly directed attentional focus. Healthy elderly, therefore, appear to mostly use the same cognitive processes as the young, just not as effectively. In AD on the other hand, the drop in WM capacity and performance appears to be due to different causes, for example, disease related functional and anatomical impairments. WM decline also tends to be more severe in AD. These behavioural hypotheses can be tested using functional magnetic resonance imaging (fMRI) working memory paradigms.

Through fMRI, it is possible to detect abnormalities in the activation patterns of patients with AD when compared to normal ageing individuals. People that are in the preclinical stages of AD should be expected to have malformed patterns of brain activity underlying the behavioural deficits. These differences may vary from increases in activation (compensatory effects) to decreases or absences of activation in task relevant areas. Both of these effects are likely to be due to early disease related pathology and/or genetic influences. Differences should be robust in middle-aged individuals with preclinical AD, as confounds such as the physiological effects of age would not be as prominent (compared to the very elderly) and if healthy, a high level of cognitive functioning would be expected. This approach, now confined to research, might be translated into clinical application and provide a way to increase confidence in clinical diagnosis very early in the disease process.

In this chapter behavioural and functional neuroimaging studies on the effects of normal and pathological ageing on working memory will be reviewed. Original results of fMRI studies demonstrating the differences in brain activation patterns between young and elderly people and younger and older patients with AD will also be included. A prospective validation study of diagnostic techniques of this kind in individuals who experience mild cognitive impairment who have a greater risk than the normal ageing population of developing AD will also be presented.

Chapter 3 – Literature data support the notion that Alzheimer Disease (AD) patients show some sort of cognitive reserve capacity that can be exploited in cognitive training. In fact, recently some randomized controlled trial have demonstrated the efficacy of cognitive stimulation treatments in order to improve cognitive status and quality of life in people affected by dementia (Spector, 2003; Olazaran, 2004). On the other hand, in AD clinical heterogeneity is the rule, not the exception, and the disease is invariably progressive. For these reasons, cognitive rehabilitation interventions must be accurately tailored to the clinical characteristics of the patients. It must also be considered that AD affects family as well as the patient, and these interventions must take into account the needs of both patients and caregivers. Interventions must try to reduce disability, preserving residual cognitive, affective and physic abilities as long as possible. A multidimensional evaluation, taking into account residual cognitive and functional abilities, the possible presence of psychobehavioural disturbances, of associated general illnesses, and of the familiar and social support is necessary to establish reasonable goals for the cognitive rehabilitation program.

Chapter 4 – Although degenerative diseases of the central nervous system, including Alzheimer's disease (AD), have an increasingly high impact in aged population, their association with Helicobacter pylori (H. pylori) infection has not as yet been thoroughly researched. This issue has only recently been addressed by two studies. A higher seropositivity for anti-H. pylori-specific IgG antibodies was reported in AD patients than in age-matched controls. Moreover, based on the histological analysis of gastric mucosa biopsy for the documentation of current H. pylori infection, a higher rate of infection was reported in AD patients compared to anemic controls. It is thus reasonable to further investigate the role of H. pylori in AD initiation, progression or susceptibility by documenting its qualitative and quantitative presence in the cerebrospinal fluid (CSF) of these patients. A prospective, non-randomized, comparative study was carried out to investigate the levels of anti-H. pylori-specific IgG antibodies in the CSF and serum of AD patients, compared with those of age-matched cognitively normal controls. CSF and serum samples were obtained from 27 patients with AD and 27 control participants. Anti-H. pylori IgG concentrations in the CSF and the serum were measured by means of an enzyme-linked immunosorbent assay. The mean concentration of anti-H. pylori-specific IgG was significantly greater in: a) the CSF of AD patients (10.53 ± 12.54 U/mL) than in controls (8.63 ± 8.01 U/mL, $p=0.047$), and b) the serum of AD patients (30.44 ± 33.94 U/mL) than in controls (16.24 ± 5.77 U/mL, $p=0.041$). Anti-H. pylori IgG antibodies in the CSF correlated with the degree of severity of the disease. These findings further support a role for H. pylori infection in the pathobiology of AD.

Chapter 5 – In cases of late-onset Alzheimer's disease (AD), there is a spatial correlation between the classsic 'cored' type of β-amyloid (Aβ) deposit and the large vertically penetrating arterioles in the cerebral cortex suggesting that blood vessels are involved in the pathogenesis of the classic deposits. In this chapter, the spatial correlations between the diffuse, primitive, and classic Aβ deposits and blood vessels were studied in 10 cases of early-onset AD in the age range 40 – 65 years. Sections of frontal cortex were immunostained with antibodies against Aβ and with collagen IV to reveal the Aβ deposits and blood vessel profiles. In the early-onset cases as a whole, all types of Aβ deposit and blood vessel profiles were distributed in clusters. There was a positive spatial correlation between the clusters of the diffuse Aβ deposits and the larger (>10μm) and smaller diameter (<10μm) blood vessel profiles in one and three cases respectively. The primitive and classic Aβ deposits were spatially correlated with larger and smaller blood vessels both in three and four cases respectively. Spatial correlations between the Aβ deposits and blood vessels may be more prevalent in cases expressing amyloid precursor protein (APP) than presenilin 1 (PSEN1) mutations. Apolipoprotein E (Apo E) genotype of the patient did not appear to influence the spatial correlation with blood vessel profiles. The data suggest that the larger diameter blood vessels are less important in the pathogenesis of the classic Aβ deposits in early-onset compared with late-onset AD.

Chapter 6 – Passive and active Aβ immunization were tested in Alzheimer's disease (AD) murine models in an attempt to provoke immune responses geared to reducing β-amyloid aggregation and cerebral β-amyloid burden. Positive results in terms of improved behavior and reduced plaque formation were found following active and passive Aβ immunization in AD transgenic mice. Pioneering trials in moderate AD cases showed variable clinical improvement and decreased β-amyloid plaques, but maintained β-amyloid angiopathy and hyperphosphorylated tau pathology. However, the trial was stopped because of the appearance of meningoencephalitis in a subset of patients. This was due to T-cell-mediated immune responses in addition to the expected antibody-related immune response. These results have prompted the development of new approaches aimed to reducing side-effects such as encephalitis and microhemorrhages, and to optimizing immunization. Together, experimental designs have delineated Aβ immunization as a potent therapeutic tool at early stages of the disease, either administered alone, or more probably, in combination with other drugs.

Chapter 7 – A number of studies have shown that oral reading ability is relatively unimpaired in patients with Alzheimer's disease (AD). Further, oral reading ability of irregular words is known to be highly correlated to intellectual function, however, there is scant information regarding that in Japanese speaking individuals with AD. The National Adult Reading Test (NART) is a reading test of 50 irregularly spelled English words that was designed as a tool to assess premorbid intellectual function. The authors recently developed a Japanese version of the NART (Japanese Adult Reading Test, JART) that utilizes 50 Kanji (ideographic script) compound words as stimuli. In the authors' initial JART development study, Mini-Mental State Examination (MMSE) scores in a group of AD patients varied from 11 to 29, suggesting that they had a very mild to moderate level of overall cognitive impairment. In the present study, the authors investigated JART-predicted IQ results in terms of overall cognitive impairment severity as measured by the MMSE. They divided a JART-standardized AD group into 3 sub-groups based on MMSE scores, as follows: very mild AD, comprised of those with MMSE scores of 24 or greater (n=11); mild AD, comprised of those with scores between 19 and 24 (n=32); and moderate AD, comprised of those with scores lower than 19 (n=27). Normal elderly (NE) individuals, examined in the authors' previous JART development study, were utilized as the control group. Using a one-way analysis of variance (ANOVA) with a post-hoc Sheffe's test, they found that the very mild AD group had a higher level of education than the mild AD, moderate AD, and NE groups. In a comparison of the very mild AD and NE groups, the former had significantly higher JART-predicted IQ results, whereas the obtained IQ values were not significantly different. These results were considered to reflect different premorbid educational and intelligence levels. In contrast, the moderate AD group, which had the same educational level as the NE group, had lower obtained IQ values than the NE group, whereas the JART-predicted IQ results did not differ. As for the mild AD group, the JART-predicted and obtained IQ results were not significantly different from those of the NE group. However, the discrepancy between JART-predicted and obtained IQ was large in the mild AD group as compared to the NE group (9.5 vs. 0.5). These results suggest that JART-predicted IQ is valid for individuals with very mild to moderate levels of AD.

Chapter 8 – Although semantic memory impairment is well-documented in patients with Alzheimer's disease (AD), it remains unclear if this neurodegenerative disease differentially affects semantic domains. Most studies have found that AD patients show differential impairments in their knowledge for living things (e.g. animals), a minority have also reported nonliving thing deficits (e.g. tools), while some have also found no evidence of category-specific effects at all in AD patients. In a longitudinal study, the authors observed the naming performance of a group of AD patients twice across an interval of one year. They investigated whether categorical effects or intrinsic variables (such as age of acquisition, familiarity, name agreement or visual complexity of the items) have a greater impact on naming performance. They conclude that intrinsic variables are better predictors of naming performance in both, AD and healthy participants, rather than the categorical status of the items.

Chapter 9 – Distinguishing between the various degenerative dementias often poses a diagnostic dilemma for clinicians. This problem is a particular concern in the accurate assessment of the middle-aged patient. A growing body of research is establishing that nearly one quarter of degenerative dementias, particularly those with a presenile onset, can be caused by diseases variously termed Pick's disease, frontotemporal dementia, primary progressive aphasia, and semantic dementia. Thus, distinguishing these various syndromes from the more common causes of dementia, such as Alzheimer's disease, is critical for making appropriate treatment decisions and accurately communicating prognosis with patients and caregivers. Thus, this chapter reviews the literature on the various degenerative dementias that often present in middle age. This review highlights the obstacle of distinguishing these various dementias from one another using general cognitive screens and neuroimaging, particularly at the early stages of disease onset. Results from a study are then described which illustrate that category and letter fluency tasks may be more helpful in distinguishing various dementia syndromes from normal controls and from one another. These fluency tasks may outperform more general cognitive screens that are typically used to assess dementia. In summary, this chapter expands and improves upon the currently accepted methodology used in the diagnosis of dementia, particularly in the middle-aged patient.

Chapter 10 – A diagnosis of possible or probable Alzheimer's Disease has repercussions at any age, however, coping with this diagnosis at mid-life can be particularly challenging. This chapter explores the coping experiences of a middle-aged couple over a period of six months. A phenomenological hermeneutic approach to analyzing the interviews reveals the individual as well as the shared impact of the disease in their lives. Experiences with Alzheimer Disease are typically portrayed either from the caregiver's perspective or the care-recipient's perspective. This chapter focuses on the longitudinal impact of living with a diagnosis of AD from a couple's perspective. The analysis reveals the impact of the diagnostic process from both a caregiver and a care-receiver's perspective and the longer term impacts on self image, adaptation, resilience, and coping to questions about relationships with spouse and others, to care, the meaning of the disease, and existential meaning. This chapter can provide insight for couples in middle-age who are learning how to cope when one of them is diagnosed with dementia of the Alzheimer Type.

Chapter 11 – The prevalence of dementia in China, manifest as Alzheimer's disease (AD) and/or vascular dementia (VaD), is comparable to that of Western countries. Overall, AD has become the most common subtype of dementia in China, yet it is interesting to note that the diagnosis of AD is significantly lower than that of VaD, specifically in middle-aged (younger than 65) men. In this paper, the authors aim to highlight the potential causes of early onset dementia in order to emphasize the importance of improving diagnosis, treatment, and prevention of these forms of brain disease.

Epidemiological studies show the prevalence of cardiovascular diseases in middle-aged Chinese populations, especially males, has increased significantly in the past 30 years. Evidence suggests that various forms of cardiovascular disease, such as hypertension, diabetes, and cerebrovascular disease, may contribute to the development of dementia, yet there is a risk of underdiagnosis of AD in middle-aged men. Clinical physicians tend to pay much more attention to elderly, rather than middle-aged persons suffering from dementia. Also, there is greater access to computed tomography or magnetic resonance imaging for VaD (50.9%) compared to AD (6.8%). These imaging methods are sensitive to early detection of all forms of dementia. While apolipoprotein E (ApoE) remains the best-established risk factor for detecting late-onset AD, studies are progressing on finding genetic evidence for detecting early onset AD. The possibility of suffering from dementia in midlife may be increased by the vascular risk factors of dementia. It is essential that more efforts be employed to identify the genetic, biochemical, neuroimaging and clinical markers for early detection and treatment of dementia in clinical practice.

Chapter 12 – Dementia and Alzheimer's disease in particular is fast becoming a major health issue in many countries where life expectancy is increasing and chronic non-communicable diseases have replaced infectious disease as the major cause of morbidity and mortality. To date a cure for Alzheimer's disease is yet to be found and the best that can be hoped for is to slow down the progression of the disease and improve the quality of life of the individual. These temporizing measures would postpone the onset of the final and debilitating stages of the disease. Interventions may be simple but profound. For example, encouraging results have been seen in pre-morbid and affected individuals in whom an active an cognitively-stimulating lifestyle has been facilitated. With this background it is easy to appreciate the need for early detection and intervention, justifying the spirited search for biomarkers. Predicting Alzheimer's disease is problematic due to the very nature of the disorder as clinical features only become apparent following a period of insiduous but substantial cell loss. Thus there is a need for biomarkers to flag early cell death as this may allow for treatment interventions which could arrest the neuropathological processes.

There are different types of biomarkers currently under investigation: ones that can predict susceptibility for dementia, those that can be used for a diagnosis, those that can help in the follow up of the patient i.e. monitor the progression of the disease, and finally those that can be useful in prognosis. Though the vast research effort has been directed towards finding a reliable diagnostic biomarker, no candidate investigated has satisfied all the recommended criteria thus far. To this end the object of this chapter is to review prospective biomarkers for Alzheimer's Disease. The chapter will focus on, cerebrospinal fluid (CSF) and serum biomarkers, genetic indicators and imaging techniques. At the conclusion of the chapter the reader will appreciate the great challenges investigators are faced with in designing a biomarker for this complex neurodegenerative disorder. At the same time it will become apparent that even though some of the candidate biomarkers are not ideal, they may have some utility in distinguishing pathologies associated with Alzheimer's disease from those of other dementias. Finally, as suggested by this review and others- combinations of biomarkers may increase antecedent, diagnostic and prognostic capacity.

Chapter 13 – Early-onset dementia (EOD) refers to those patients with dementia onset before the age of 65 years. In most, but not all, studies the most frequent EOD of AD accounts for 20–34% of the patients, Despite a plurality of AD, the proportion of EOD patients with AD is far less than for late-onset dementia (LOD). AD accounts for about two thirds of all dementias for LOD, but only about one third of all patients with an early age of onset.

In China, there is no detailed data about the frequency of early-onset AD. The patients were very rare in clinical activity. The authors followed up a patient with early-onset AD for twenty-two months, and used diffusion tensor imaging (DTI) to study the brain of the patient to assess the progression of the disease.

Diffusion tensor imaging (DTI) is a magnetic resonance imaging (MRI) technique that can be used to characterize the orientational properties of the diffusion process of water molecules. Application of this technique to the brain has been demonstrated to provide exceptional information on white matter architecture. Usually, the information is conveyed into two types of parameters: mean diffusivity (D) which is a measure of the average molecular motion independent of any tissue directionality and is affected by cellular size and integrity, and the fractional anisotropy (FA), which is one of the most used measures of deviation from isotropy and reflects the degree of alignment of cellular structures within fiber tracts, as well as their structural integrity. There are no articles available about using DTI in a longitudinal study of AD. The authors investigated the dynamic change of the D value and FA value in the brain of this patient.

Chapter 14 – The Chronic Progressive Dementization, (CPD), the scientific name of that vulgarly called Alzheimer, is a quite different question than depression, different types of psychosis and obviously of sometimes surprising behaviors of the normal aging, and in the long run much more serious.

Although the final phase of cerebral disintegration is similar, there are two types of processes: the one that occurs in young adults or greater adults, and another different one that it happens in very greater adults, around 80 years or more. In these, at the final phase the problem it is "simply" the loss of the vital motivation, the exhaustion of desire to continue living. Abandonment of dreams, as Miguel de Unamuno would say on the cession of such dreams that Don Quixote in favor of Sancho did, and then, obviously, dying.

Persons with risk for a CPD (Alzheimer) are those that generally have an introverted personality, few and restricted social relations, with and isolation tendency, coping deficit for difficulties and losses, tendency to depend on others, to had constructed their personal identity in the shade of another one (the woman of the doctor, the husband of…) or some other equivalent transference, tendency to be obstinate to proper painful events or of the other's life, which is diagnosed in general like depression.

Then, in any way it touches to anyone.

There is nothing of chance's dependence, neither suddenly nor no magician in it. Logically with advance into years the probability that these people suffer a painful loss increases, obviously, like everybody. With its coping deficit the risk increases enormously when they have a painful loss, for example her husband who gave or lent the personal identity, or a son or daughter who gave sense to their life, of their work that justified the existence to him, of their corporal and mental capacity to which he had bet or concentrated, and when not counting on a familiar network and a social network that stopped its fall after the duel impossible to elaborate and to go on, the person collapses.

It is the beginning of the aim. It can have 40 years old (the younger case than the authors have was a woman of 38 years), or 80 years old. It does not related to aging, but only that when they advance the years is more probable that the authors suffer painful losses. Until this moment its brain is totally normal, does not show absolutely anything abnormal and is totally useless to want to see something in images or less even in electroencephalograms, that it is something so coarse and inadequate as a toad arrives of a luxurious piano of tail.

The landslide of the person, its "delivery" as much in the dictionary of the Real Spanish Academy like in the original dictionaries of all the languages, is expressed in the idea to wish to die, in the fixation of the attention in its own one and wished death. Then the abnormal thing begins, the unnatural thing, the destructive thing, because in fact we are programmed biologically, ancestrally, for all the opposite, as it is to explore, to fight, to defend to us, to hunt (in the literal sense and the symbolic sense), to attack, to ask to us, to inquire to us, and the authors' attention concentrated in each objective part of a basic alert status that we never lose, except for when we slept very well. We are not programmed to give to us tamely, as it is not it in any animal.

Chapter 15 – Despite most cases of Alzheimer's disease (AD) are sporadic, about 3-5% are inherited in an autosomal dominant fashion, and are characterized by an early onset. It has become clear from phenotypic analyses of familial AD forms versus sporadic cases that these two forms are phenotypically highly similar and often indistinguishable, except for the earlier age at onset. Autosomal dominant forms are characterized by mutations in three genes: Amyloid β precursor protein (β-APP), Presenilin 1(PSEN1) and Presenilin 2 (PSEN2) genes. The mutations in Amyloid Precursor Protein (APP) occur at its cleavage sites, thus altering APP processing such that more pathogenetic Aβ42 peptide is produced. PSEN1 and PSEN2 represent a central component of γ-secretase, the enzyme responsible for liberating the C-terminal fragment of APP. Mutations in presenilins also alter APP, leading to an increased production of Aβ42. Another degenerative dementia with an onset about 50-60 years is Frontotemporal Lobar Degeneration (FTLD). In 1994 an autosomal dominantly inherited form of Frontotemporal Dementia (FTD) with parkinsonism was linked to chromosome 17q21.2. Subsequently, other familial forms of FTD were found to be linked to the same region, resulting in the denomination "frontotemporal dementia and parkinsonism linked to chromosome 17" (FTDP-17) for this class of diseases. All cases of FTDP-17 have so far shown a filamentous pathology made of hyperphosphorylated tau protein. Although many FTD families exhibit MAPT mutations, in some cases these mutations did not occur suggesting that other, related genes on chromosome 17 also cause FTD in an autosomal-dominant manner. Subsequently, region within the 3.53 centimorgan critical region defined by haplotype analysis in reported families was examined. Several pathogenic mutations were therefore found in progranulin gene (PGRN), harbouring a new causative gene in FTLD pathology. PGRN is a widely expressed growth factor, which plays a role in multiple processes including development, wound repair and inflammation by activating signalling cascades that control cell cycle progression and cell motility. Its role in neurodegeneration is at present under investigation.

As regards sporadic forms, genetic factors play a role in determining the age at disease onset. The gene mainly related to the sporadic forms of AD is APOE, which is located in chromosome 19 and was initially identified in 1991 as a risk factor for AD. In addition, the APOE 4/4 genotype seems to correlate with an earlier onset of the disease.

In this chapter, these genetic studies recently carried out will be described and discussed in detail.

Chapter 16 – The authors evaluated, from April 2001 to March 2007, the sensitivity and specificity of their French version of the Addenbrooke's Cognitive Examination (ACE), to detect dementia in the less than 66 year-old patient's population attending their outpatient's memory clinic. Validation of the French ACE has already been published but not assessed specifically on younger patients. The 149 included subjects had at least six months of follow-up. The diagnosis of a specific dementing illness was based on the consensus of the neurologist and neuropsychologists in the team. In this population of young patients, the sensitivity for diagnosing dementia with an MMSE score $\leq 24/30$ was 59,5 %. The sensitivity of an MMSE score $\leq 27/30$ was 83,8 % with a specificity of 88,6 %. The sensitivity of an ACE score $\leq 83/100$ was 86,5 % with a specificity of 86 %, and the sensitivity of an ACE score $\leq 88/100$ was 94,6 % with a specificity of 74,6 %. Three hundred thirty-nine patients older than 66 year-old were then selected identically. In this older population, the sensitivity for diagnosing dementia with an MMSE score $\leq 24/30$ was 40,2 % while the sensitivity of an MMSE score $\leq 27/30$ was 67,1 % with a specificity of 73,9 %. The sensitivity of an ACE score $\leq 83/100$ was 84,6 % with a specificity of 73 %, and the sensitivity of an ACE score $\leq 88/100$ was 94,4 % with a specificity of 47,8 %. The authors conclude that the French version of the ACE remains a very accurate test for the detection of dementia in the youngest but that its benefit in comparison to MMSE is more intense in the older population.

In: Alzheimer's Disease in the Middle-Aged
Editor: Hyun Sil Jeong, pp. 1-66

ISBN: 978-1-60456-480-8
© 2008 Nova Science Publishers, Inc.

Chapter 1

MILD COGNITIVE IMPAIRMENT: CURRENT TRENDS FOR EARLY DETECTION AND TREATMENT

Jena Kravitz[*1], *Jeanne Kim*[*2], *Achinoam Faust-Socher*[*3], *Steven Rogers*[*4] *and Karen Miller*[*5]

[1] UCLA Semel Institute; Aging and Memory Research Center;
[2] UCLA-Semel Institute, Suite 88-201; Los Angeles, CA 90024;
[3] UCLA-Semel Institute, Suite 88-201;Los Angeles, CA 90024;
[4] Westmont College; 955 La Paz Road; Santa Barbara, CA 93108;
[5] UCLA-Semel Institute, Suite 88-201; Los Angeles, CA 90024

ABSTRACT

There is significant research suggesting that Alzheimer's disease (AD) initially begins as a stage of cognitive decline that is referred to as mild cognitive impairment (MCI). Individuals with MCI demonstrate cognitive deficits that are in excess of normal aging, but that are not yet sufficient for the diagnosis of AD. This chapter presents a comprehensive overview of the epidemiology and current clinical criteria for MCI, how it differs from normal aging and dementia, the subtypes of MCI, and some of the recent theories about its neuropathological underpinnings. To aid in the early detection of MCI, clinicians and researchers are increasingly relying on neuropsychological assessment, genetic testing, and the use of neuroimaging. The latter includes region-of-interest (ROI) approaches on MRI, FDG-PET imaging to measure neuronal loss and neuropathological hallmarks, and FDDNP-PET imaging of amyloid and tau. This chapter also discusses the efficacy of MCI treatment and the most appropriate methods for clinical intervention. This includes discussing the current research on pharmacological, healthy lifestyle, and cognitive interventions. Because of the risk that those with MCI will progress to AD, this

[*] jenakravitz@yahoo.com
[*] jeannekim@mednet.ucla.edu
[*] achinoam.socher@gmail.com
[*] sarogers@westmont.edu
[*] kmiller@mednet.ucla.edu

review may be particularly important for detecting, diagnosing, and treating cognitive difficulties in the growing number of aging individuals experiencing MCI.

In our current neuropsychiatric climate, there no longer exists a discrete dichotomy between dementia and non-dementia among older adults, but rather many shades of gray representing differing levels of memory and cognitive impairments. In response to this, there has been a relatively recent surge in geriatric research towards gaining further understanding about the early stages of dementia and the clinical phenomenon that exist prior to onset. Increased attention has been particularly devoted to a pre-diagnostic stage referred to as mild cognitive impairment (MCI), with the most recent focus on early detection, lifestyle modifications, and both pharmacological and non-pharmacological interventions for MCI. Given the growing older adult population and the rising interest in longevity, it will be critical for clinicians to be familiar with this emergent area of science. This chapter will review the most current literature on diagnostic issues in MCI, early detection of MCI via neuropsychological and biological markers, and potential biological and cognitive treatment interventions for MCI.

NORMAL AND PATHOLOGICAL AGING

Normal Aging

To understand MCI, it may help to start with a quick review of the cognitive changes that accompany normal aging. As with all aspects of MCI, normal aging is not a homogeneous concept. Any attempt at defining normal aging requires the consideration of a vastly large group of characteristics that span across decades of cognitive, psychological, and physical changes, which only increase with age (Anstey and Low, 2004; Christensen, 2001; Christensen et al., 1999; Ylikoski et al., 1999). Normal aging is best explained in terms of generalities, so that comparisons can be made when individuals sense that they are not keeping pace with their peer group. A common complaint attributed to aging is a decline in memory. Reviews have suggested that memory disturbances occur in 22-56% of community-dwelling older adults (Drachman, 2006), with declines becoming most evident after age 40 (Corral et al., 2006; Schaie, 1994). Specifically, changes occur in working memory, recent long-term memory, episodic long-term memory, encoding and retrieval, and prospective memory, with the greatest compromise in the manipulation and learning of new information (Rogers et al., 2007). On the other hand, remote long-term memory, semantic memory, and procedural memory remain relatively intact; these abilities are generally automatic and may require less effort to recall (Rogers et al., 2007). A second area of cognitive complaint among those with normal aging is a decline in the speed of information processing and reaction time. These declines appear as early as 30 years (Corral et al., 2006), with a 20% drop by 40 years, and a 40-60% drop by 80 years (Christensen, 2001). However, immediate and simple attention for conversations and tasks remain relatively intact (Salthouse and Babock, 1991; Sliwinski and Buschke, 1999). A third area of decline is in executive functioning, which begins around age 40 (Corral et al., 2006; Gunstad and Brickman, 2006). Executive skills that involve divided attention, inhibition, set shifting, and inability to discriminate relevant from irrelevant information have been found to be affected by age (Lezak, Howieson, and Loring, 2004). In contrast, some forms of abstract verbal reasoning and nonverbal problem-solving can remain relatively preserved with age, particularly if the task is simpler and practiced

(Lezak et al., 2004; Royall et al., 2005). Overall, the ability to acquire new concepts and adapt to new situations appears more vulnerable to decline (fluid intelligence), while accumulated knowledge and expertise remains relatively stable (crystallized intelligence) (Anstey and Low, 2004).

Neurophysiological and neuroanatomical changes observed in normal agers are also widely heterogeneous and somewhat coincide with functional changes, although this not uniformly true. The average brain weight declines by about 2-3% per decade after 50 years, with a 10% loss by age 80 relative to young adults (Drachman, 2006). On average, cortical atrophy provides for a 4.25% annual rate of ventricular expansion (Guttman et al., 1998; Raz and Rodrigue, 2006). Areas most vulnerable to atrophy are the hippocampus, anterior dorsal frontal lobe, and select subcortical structures, such as the thalamus and basal ganglia (Lezak et al., 2004), as well as shrinkage of cortical white matter (Jernigan et al., 1991). On a cellular level, senile plaques and neurofibrillary tangles accumulate and result in neuronal loss (Guttman et al., 1998; Jernigan et al., 1991). Reduced metabolic activity has been found in certain areas, such as the prefrontal and temporal lobes (Krausz et al., 1998), along with the slowing of background alpha-rhythms, also in the temporal regions (Babiloni et al., 2006). In general, the aging brain appears to follow a pattern of loss proceeding from anterior to posterior regions on both the macro- and micro-levels (Rogers et al., 2007).

Table 1. Clinical terms and timeline for cognitive impairment without dementia (Mariani, et al., 2007; DeCarli, 2003; Panza, et al., 2005)

Term	Initial description	Year	Diagnostic criteria
Benighn Senescent Forgetfulness (BSF)	Kral	1962	Stable, nondisabling memory deficit with inability to recall data and parts of experiences like name, date, place.
Mild cognitive decline and mild cognitive impairment (MCI)	Reisberg, et al.	1982	Global Deterioration Scale (GDS) score of 3.
Limited cognitive disturbance	Gurland, et al.	1982	Comprehensive Assessment and Referral Evaluation (CARE)
Age-associated memory impairment (AAMI)	Crook, et al.	1986	Subjective memory impairment with objective memory impairment compared with that of a young adult
Minimal dementia	Roth, et al.	1986	Cambridge Mental Disorders of the Elderly Examination (CAMDEX)
Late-life forgetfulness (LLF)	Blackford and LaRue	1989	Age-associated memory impairment plus age-adjusted deficits in four or more specific cognitive tests
Mild Cognitive Impairment (MCI)	Zaudig	1992	MCI refined and based on DSM-III-R and ICD-10 criteria.
Mild cognitive decline (MCD)	ICD-10	1993	Impairments in cognitive tests of learning, memory, or concentration secondary to defined illness
Possible dementia prodrome (PDP) or quetionable dementia	Morris, et al.	1993	Scoring 0.5 on Clinical Dementia Rating scale by Consortium for the Establishment of Registries in Alzheimer's Disease (CERAD)

Table 1.(Continued)

Term	Initial description	Year	Diagnostic criteria
Ageing-associated cognitive decline (AACD)	Levy	1994	Age-adjusted impairment on any cognitive task
Mild neurocognitive decline and Age-related Cognitive Decline (ARCD)	DSM-IV	1994	Impairments in memory, learning, perceptual-motor, linguistic, or executive functioning
Cognitive impairment-no dementia (CIND)	Graham, et al.	1997	Impairments in memory, learning, perceptual-motor, linguistic, or executive functioning in the absence of clinically defined dementia
Mild Cognitive dysfunction (MCD)	Johansson and Zarit	1997	Dysfunction according to five cognitive tests
Mild Cognitive Impairment (MCI)	Petersen, et al.	1999 and 2001	Subjective complaint of memory impairment with objective memory impairment adjusted for age and education in the absence of dementia. The definition was then expanded to include four clinical MCI subtypes.
Subclinical cognitive impairment	Ritchie, et al.	2000	Scoring below a specific score on the Deterioration Cognitive Observee, a test sensitive to early change in cognitive functioning.
Cognitive impairment, no dementia (CIND)	DeRonchi, et al.	2005	Scoring 2 or more SD below the mean score of MMSE, corrected for age and education, calculated among the non-demented people.
Mild Cognitive Impairment (MCI)	Portet, et al.	2006	New diagnostic procedure for MCI by MCI Working Group of the Eropean Consortium on Alzheimer's Disease

Diagnostic Criteria for Mild Cognitive Impairment

As shown in Table 1, there have been many names and definitions proposed for progressive cognitive decline in the absence of dementia. In recent years, investigators have struggled to define the nebulous juncture between normal aging and dementia. Currently, the criteria of Petersen and colleagues (1999, 2001) are the most widely used in operationalizing clinical standards for diagnosis. Although these have not been established as standards set by a professional body, there is general consensus that the following criteria must be met for a diagnosis of Mild Cognitive Impairment (MCI):

1) cognitive complaint (usually memory), preferably corroborated by an informant;
2) cognitive impairment (usually memory) for age and education
3) essentially normal general cognitive function

4) largely preserved activities of daily living
5) absence of dementia

These are criteria are based solely on clinical evaluation. An MCI diagnosis cannot be made without clinical judgment (Kelley and Petersen, 2007).

The first criterion is an individual's complaint of mild cognitive symptoms. If possible, corroboration should be obtained by an informant, who can validate the concern and may be more reliable. Interviewing someone close to the individual often provides the only clue to deficits that may be more subtle (Rosenberg et al., 2006). The second criterion requires data collection through neuropsychological test results, utilizing normative data matched to the individual's age and education. Cognitive deficits in any domain would satisfy this requirement, although memory deficits are most common (Petersen, 2004). Kelley and Petersen (2007) warn against using neuropsychological tests alone to establish a case for MCI, since all the criteria mentioned above should inform the diagnosis. They suggest that arbitrary neuropsychological cut-offs without considering all the criteria eliminate the reliable and predictive value of an MCI diagnosis. There is considerable variance in the use of neuropsychological tests for diagnosis due to a lack of consensus on the types and number of cognitive tests to use, as well as the particular thresholds to consider (Mariani et al., 2007), not to mention measurement errors, lack of appropriate norms, and differences in sensitivity and specificity. Petersen and colleagues (1999) initially suggested a guideline of 1.5 standard deviations (SD) below age-matched norms, but specific tests of delayed recall, executive functions, and selective attention have been found to better predict the conversion of MCI to dementia, although even these usually have a sensitivity and specificity lower than 70% (Mariani et al., 2007). Therefore, 1.5 SD should only be used as a guideline and not a cut-off for diagnosing MCI. In fact, individuals who have declined from their higher pre-morbid functioning may be appropriate for an MCI diagnosis even if their test scores fall within normal range for the general population (Kelley and Petersen, 2007). It may be more effective to ascertain cognitive status by longitudinally following cognitive performance over time (e.g., 6 months to 2 years) (Collie et al., 2002; Portet et al., 2006).

The third criterion is that gross cognitive functioning is generally intact, not discounting the aforementioned cognitive complaints. Subtle deficits may emerge on closer inspection, but these cannot be of sufficient severity to suggest dementia or significant interference with daily functioning (Kelley and Petersen, 2007). Petersen and colleagues require this judgment to be clinical, as there are no standard ways of determining this.

The fourth criterion is intact activities of daily living (ADL). Again, there are no objective criteria to measure this. The International Working Group on Mild Cognitive Impairment (Winblad et al., 2004) suggests that basic ADL's are typically preserved, but there may be minimal impairment in instrumental ADL's (IADL). One study showed more IADL impairment in MCI individuals than in controls for tasks such as shopping, self-administration of drugs, and handling economic decisions (Bennett et al., 2006). The limitations were in everyday tasks that involved memory or complex reasoning, but their basic ADLs were normal. It was found that the inclusion of IADL restriction improved the prediction of dementia, as well as the stability of the MCI condition over time (Bennett et al., 2006; Perneczky et al., 2006). The fifth and final criterion is the absence of overt or probably dementia, as typically indicated by a generally intact Mini-Mental Status Examination (MMSE).

Recently, new diagnostic criteria have emerged from the European Consortium on Alzheimer's Disease Working Group on MCI (Portet et al., 2006). These criteria also emphasize the importance of the clinical evaluation, combining neuropsychological data and a family interview. The criteria include:

(1) cognitive complaints from patients or their families,
(2) the report by a patient or informant of a decline in cognitive functioning relative to previous abilities during the past year,
(3) cognitive disorders as evidenced by clinical evaluation (impairment in memory or in another cognitive domain)
(4) absence of major repercussions in daily life (the patient may, however, report difficulties concerning complex day-to-day activities)
(5) absence of dementia.

The European Consortium also emphasizes other features. They no longer focus exclusively on the domain of memory, and clinical impressions are given greater weight because longitudinal studies have shown that clinicians' judgments are surprisingly valid, accurate, and predictive of diagnosis (Tschanz et al., 2006). The individual's cognitive complaint is also seen as both quantitative and qualitative. They also emphasize difficulties with complex day-to-day activities or IADL's. Moreover, the group advocates the administration of questionnaires about function in the past year or repeated neuropsychological batteries at six months. They state that none of the tests are obligatory and that a cut-off is not used. The International Working Group on Mild Cognitive Impairment (Winblad et al., 2004) formulated similar recommendations that emphasize: (1) the individual is neither normal nor demented; (2) the presence of cognitive decline as shown by objective measures, or by self-report or informant in conjunction with objective measures; (3) ADLs are preserved and complex IADLs are intact or minimally impaired.

Subtypes of MCI

MCI is divided into four subtypes that depend on the number of domains affected and whether there are deficits in memory: (1) amnestic, single domain; (2) amnestic, multiple domain; (3) non-amnestic, single domain; (4) non-amnestic, multiple domain (Kelley and Petersen, 2007). The overall subtypes have only been validated in one epidemiological study to date (Busse et al., 2003), but these distinctions are critical since studies have found that amnestic types have an increased rate of progression to clinically probable Alzheimer's disease (AD) (Petersen et al., 2001). This progression of amnestic subtype to AD has been the most investigated and validated, though with varying rates (Grundman et al., 2004; Luis et al., 2003; Petersen et al., 1999). There are mixed results on what type of MCI leads to what type of dementia (Kelley and Petersen, 2007), some of which is likely owing to the diverse etiology of MCI, which can be degenerative, vascular, psychiatric, traumatic, or secondary to a medical condition. Intuition suggests that amnestic subtypes progress to AD and non-amnestic types progress to other dementias such as frontotemporal and Lewy body dementia, but the research is not yet definitive on the conversion of non-amnestic types of MCI (Kelley and Petersen, 2007). There have also been proposed subtypes of MCI based on clinical categories of dementia (e.g., MCI-AD, vascular MCI, MCI-Parkinson's disease) (Luis et al., 2003). For example, single non-amnestic MCI individuals have been found to have higher prevalence of ischemic heart disease and transient ischemic attacks/stroke, higher Hachinski ischemic score, and higher prevalence of white matter lesions on computer tomography/ magnetic resonance imaging scans when compared to amnestic MCI (Mariani et al., 2007). However, the utility of these more refined subtypes is questionable because it is unclear whether this vascular subtype profile progresses to vascular dementia.

Epidemiology of MCI

Most of the variability in the epidemiological descriptions of this population is likely due to varying definitions of MCI rather than varied characteristics of studied populations. Depending on the study, the prevalence of MCI and its subtypes range from 2-53% for people over 60 years old (DeCarli, 2003; Panza et al., 2005). The incidence rate is also varied with a range of 8-77 per 1000 people over 60 (Panza et al., 2005). It also depends on the type of population or sample selected. Progression to dementia is higher in clinic-based studies, ranging from 10-15%, and lower in population-based studies, ranging from 5-10% (Bruscoli and Lovestone, 2004; Marianai 2007). It has been suggested that since community participants are volunteers and thus self-selected, the true rate of conversion is likely even lower (Bruscoli and Lovestone, 2004). In fact, the conversion rate for community clinics is roughly twice that of the general population. Some suggest that people seeking help for memory problems have a high risk for dementia, confirming that the subjective memory complaint criteria is one of the strongest predictors of dementia (Jonker et al., 2000). Another reason for the heterogeneity in epidemiology is that earlier studies were based on a stringent definition of MCI, which mostly consisted of the amnestic subtype versus a more general definition of MCI in current studies (Portet et al., 2006). Many of these studies also do not take into consideration that MCI can remain stable or even reverse, with a 20-25% rate of reversion from MCI to normal (Panza et al., 2005).

One generally consistent finding is that amnestic and multiple domain subtypes have a high likelihood of progression to AD. The annual rate of conversion for amnestic MCI to AD generally ranges from 2-31% per year (Bruscoli and Lovestone, 2004), which is considerably higher than the conversion rate of 1-2% per year for age-matched non-MCI individuals (Bennett et al., 2005). One study showed that 75% of those previously diagnosed with MCI went on to develop AD, but the other 25% developed other dementias (Jicha et al., 2006). Although amnestic MCI is generally predictive of AD, this does not occur in all cases (Kelley and Petersen, 2007). Individuals with non-memory forms of MCI are assumed to convert more frequently to non-AD dementia, but this remains uncertain. Amnestic subtypes have converted to both AD and non-AD dementias, and many individuals have developed AD from non-amnestic MCI (Mariani et al., 2007). This again demonstrates the low positive predictive value of the subtypes, which restricts their clinical significance (Fisk et al., 2003). Even the diagnostic accuracy of MCI criteria used in drug trials was shown to be low to moderate (Visser et al., 2005). This has led Petersen's criteria to be criticized for not allowing homogeneous populations to be defined, both in terms of the subtypes of MCI and their mode of progression (Portet et al., 2006).

Moderating Variables

It is important to note, however, there is considerable heterogeneity in the symptoms of those in the preclinical or early stages of MCI. Age is certainly one of the biggest moderating variables, with greater heterogeneity in cognitive performance associated with advancing age. As mentioned previously, there are some common trends for age-related declines in memory, processing speed, and executive functioning, but relative to their younger counterparts, older adults experience greater cognitive variability with age (Anstey and Low, 2004; Christensen, 2001; Christensen et al., 1999; Ylikoski et al., 1999). In fact, both age and race have been found to be significant predictors of memory performance, even after factoring for education, depression, gender, and memory complaints. In one study on ethnic differences in memory performance (McDougall et al., 2007), 44% of African Americans and only 25% of Caucasian Americans had moderate to serious memory impairments. Overall, the African American group, who had lower educational attainment with lower baseline cognition and memory performance, was more was more likely to have impaired memory performance. Similarly, a comparison of American and Chinese populations showed that despite their lower educational level, Chinese participants with MCI were 1.7 times *less* likely to progress to AD and 2.3 times *more* likely to progress to vascular dementia within three years of diagnosis (Xu et al., 2004). The data suggest that progression rates from MCI to dementia may vary considerably between countries and ethnicities.

Many medical conditions also convey greater risk for MCI, particularly those conditions associated with risk for cardiovascular disease. Hypertension, hyperlipidemia, diabetes, and depression are all risk factors for impaired cognition in later life and in MCI (Verhaeghen, Borchelt, and Smith, 2003). In particular, high blood pressure potentiates the effects of aging on brain structure, including exacerbating white matter abnormalities, hippocampal atrophy, and both anterior and posterior changes (Raz and Rodrigue, 2006). Hyperlipidemia, which is particularly elevated by a diet high in low-density lipoprotein, increases cerebral atrophy and beta-amyloid deposition in the brain (Fillit et al., 2002). Both hyperglycemia and hypoglycemia are associated with impaired cognitive function, and the deleterious effects of depression on cognitive function are evident in the finding that it is the most common cause of reversible cognitive impairment in older adults (Fillit et al., 2002). Moreover, maintaining an active physical and cognitive lifestyle that ensures physical exercise, avoids vitamin deficiencies, and maintains cognitive vitality may reverse or slow the cognitive declines of MCI (Andel, Hughes, and Crowe, 2005; O'Hara et al., 2007; Small et al., 2006; Willis et al., 2006), including improving cognitive speed and executive control. Even playing board games and reading can lower one's risk for cognitive impairment (Wang et al., 2006). Granted, even healthy elderly adults will show age-related cognitive decline on some measures (Lezak et al., 2004) but controlling and treating these medical conditions, particularly those related to cardiovascular integrity, may slow rate or decrease their vulnerability to mild cognitive impairment.

Another factor that seems to influence heterogeneity in mild cognitive impairment is the educational differences between older adults. Advanced education may have a protective effect against cognitive decline. Some have suggested that this protection is restricted to crystallized intelligence, memory, and gross cognitive functioning (MMSE) (Christensen, 2001), but regardless of domain, there are generally faster rates of decline among those with less education. Education may convey more protection against MCI because it provides more cognitive reserve, which generally refers to the brain's ability to effectively use or recruit alternative networks and rely on different cognitive strategies when necessary. Among the areas that contribute to cognitive reserve are education and skills involving intensive, well-designed practice, which preserve regions that would otherwise undergo decline in mild cognitive impairment. This preservation may occur due to brain plasticity, the effects of education and experience on synaptic density, or the faster cognitive development and lifelong mental stimulation associated with the effects of education. Perhaps this explains why those with greater education perform better on tests of attention, memory, and global functioning, whereas low education may reduce the margin of intellectual reserve (Ardila, Ostrosky-Solis, Rosselli, and Gomez, 2000).

EARLY DETECTION AND IDENTIFICATION OF MCI

Despite some of the putative problems with the diagnosis of MCI, converging lines of evidence are showing that it has considerable value as both an independent diagnostic entity and as a potential harbinger of incipient dementia. This has contributed to increased interest in understanding, detecting, and identifying MCI in its earliest stages, when intervention and prediction might be most valuable for those who are either recently diagnosed or at risk for developing it. In an attempt to identify risk factors and early clinical features of MCI, researchers have uncovered several preclinical markers and prodromal symptoms.

Neuropsychological Markers

Among these markers are distinct, albeit subtle, cognitive deficits that appear before the complete, clinical symptoms of MCI emerge. Considering that MCI is largely a neuropsychological diagnosis, it is not surprising that cognitive symptoms are among the earliest symptoms (Morris et al., 2001). The exact profile of cognitive difficulties in the early or preclinical stages of MCI likely depends on the subtype of MCI in question (e.g., amnestic versus non-amnestic MCI), but much of the emerging research suggests that standard neuropsychological measures in multiple domains demonstrate strong sensitivity to the detection of cognitive dysfunction in the early stages of MCI. For example, there appears to be overall global deficits (Backman Jones, Small, Aguero-Torres, and Fratiglionni, 2003), progressive and profound impairment in episodic memory (Almkvist and Winblad, 1999; Amieva et al., 2005; Arnaiz and Almkvist, 2003; Blackwell et al., 2004), and deficits in executive abilities (Albert, Blacker, Moss, Tanzi, and McArdle, 2007; Bellevielle, Chertkow, and Gauthier, 2007; Chen et al., 2000, 2001; Saxton et al., 2004; Silveri, Reali, Jenner, and Puopolo, 2007), that are manifestations of incipient MCI. According to a recent meta-analysis of 47 studies, certain cognitive areas may be differentially affected, with the greatest deficits in verbal memory, executive functioning, and perceptual speed, followed by more moderate difficulties in language, visuospatial functioning, and attention (Backman, Jones, Berger, Laukka, and Small, 2004, 2005). There is even some research suggesting that subtle asymmetric cognitive changes may characterize the neuropsychological profile of those in the preclinical stages of MCI. Imaging studies have revealed a higher incidence of asymmetric structural and metabolic changes in at-risk individuals (Bigler et al., 2002), with atypical asymmetries in medial temporal and parietal regions for those at risk (Reiman et al., 1996; Small et al., 1995). These asymmetries may be the prelude to the larger lateralized cognitive deficits between verbal and nonverbal test scores seen among those with AD (Bugiani, Constantinidis, Ghetti, Bouras, and Tagliavine, 1991).

The actual course and progression of this prodromal cognitive dysfunction can vary, depending on the subtype of MCI (Busse, Hensel, Guhne, Angermeyer, and Riedel-Heller, 2006). Cognitive decrements have been discovered three to nine years (Backman et al., 2003; Small et al., 2000; Saxton et al., 2004; Amieva et al., 2005) prior to the clinical diagnosis of AD. This suggests that the course from normal aging to MCI and dementia can be extensive. Typically, the deficits associated with MCI remain relatively stable and plateau until three to six years prior to diagnosis of dementia, after which individuals undergo a precipitous decline in global cognitive functioning, memory, and executive functioning, that ends with diagnosis of dementia (Amieva et al., 2005; Backman et al., 2003, 2005; Caselli et al., 2004; Cerhan et al., 2007; Fabrigoule et al., 1998; Fox, Warrington, Seiffer, Agnew, and Rosser, 1998; Galvin et al., 2005; Small et al., 2000; Smith, Pankratz et al., 2007). At each stage, neuropsychological measures of multiple cognitive domains can be useful for differentiating between normal aging and the prodromal phase of MCI.

Neuropathology

There is little data regarding the neuropathology of MCI versus dementia. In the case of Alzheimer's disease, the typical neuropathology involves senile plaques of beta-amyloid proteins and neurofibrillary tangles (NFT) from hyperphosphorylated tau proteins. Any lesions of this type would support the hypothesis that MCI is a prodromal stage for AD. One study showed more than half of those with MCI met the National Institute on Aging-Reagan criteria for AD, and a third also had cerebral infarcts, suggesting that both neurodegenerative and vascular features may account for the clinical picture of MCI (Bennet et al., 2005). Another study found that those with amnestic MCI did not completely fulfill the neuropathic criteria for AD, but still appeared to be in a transitional state towards AD (Petersen et al., 2006). The patients had argyrophilic grain disease, hippocampal sclerosis, and vascular lesions, in addition to the hallmark AD signs of plaques diffusely in the neocortex and tangles in medial temporal lobe structures. This is consistent with the findings of Markesbery and colleagues (2006), who suggest that neurofibrillary tangles are more prominent in MCI and peak in individuals with early AD, whereas amyloid deposits accumulate at their peak in the later stages of dementia. Furthermore, in an autopsy study, individuals classified as MCI were more similar in terms of neuritic plaques to early AD than normal controls (Riley et al., 2002).

In similar fashion, the brains of those in the early or preclinical stages of MCI undergo changes in hypometabolism and volume. Interestingly, those in the preclinical stage present with mild atrophy and hypometabolism in the brain regions typically affected in clinical AD, namely atrophy of the medial temporal lobes and hippocampus, as well as hypoperfusion in bilateral parietotemporal, frontal, and posterior cingulate areas (Almkvist and Winblad, 1999; Chong and Sahadevan, 2005; Herholz et al., 2002). A review of 91 imaging studies suggested that the most common findings were temporal lobe changes, particularly in the entorhinal cortex and hippocampus, followed by changes in the parietal and frontal lobes (Twamley et al., 2006). Others have also found global cerebral atrophy and ventricular enlargement (Adak et al, 2004; Chong and Sahadevan, 2005), medial temporal lobe atrophy and hypometabolism (Bouwman et al., 2007; Mosconi et al., 2006, 2007); and decreased volumes in the entorhinal cortex and hippocampus (Chong and Sahadevan, 2005; Convit et al., 1997; Smith et al., 2007). As this suggests, parietal and frontal alterations are common among those in the early or preclinical stages of MCI, but the medial temporal lobe experiences the greatest change, with some research even suggesting a loss of 14% of the volume in the hippocampus relative to normal controls not at risk for MCI (Convit et al., 1997; Smith et al., 2007).

Neuroimaging for Detection

Despite this heterogeneity, several useful adjuncts to neuropsychological testing have been used for detecting these early or preclinical stages of MCI. Magnetic resonance imaging (MRI) can measure the volumes of specific brain structures and thereby distinguish normal aging from MCI and AD. Many of those using MRI techniques rely on the region-of-interest (ROI) approach to measure volumes of the medial temporal lobe as a means to estimate neuronal loss. Typically, this is a standardized manual method that involves drawing regions of interest on MRI images by outlining the desired structures, such as the temporal lobes, and then excluding the pixels that fall within a predetermined threshold. The volumes of the temporal lobe structures are then estimated from the pixel counts over the slices chosen for these measurements. One of the benefits of this approach is the ability to discern the level of neuronal loss secondary to volume reductions and atrophy. However, this comes at the cost of intensive preprocessing labor, specifically dedicated software, and the intense training and inter-rater reliability needed for ROI analysis.

Structurally, MRI studies suggest atrophy of the entorhinal and hippocampo-amygdala regions that are intermediate between normal aging and AD (Schott et al., 2006). The rate of medial temporal lobe atrophy was shown to be the most significant predictor of conversion from normal aging to MCI, with 91% specificity and 85% sensitivity (Rusinek et al., 2003). Some of this atrophy may be related to a disruption of parahippocampal white matter fibers, which partially disconnect the hippocampus from incoming sensory information (Stoub et al., 2006). This mesial temporal and cortical volume loss occurs in both amnestic and multiple domain MCI, but the amnestic subtype has more severe involvement of the mesial temporal structures and less of the neocortical heteromodal association cortices than the multiple domain types (Bell-McGinty et al., 2005).

An alternative to this ROI approach has been positron emission tomography (PET) using the F-fluorodeoxyglucose (FDG) ligid. Similar to the ROI approach on MRI, FDG-PET can measure the extent of neuronal loss among those in the early or preclinical stages of MCI, but its particular method of action involves measuring changes in brain metabolism. Specifically, it estimates local cerebral metabolic rates of glucose consumption, providing information on the distribution of neuronal death and synapse dysfunction in vivo (Mosconi, 2005). In fact, Silverman et al. (2001) found 93% sensitivity and 76% specificity for distinguishing between normal aging, MCI, and AD using FDG-PET. Measurement of medial temporal lobe metabolism alone provides 74% accuracy in distinguishing between normal controls and MCI (Mosconi et al., 2006). PET studies have also found that the use of PET to detect reduced glucose metabolism in the hippocampus significantly improves diagnostic accuracy for MCI relative to the use of MRI (85% versus 73%) (De Santi et al., 2001). Furthermore, de Leon and colleagues (2001) found significantly lower brain glucose metabolism in MCI relative to controls in the entorhinal cortex (17%), hippocampus (7%) lateral temporal oboe (8%), and dorsolateral frontal cortex (10%). These enabled prediction of decline from normal aging to MCI with 84% accuracy, which illustrates the improved accuracy of FDG-PET over MRI methodology.

A more recent PET approach is the in vivo imaging of amyloid plaques using FDDNP, a highly lipophilic fluorescent molecule recently developed at UCLA (Small et al., 2006). Before this approach, it was thought that plaques and tangles could only be clearly assessed at autopsy or biopsy, but FDDNP is a distinct radioactively labeled marker of cerebral amyloid and tau proteins. Due to its high lipophilicity, it readily crosses the blood-brain barrier, and its method of action involves targeting the Aβ1-40 fibril, which is an Aβ peptide produced from the cleavage of amyloid precursor protein. Aβ1-40 seems to show a particular affinity toward aggregation in the form of plaques and tangles (Sair, Doraiswamy, and Petrella, 2004), so FDDNP specifically labels plaques, and to lesser extent, NFTs in brain slices. Recent research shows that this method correlates well with MMSE scores, as well as FDG-PET and MRI findings, with areas of greater binding corresponding to areas of decreased glucose metabolism and atrophy (Sair et al., 2004). There is even superior binding for FDDNP relative to FDG in the temporal, parietal, and frontal regions of those with MCI, suggesting that FDDNP can distinguish between AD, MCI, and normal aging (Small et al., 2006). However, more research needs to be done to appreciate the full extent of its ability to detect the preclinical stages of MCI.

Biomarkers

There are also some particular biomarkers that have been implicated in the early stages of MCI. Those who have a copy of the ApoE ε4 allele appear to be at increased risk for developing MCI (Grundman et al., 2004). Apolipoprotein E alleles are polymorphic proteins that direct lipid metabolism and are directly involved in transporting blood cholesterol and inducing synaptic plasticity. They are also related to the deposition of amyloid and formation of neurofibrillary tangles in brain (Twamley et al., 2006). The ApoE gene is found on chromosome 19 and has three alleles (ε2, ε3, and ε4), with ApoE ε4 occurring in only 14-16% of the population and often leading to sporadic and late-onset familial AD (Driscoll et al., 2005; Saunders et al., 1993; Poirier et al., 1995). However, even among older and elderly adults with MCI, the presence of the ApoE ε4 allele seems to have a negative impact on cognition (Alexander et al., 2007; Heun et al., 2006). In particular, the ApoE ε4 allele has been associated with a more rapid decline in memory (Bondi et al., 1999; Caselli et al., 2004; Fleisher et al., 2007; Mayeux et al., 2001), but there is some ambiguity and inconsistency about its impact on other cognitive domains. In some cases, no other cognitive areas have been impacted for carriers of the ε4 allele (Bondi et al., 1999), leading to the contention that it has a preferential effect or impact on episodic memory (Snowden et al., 2007). Other research, however, shows greater heterogeneity in memory and verbal skills (Wetter et al., 2006), deficits in prospective memory (Driscoll et al., 2005), and impaired attention and executive skills over time (Albert et al., 2007; Parasuraman et al., 2002; Rosen et al., 2002). These more pervasive effects are consistent with a recent meta-analysis showing that those with ApoE ε4 had significantly lower global cognitive functioning, episodic memory, and executive functioning relative to non-ε4 carriers (Small et al., 2004).

The pathological activity of the ε4 allele seems to be related to its interference with the clearance of β-amyloid peptide from the brain, leading to more rapid accumulation of neuritic plaques of aggregated amyloid protein, intracellular neurofibrillary tangles, hyperphosphorylated tau protein, reduced cholinergic activity, and increased density of senile plaques (Albert et al., 2007). This results in impaired cholinergic basal forebrain, hippocampal, and thalamocortical networks (Babiolioni et al., 2006), as well as smaller hippocampal volumes (Lind et al., 2006) and reduced cerebral metabolism and blood flow in temporal and parietal cortices (Parasuraman et al., 2002). In fact, these levels and patterns are qualitatively similar to those clinically diagnosed with AD.

However, there is some controversy regarding the utility and ethics surrounding genetic testing early in the diagnostic process. Even though there is a distinct relationship between the ApoE ε4 allele and one's risk for AD and MCI, neither the presence nor absence of ApoE ε4 offers diagnostic certainty (McConnell et al., 1999). It may convey information about one's level of risk, but it cannot currently determine whether or not someone will develop MCI or AD, which raises questions about its practical value, sensitivity, and specificity. For those who do pursue it and test negative for ApoE ε4, genetic testing may alleviate some distress or facilitate a false illusion of hope. Alternatively, if the results are positive, this finding can elevate some preparedness, but it can also incur a level of fear and psychological distress that could ultimately be unwarranted. Either finding has implications for patients' employment, insurability, and right to awareness. Therefore, patients and physicians alike must struggle to decide if genetic testing would supply enough information to change their decisions regarding their current and future care. Most physicians agree that it should not be performed in asymptomatic individuals, or with individuals who have family members with sporadic AD. Nor should it be provided without adequate pretest and post-test counseling, education and support. It may be most helpful in cases where there is a positive family history of early-onset dementia and where there is a convergence of evidence to suggest a strong likelihood of AD. However, even this should be done in the context of a multidisciplinary team that understands the implications, risks, and limitations of the proposed genetic tests.

Another biomarker is the tau protein in cerebrospinal fluid (CSF). Tau is one of two proteins that accumulates abnormally in MCI and AD, and it may directly contribute to the development of one of the hallmark features of MCI and AD, namely neurofibrillary tangles. These NFTs contain paired helical filaments, which are formed by the abnormal aggregation of hyperphosphorylated tau. Normally, tau is a microtubule-associated intracelluar protein, but when it is hyperphosphorylated, it loses it ability to participate in assembling and stabilizing the microtubule of the axon. This results in the breakdown of the neuron and abnormally elevated tau levels in CSF (Almvist and Winblad, 1999). The NFTs that form secondary to the aggregated tau interfere with the integrity of axonal structure, including neuronal dysfunction and destruction of synapses and neurons. Measuring tau, which typically requires a lumbar puncture followed by a CSF assay, may therefore reflect the extent of neuronal and axonal damage.

Among those with MCI, the elevations of tau are typically higher than normal controls and lower than those with AD (Andreasen et al., 1998, 2001; Okamura et al,. 2002). Most of this elevation is detected in the hippocampus and other medial temporal regions that are responsible for corresponding difficulties in memory. Therefore, an increase in CSF tau may represent early pathogenesis and a biomarker for later MCI. The primary downside to relying on this biomarker, however, is that it is not directly associated with the clinical features of MCI. There has been little evidence supporting a direct relationship between tau levels and cognitive functioning (Andreasen et al., 1998). Instead, the relationship has been indirect, between tau levels and the NFTs that are implicated in neuronal loss and cognitive decline.

CLINICAL EVALUATION

Diagnosing an individual as MCI and determining the appropriate subtype requires a thorough clinical interview, although the suggested examination procedures have not yet been standardized. First, it is widely recommended that the interview should include the individual's detailed history verified by an informant, as well as a mental status examination within a general neurological examination. The most common mental status measures such as the MMSE (Folstein, 1975), Modified Mini Mental Status Exam (3MS; Teng et al., 1987), and the Kokmen Short Test of Mental Status (Kokmen et al., 1987) are not sensitive enough for MCI. Those with MCI can get 26-28 total points on the MMSE and still be considered normal most of the time (Kelley and Petersen, 2007). As an alternative, the the Montreal Cognitive Assessment (MoCA; Nasreddine et al., 2005), which was originally designed for detecting MCI, is a brief cognitive screening tool with high sensitivity and specificity for individuals with normal MMSE. Li and colleagues (2006) even suggest that a simple informant screening that covers memory and IADLs is able to differentiate MCI and mild AD from normal aging with high accuracy, sensitivity, and specificity. This screening can effectively combine a single-item informant report of memory problem and a few items on ADLs

To detect memory impairment among those with MCI, Knopman and Ryberg (1989) suggest using a test called Delayed Word Recall (DWR). It was designed specifically to maximize the likelihood of poor performance in patients with AD and minimize the likelihood of poor performance in normal elderly subjects. The DWR uses elaborative processing of to-be-remembered words and delayed free recall. The overall predictive accuracy of the DWR was 95.2%. Similarly, the word list from the Consortium to Establish a Registry for Alzheimer's Disease (CERAD-CWL; Morris et al., 1988) evaluates long-term verbal recall and was shown to be highly sensitive to MCI, with accuracy, sensitivity, and specificity rates between 89-98% (Shankle et al., 2005). The Buschke Selective Reminding Test (Buschke and Fuld, 1974) is a lengthier and more challenging word list test that can detect recall deficits before functioning is compromised (Rogers et al., 2005). The only drawback to this test is its complex administration.

Regardless of the tests that are used, they must be challenging enough to detect subtle changes in cognition. Tests of general cognitive function such as the MMSE and full-scale IQ offer no differentiation between MCI and normal populations. Similarly, tests that specifically target memory functions of delayed verbal and nonverbal recall have been shown to identify

MCI as more similar to mild AD (Petersen et al., 1999). Therefore, comprehensive neuropsychological evaluations that are sufficiently challenging can provide differential diagnosis between MCI subtypes to determine what domains are functionally affected. Often, the deficit in a specific stage of learning or pattern of memory deficits can be determined, which can inform the type and severity of impairment.

Various laboratory tests should also be considered to rule out other medical conditions that may be impacting cognition (Rosenberg et al., 2006). Electrolytes, complete blood count, vitamin b12, thyroid function, syphilis serology, computerized tomography (CT), and/or MRI are recommended. Other tests for determining sedimentation rate, drug level, HIV, lyme serology, urinalysis, 24-hour urine for heavy metal, cerebrospinal fluid, electrocardiogram, ecetroencephalogram, PET, or SPECT are optional, but can rule out significant illnesses. In addition, there is evidence that the combined use of two or three genetic, biochemical, or imaging techniques is more powerful than any one alone in predicting MCI (de Leon et al., 2004). Thus, the Alzheimer's Disease Neuroimaging Initiative (ADNI) was formed to identify the combination of established biomarkers with the highest diagnostic and prognostic power (Mueller et al., 2005). Ideally, a diagnosis should be made by a specific neuropsychological evaluation, and confirmed by laboratory tests and brain imaging (Burns and Zaudig, 2002).

Neuropsychiatric symptoms are not included in the diagnostic criteria but should be included in the evaluation due to overlapping features described in MCI. Much like the neuropsychiatric profile of AD, the frequency of neuropsychiatric problems in MCI is between 29-85% (Rozzini et al., 2007; Apostolova and Cummings, 2007; Lyketsos et al., 2002). The most common symptoms in both conditions are anxiety, depression, apathy, irritability, agitation (Chan et al., 2003; Feldman et al., 2004; Forsell et al., 2003; Geda et al., 2004; Hwang et al., 2004; Lyketsos et al., 2000). Another study found many symptoms in MCI individuals, including 33% with depression and anxiety, 22% with apathy, 20% with irritability, and a greater association with severe somatic comorbidity and functional disability (Mariani et al., 2006). Depression, in particular, has been shown to be a predictor for cognitive decline and an independent risk factor for MCI (Barnes et al., 2006; Bassuk et al., 1998; Yaffe et al., 1999). Depression predicted faster cognitive deterioration in amnestic MCI, increasing the risk of conversion (Modrego and Ferrandez, 2004). Psychosis also independently increases one's risk for MCI (Monastero et al., 2007), and converters to AD have been shown to have a higher frequency of apathy than nonconverters (Robert et al., 2006). It is important to note, however, that neuropsychiatric symptoms may be precursers not only to AD, but also to frontotemporal dementia and Lewy body dementia (Gauthier et al., 2006).

Clinical Limitations in Early Detection Procedures

When considering the early detection of MCI, it is important to realize that the diagnostic utility of both neuropsychological testing and neuroimaging are limited by the inherent difficulty in predicting when individuals will convert to dementia. This makes it difficult to adequately discern what differentiates the early and late stages of MCI, and when individuals cross over into dementia. Other neurological and psychological conditions can also mask as the symptoms of MCI. Depression presents with a similar profile of hypoperfusion on PET imaging (Almkvist and Winblad, 1999); tau elevations are not specific to MCI and can be elevated in other neurodegenerative diseases (Arai et al., 1997); and many brain volume and metabolism reductions are not disease-specific (de Leon et al., 2004). As a result, each of these markers alone may not be an accurate baseline predictor of MCI. Instead, the greatest accuracy in detection may come from a multi-perspective approach that combines neuropsychological testing with neuroimaging to improve diagnostic accuracy for predicting MCI.

These limitations not withstanding, there is increased need to accurately detect and identify the early, preclinical phase of MCI. Understanding these factors can lead to better sensitivity and specificity in screening someone's risk for dementia, while simultaneously increasing the quality of life among the afflicted and minimizing the financial burden for society and the psychological burden for caregivers. It will also promote our understanding of the course of the disease and better aid patients and families in decisions regarding healthcare.

PHARMACOLOGICAL INTERVENTIONS IN MCI

While many pharmaceutical companies and scientific researchers are examining compounds that may be neuroprotective against AD, there is still no FDA-approved treatment for MCI. As such, the only substantial pharmacological treatment options are borrowed from efficacy evidence in AD and related memory disorders (Allain et al., 2007). Based on the assumption that MCI and AD share the same pathological pathways, it may seem logical to treat MCI patients with AD-targeted medication. On the other hand, some of the therapeutic targets in MCI are different from those of AD patients, as they still have more cognitive and probably neuronal reserve, which may benefit from additional agents. This makes it important to review the current literature regarding the possible effect of several medications in the treatment for MCI.

Acetylcholinesterase Inhibitors

Donepezil, rivastigmine, and galantamine are cognitive enhancing drugs that increase the availability of the body's level of the neurotransmitter acetylcholine by inhibiting the enzyme that breaks down this neurotransmitter. Brains of individuals with AD exhibit decreased levels of acetylcholine (Small et al., 2004), which makes acetylcholinesterase inhibitors (AChEI) a common treatment for mild to moderate forms of AD (Doody et al, 2001). Only recently have clinical trials began to evaluate the efficacy of AChEI in MCI. In a 24-week multi-center, double-blind, randomized, placebo-controlled group trial (RCT), Salloway and colleagues (2004) evaluated the effects of donepezil on cognitive functioning in a sample of 269 amnestic MCI individuals. Findings indicated significant improvements in the donepezil group relative to the control group on global measures of cognitive functioning, immediate and delayed contextual verbal memory, working memory, and subjective measures of memory improvement. Another large RCT examined the efficacy of donepezil versus vitamin E and placebo groups over the course of three years in an effort to measure conversion time to possible or probable AD (Petersen et al., 2005). Of the 539 subjects with amnestic MCI who had completed the trial, almost 40% (212 subjects) had progressed to dementia within three years. More specifically, there was a significant positive effect on conversion time and performance on objective cognitive measures for the first 18 months of the study in the donepezil treatment group, but no effect in the vitamin E group. All three groups, however, eventually converged in their transition to AD within the latter portion of the study. Overall, this research suggests that AChEI medications may prove to be beneficial in delaying progression from MCI to AD, and they are certainly more efficacious than vitamin E supplements alone. However, additional clinical trials are essential for further confirmation.

Another AChEI medication, galantamine, has been evaluated in two 24-month randomized, double-blind, parallel placebo-group controlled studies (van de Pol et al., 2007) and in one smaller randomized and double-blind study (Koontz and Baskys, 2005). Results from the van de Pol (2007) study revealed slightly lower rates of conversion to AD in the galantamine group after two years. Additionally, improvements were also observed on measures of global cognitive functioning in the galantamine group. Koontz and Baskys (2005) reported similar findings of improvement in global cognitive functioning (via the self-reported memory functioning), and additional improvement on some tasks requiring executive functioning, working memory, and immediate recall of rote word lists. The small sample (n = 19) and homogeneity (all males) of the subjects, however, significantly limit the generalizability of the findings. To date there remains some active studies evaluating the effects of galantamine in the treatment of MCI (www.clinicaltrials.gov; please refer to the website for more information), which could provide more compelling evidence of its efficacy.

Nmda Receptor Antagonist

Several researchers (Tariot et al., 2004; Weycker et al., 2006) have found that the efficacy of AchEI drug therapy can be further augmented when combined with Namenda (memantine HCL), an NMDA receptor antagonist, that is FDA approved for AD. Tariot and colleagues conducted an RCT on 404 patients with moderate-severe AD who received memantine plus donepezil or placebo plus donepezil. Their main hypothesis was that administration of memantine plus donepezil would have clinical benefit as well as safety for the use of moderate-severe AD compared to placebo. The combined treatment had better outcomes regarding cognition, activities of daily living, and behavior than donepezil treatment alone. The results indicate that memantine treatment with donepezil is safe and effective in treating moderate-severe AD. This study was conducted following another study which demonstrated that memantine alone reduced deterioration in mild-moderate AD compared to placebo (Reisberg et al., 2003). More recently, Peskind and colleagues (2006) conducted an RCT which suggested that memantine treatment has benefits for mild-moderate AD on aspects of memory and language (Pomara et al., 2007).

This effect of memantine (Namemda) on AD is attributed to its binding to NMDA receptors in the brain, which in turn decrease their binding to the neurotransmitter glutamate and reduce overstimulation of the receptor and neuronal damage (Small et al., 2004). In addition, animal studies demonstrate that memantine can reduce oxidative damage and enhance cognition in healthy aged rats, as well as the transgenic mouse model for AD (Dias et al., 2007, Minkeviciene et al., 2004). Currently, there are no RCTs on memantine and MCI, but hopefully this treatment option will be investigated in the future.

Non Steroidal Anti-Inflammatory Drugs (Nsaids)

Inflammation is thought to be one of the underlying mechanisms of AD. The NSAIDs are a group of drugs that inhibit the body's inflammatory response by impeding cyclooxygenase, an important enzyme in the inflammatory pathway. These drugs are so effective in mediating the inflammatory response that they are used in the treatment of such inflammatory diseases as rheumatoid arthritis (Baraf, 2007). Several epidemiological studies suggest that the use of anti-inflammatory drugs can improve cognitive function and may have a protective effect against AD (Hayden et al., 2007; Rich et al., 1995; Szekely et al., 2004). Animal studies have demonstrated the positive impact of NSAIDs in their ability to affect the amyloid pathology in the brain by lowering amyloid β peptide levels, separately from its cyclooxygenase or anti-inflammatory activity (Weggen et al., 2001). The Cache County study is a longitudinal study that examined the effects of NSAIDs on cognition over the course of eight years and hypothesized that starting treatment earlier in life may have a greater effect on enhancing cognition (Hayden et al., 2007). The findings suggest that long term treatment with NSAID starting in mid-life has a significant effect on preserving cognitive functions in the elderly. This effect has shown to be more prominent among ApoE ε4 carriers (Hayden et al., 2007).

However, not all the data in the literature supports the use of NSAIDs for the treatment of AD. A RCT study examined the potential of two NSAIDs for the prevention of AD. The participants, aged 70+, were randomly assigned to receive celecoxib, naproxen sodium, or placebo. However, the study was discontinued after an average duration of 20-months because of significantly increased cardiovascular risk with celecoxib (ADAPT Research Group 2006, 2007). The results failed to prove the hypothesis that NSAIDs may reduce the incidence of AD (ADAPT Research Group, 2007). As a result, it is too soon for clinicians to recommend NSAID treatment for patients with MCI based on observational studies alone. There is still a need for additional research regarding this treatment option (Scharf et al., 2007).

Statins

The statins are a group of drugs with lipid lowering properties. They interrupt the cholesterol synthesis in the liver, which results in lower levels of cholesterol in the blood (Small et al., 2004). Therefore statins can treat hypercholesterolemia (excess cholesterol in the blood) and help in the prevention of cardiovascular disease (Adabag et al., 2007; Arca et al., 2007). The possible connection between vascular disease and AD fueled investigators' interest in the possible associations between cholesterol and AD (Casserly et al., 2004; Wilson et al., 1994). Several clinical studies have tried to examine the effect of different statins on amyloid β in normal aging as well as AD patients (Sparks et al., 2000, Simons et al., 2002). The AD Cholesterol Lowering Treatment trial (Sparks et al., 2000, 2006) was an RCT that examined the effect of atrovastatin on mild-moderate AD. The participants had the diagnosis of possible or probable AD and were randomized to receive once daily treatment of atrovastatin or placebo for one year. The study showed that atrovastatin reduced cholesterol levels and had a positive effect on the cognitive and behavioral scales of AD, such as the

MMSE, ADAS-cog (a rating scale for AD), and clinician's global impression of. These results imply that atrovastatin may be used as a possible treatment for AD.

Other studies examined the possible mechanisms that are involved in the connection between statins and AD (Jarvik et al., 1995; Li et al., 2006; Sparks et al., 1994). For example, Sparks and colleagues (1994) found elevated amyloid β levels in New Zealand white rabbits after feeding them a cholesterol rich diet, whereas amyloid β levels returned to normal after resuming a balanced diet. This study suggests that cholesterol lowering might include inhibition of amyloid production. It is not clear, though, whether lowering peripheral levels of cholesterol affects brain cholesterol (Kivipelto et al., 2005). Other studies suggest neuroprotective, antioxidant, and anti-inflammatory effects of statins on AD (Cucchiara et al., 2001; Darvesh et al., 2004). More research is needed to investigate the relationship between statins and AD and its implications for treatment of AD and MCI.

Estrogen Replacement Therapy

Estrogen is hypothesized to have an important protective role against age-related deterioration of cognitive functions (Sherwin, 2007). Estrogen is a key player in several biological pathways, and estrogen receptors are expressed in several brain regions that are involved in the process of learning and cognition (Aennle et. al., 2007; McEwen, 2002; Rocca et al., 2007).

To date, the largest study aimed at investigating the long-term cognitive effects of HRT is the Women's Health Initiative Memory Study (WHIMS), an ancillary study to the Women's Health Initiative (WHI, 2002). Those who had hysterectomies were randomized into the conjugated equine estrogen (CEE) vs. placebo arm, whereas those with intact uteri were randomized into the arm comparing CEE + medroxyprogesterone (MPA) with placebo. Unfortunately, due to unforeseen health risks associated with HRT, both arms of the WHI were terminated before completion (WHI, 2004). Furthermore, contrary to expectations, data from the WHIMS revealed that women who received CEE + MPA had an increased risk of cognitive decline compared to the placebo group, with a similar trend among the CEE-only users, although it did not reach statistical significance (WHI, 2004). In addition, pooled data from both study arms resulted in a strikingly higher rate of dementia among hormone users relative to the placebo groups (92 vs. 50 participants), including a higher rate of MCI (169 vs. 127 participants). In addition, the Women's Health Initiative Study of Cognitive Aging (WHISCA), which utilized the data of 1416 women from the CEE + MPA arm of the WHIMS, found that the CEE + MPA group declined faster on a measure of verbal learning (Resnick et al., 2004). These results were interpreted as further evidence of specific cognitive decline in women taking HRT.

Despite the large scale and long duration of the WHI and its ancillary studies, it soon became clear that they were beset by a number of serious limitations. First, researchers collapsed all dementias into a single category that included AD, vascular dementia (VD), Parkinson's dementia, and frontal lobe dementia. Second, it has been suggested that the higher rates of dementia among the hormone treatment groups may have been due to vascular disease (Schmaker et al., 2004). In addition, more than half of the WHIMS participants were non-compliant with their hormone regimen at some point in the study (Craig et al., 2005). A fourth, and rather serious limitation, especially with regards to the WHISCA, was that diagnoses were never ascertained for about 40% of participants who were determined to have impaired neurocognitive functioning based on a cognitive screening measure. There were also issues of delayed data collection (three years after randomization), a lack of pretreatment measures for cognitive ability [implicating that many women were impaired cognitively prior to initiating hormone replacement therapy (HRT)], methodological problems in data collection and statistical analysis, and the inappropriateness of starting women on HRT who are significantly past menopause (Machens et al., 2003). In summary, the WHI and WHIMS may not be the most definitive or robust study for understanding the impact of estrogen on cognition or dementia.

Since the termination of the WHIMS, the case for HRT in reducing the risk of AD and improving the cognitive functioning of postmenopausal women has continued to gain support via RCTs and epidemiological studies. RCTs using 17β-estradiol (E2) have shown the most beneficial effects, particularly on information processing (Anderer et al., 2004), verbal fluency and attention (Kugaya et al., 2003), reaction time (Schiff et al., 2005), and other cognitive abilities (Saletu et al., 2003). Most recently, a two-year longitudinal study showed that lower baseline levels of endogenous estradiol were associated with a greater chance of decline on a cognitive screening measure and a test of verbal learning and memory (Yaffe et al., 2007). This led the authors to suggest that there is an ideal range of exogenous estradiol that can help prevent cognitive decline, and that those with lower endogenous levels may receive the greatest benefit. Neuroimaging studies have also been supportive. The use of estrogen replacement therapy (ERT) has been shown to improve neural processing speed (Anderer et al., 2004) and enhance cerebral metabolism (Kugaya et al., 2003; Rasgon et al., 2001), including minimizing decline in cerebral metabolism over time and possibly preventing atrophy of the hippocampus (Hu et al., 2006; Rasgon et al., 2005). Finally, several studies have indicated that HRT users are 30 to 50 times less likely to be at risk for dementia (Green and Dixon, 2002; Le Blanc et al., 2001). However, HRT is not considered a treatment for cognitive problems once diagnosed with MCI or dementia (Mulnard, Corrada, and Kawas, 2004).

Perhaps the most supportive findings for estrogen's neuroprotective effects, especially against neurodegenerative diseases, come from basic science research. While the cause of AD remains unclear, there is strong indication that β-amyloid is involved in the chain of events leading to AD neuropathology. Evidence that estrogen, E2 in particular, protects against β-amyloid-induced damage and tau-related changes have been convincing. For example, one group reported that E2 reduces the generation and secretion of β-amyloid in vitro and in vivo (mice), which led to the proposal that E2 decreases the amount of amyloid precursor protein available for production of β-amyloid (Xu et al., 2006). Findings from another group indicate that 17β-estradiol pre-treatment is effective in limiting mitochondrial dysfunction by maintaining calcium homeostasis and activation of anti-apoptotic mechanisms in protecting neurons against β-amyloid neurotoxicity (Nilsen et al., 2006).

Miller and Rogers (2007) provide a comprehensive overview of the connection between estrogen, the brain, mood, and cognition. In general, research on estrogen, cognition, and dementia suggests that women benefit most from ERT or HRT when it is started during, or soon after, menopause (Almeida et al., 2006; Sherwin, 2005). As such, HRT is not recommended as a treatment for MCI, but additional research is needed in understanding estrogen's role in preventing cognitive decline.

Testosterone

Another sex hormone, testosterone, may also have a positive effect on AD. Several epidemiological studies on healthy adults have found that lower levels of testosterone are associated with poor cognitive performance, whereas higher levels of testosterone are associated with stronger performance on tests of global cognitive functioning (Hogervost et al., 2004; Yaffe et al., 2002). Low testosterone levels have been associated with increased risk for dementia (Moffat et al., 2004), and a specific correlation between testosterone and spatial memory and spatial skills has been found in animal and human studies (Janowsky et al., 1994; Silverman et al., 1999). Cherrier and colleagues (2005) even investigated the efficacy of testosterone on cognition in a RCT. Their subjects were aged 63-85, diagnosed with either MCI or AD, and received weekly injections of either testosterone or placebo for six weeks. Significant cognitive improvements were evident in spatial memory, verbal memory, and constructional abilities in the testosterone group, but not in the placebo group. The results indicate that testosterone treatment for men with MCI and AD may have benefit in some cognitive domains. There may be several mechanisms by which testosterone affects cognition, such as binding to androgen (e.g. testosterone) receptors found in the brain, particularly in the hippocampus and the hypothalamus (Kerr et al., 1995). Another possible mechanism is by reducing amyloid β levels (Gouras et al., 2000). However, other studies failed to demonstrate the positive effects of testosterone on cognition and memory (Kenny et al., 2004; Vaughan et al., 2007), and testosterone treatment may have some safety concerns regarding prostate cancer, making additional research necessary to assess the safety and efficacy of testosterone before recommending it for patients (Small et al., 2004).

LIFESTYLE INTERVENTIONS

One of the best ways to prevent many medical problems, and the potential onset of MCI and dementia, is by maintaining a healthy lifestyle. This includes nutrition, supplements, glycemic control, stress reduction, physical exercise, and sleep. All of these lifestyle modifications present with brain-protecting properties that may allow for the prevention of cognitive decline.

Anti-Oxidants

The pathophysiology of AD involves several mechanisms, such as oxidative damage and inflammation. Oxidants, or free radicals, are molecules that are highly reactive to chemical or stress exposure. Free radicals, such as reactive oxygen particles, can be removed by a cellular defense system. When their production is increased during a process called oxidative stress, the result is DNA damage and cell death (Bradford et al., 2005). Among those with MCI, a recent study found a marked decrease in the main components of the endogenous antioxidant defense system (Mecocci, 2004). Similarly, Rinaldi and colleagues (2003) found that the plasma levels of antioxidants, as well as their activity, was lower in MCI and AD individuals when compared with controls. It is hypothesized that an increased intake of antioxidants, such as garlic extract, vitamins C and E, curcumin, ginkgo-biloba, green tea, and ginseng, may aid in decreasing the risk of developing AD.

Unfortunately, well-designed clinical trials on antioxidants are scarce, creating conflicting evidence regarding the use of antioxidants in the prevention and treatment of dementia (Bradford et al., 2005). For example, in the Rotterdam prospective cohort study, which examined the association between dietary intake of antioxidants and the risk for AD, it was reported that a high intake of vitamins C and E may aid in the prevention of AD (Engelhart et al., 2002). In contrast, a recent RCT for those with MCI examined the effects of donepezil versus treatment with vitamin E and placebo (Petersen et al., 2005). Only donepezil therapy was associated with a reduced rate of progression to AD during the first 12 months of treatment; vitamin E had no benefits for those with MCI.

Nutrition and Supplements

A primary factor associated with age-related cognitive decline is nutrition. While the benefits of a balanced and nutritious diet are widely known, there is significantly less attention dedicated to vitamins and nutritional supplements. To date, several studies have analyzed the effect of various food ingredients on the prevention of cognitive decline in MCI. The following section will address the effects of integrating supplemental nutrients, as well as combinations of nutrients, in the context of preventing pathological aging.

Fruits and vegetables represent a form of antioxidant that also contains vitamins and polyphenols, which are abundant micronutrients whose chemical structure consists of hydroxyl groups on aromatic rings (Manach et al., 2004). Polyphenols have been identified on edible plants and have antioxidant properties as well as a probable role in the prevention of diseases associated with oxidative damage, such as AD (Scalbert et al., 2005). In a prospective study conducted among Japanese Americans (Dai et al., 2006), researchers found that frequent consumption of fruit and vegetable juices was associated with a significantly reduced risk of AD. However, this finding could not be exclusively explained by the role of the antioxidant vitamins, and suggests that other active ingredients, such as the antioxidant polyphenols, play a more significant role in protecting against dementia.

Most recently, dietary research relevant to AD has noted an association with the spice curcumin. Used as a yellow curry spice, curcumin is derived from tumeric and used as a food preservative and herbal medicine in India, a country where the prevalence of AD is significantly lower than the United States. Curcumin is a potent polyphenolic antioxidant and a powerful anti- inflammatory agent. In addition, it has an anti-amyloidogenic effect (recall that amyloid is a protein accumulated in the brains of AD patients, and is considered one of the pathologic hallmarks of the disease). Lim and colleagues (2005) reported that mice who carry a genetic form of AD (referred to as APPSw), and who received a relatively low dose of curcumin, had reduced levels of inflammatory markers in their brains than mice who had not received the spice. Furthermore, levels of insoluble β-amyloid, soluble β-amyloid, and plaque burden were also decreased in the brains of these mice, providing further evidence of curcumin's potential benefit. Ng and colleagues (2006) examined the association between curry consumption and cognition in non-demented Asian subjects aged 60 and older. Participants who consume curry "occasionally" or "often and very often," as compared with "never or rarely," had significantly better scores in the MMSE test. These findings may support the hypothesis that curry consumption is associated with stronger cognitive functioning. However, there is still lack of information regarding the association between curry consumption and MCI or AD.

Fatty acids, such as omega-6 and omega-3, are essential parts of our diet. The fatty acid omega-3 (e.g. docosahexaenoic acid, or DHA), can provide neuroprotection via several mechanisms. According to Small and colleagues (2004), these mechanisms include: (1) increasing the level of the neurotransmitter acetylcholine in the brain, which is relatively low in the brains of AD patients, (2) assisting in the prevention of neuronal death due to its antioxidant effects, and (3) minimizing inflammation in the brain. The results of several epidemiological studies suggest a reduced risk of AD with low dietary intake ratios of omega-6 and omega-3 fatty acids (e.g., Morris et al., 2003). Research utilizing a transgenic mouse model to examine the effects of dietary DHA (omega-3) on pathological AD markers indicated that dietary DHA intake can have a significant effect on β-amyloid levels and thus suggests that DHA intake may reduce the risk for AD (Lim et al., 2005).

Glycemic Control

A common view holds that sugar is like "fuel to the brain;" however, too much fuel may have negative effects. There is some evidence suggesting that diabetic patients exhibit impairments in recent memory (Biessels et al., 2001). Other studies show mild cognitive deficits in people who have impaired glucose tolerance, a condition that often precedes diabetes (Messier et al., 2003). However, in type 2 diabetic patients younger than 70 who achieve good glycemic control, the disease has a minor effect on cognitive functioning. The specific mechanisms underlying the progressive cognitive decline in individuals with impaired glucose tolerance remains unclear. Convit and colleagues (2003) tried to characterize glucose regulation and its implications on brain structure and function in 30 non-diabetic middle-aged and elderly individuals. The researchers revealed an association between glucose regulation and the volume of the hippocampus. Non-diabetic subjects with impaired peripheral glucose regulation were more likely to have reduced memory performance and smaller hippocampal volumes. There was no evidence for the same association between poor peripheral glucose regulation and the volume of other brain regions. This finding might be related to higher hippocampal vulnerability, different than other brain regions, since it is highly susceptible to damage caused by hypoglycemia and hypoxia (Ng et al., 1989).

Healthy Diet and Caffeine

With a rising concern and awareness for longevity and cognitive health in older age, researchers have begun to consider the neuroprotective impact of diet and nutrition. Previous studies examining the effects of nutrients as neuroprotective agents in AD have generally evaluated the impact of single nutrients; however, the typical daily diet consists of various combinations of these nutrients. Keys and colleagues (1968) described a diet rich in fruits, vegetables, cereals, legumes, and fish (high omega-3 concentration), accompanied by a substantial intake of unsaturated fatty acids (e.g. olive oil). This diet, known as the Mediterranean Diet (MeDi), has been positively associated with good health and is largely based upon a low intake of saturated fatty acids, low to moderate intake of dairy products, low intake of meat and poultry, and moderate intake of alcohol, mostly in the form of wine consumed with meals. Scrameas and colleagues (2006) examined the association between the MeDi and the risk for AD. In their study, 2,258 non-demented individuals were prospectively evaluated every 1.5 years. Results from their study indicated that better adherence to the diet may lead to a reduction in the risk for AD and that the reduction in the risk is dose dependent. Moreover, in an adjusted model analysis, none of the individual components (meat, dairy, vegetable, cereal etc.) of the MeDi exhibited a significant effect of protection against AD. These findings support the hypothesis that a composite dietary pattern, such as the MeDi, has a greater beneficial effect on AD prevention than a single component or nutrient. Additionally, many nutrients such as antioxidant vitamins (C and E) or phenols are found in high concentration in the MeDi, and may offer some protection against the pathological aging process.

With over 80% of the world population's dependent on coffee and tea, caffeine has been referred to as the most commonly used psychoactive substance in the world (Kendler and Prescott, 1999). Caffeine has many positive effects on the brain, including effects on mood (Fredholm et al., 1999), attention and subjective alertness (Rogers et al., 2008), and motor output and information processing (Dixit et al., 2006). Some of these studies have also suggested a neuroprotective effect of caffeine on the brain. For example, a prospective study by Ritchie and colleagues (2007) examined the relationship between coffee consumption and cognitive decline. They found that the protective effect of caffeine consumption was only observed in women and had the greatest impact on verbal skills, which was evident by a reduced decline in word retrieval. In addition, the effect was dose dependent on the amount of coffee units and the degree of cognitive protection. Nevertheless, the authors did not find any impact of coffee consumption on the incidence of dementia. Even if it turned out that caffeine consumption can be protective against dementia, clinicians should remember that it can also have some adverse effects before recommending caffeine consumption to their patients. Caffeine may be associated with a higher risk for cardiovascular disease, obstetrics complications (spontaneous abortion, etc.), and psychiatric and substance abuse disorders (Higdon et al., 2006, Kendler et al., 2006).

Stress Reduction

The twenty-first century lifestyle is often associated with increased levels of everyday stress. Today's source of stress might be related to worries regarding family, finances, health, traffic, politics, etc. Stress causes our body to react in several ways that can eventually result in physiological and psychological adaptations (Esch et al., 2002). These adaptations usually involve a hyperarousal state (also known as fight-or-flight response) that is also known as the "Stress Response" (SR; Canon, 1914). Studies are suggesting that several molecules such as cortisol (from the hypothalamic-pituitary-adrenal axis) play an important role in the stress response (Negrao et al., 2000).

Stress has been demonstrated to cause deficits in learning and memory, which can be relevant for AD pathophysiology (Esch et al., 2002; Newcomer et al., 1999). There are several possible explanations for this effect of stress on cognition and AD. Hippocampal atrophy can be associated with the stress response, and it is also associated with the neurodegenerative process in AD (Mizogunchi et al., 1992). In part, corticosteroid (e.g. cortisol) secretion, which is part of the stress response, can suppress neuronal activity in the hippocampus (Hoschl et al., 2001). Moreover, inflammatory processes that are associated with AD can also be the result of stress mechanisms (Hull et al., 1996).

Esch and colleagues (2003) examined the association between a stress reduction method called the Relaxation Response (RR) and diseases related to stress, such as AD and MCI. The RR is a combination of physiological mechanisms (adaptations) which are evoked when a person ignores distracting thoughts using a repetitive mental or physical activity, such as meditation and Tai Chi (Benson, 1974). By reducing the stress response, it is believed that the RR is associated with protective effects in neurodegenerative disorders such as AD. In addition, an fMRI study on normal subjects demonstrated activation of brain regions, such as the hippocampus and cingulate gyrus, that are associated with cognitive functions during the RR (Lasar et al., 2000). When using the RR on healthy adults to examine its effects on anxiety, memory and attention, Galvin and colleagues (2006) found that a reaction time for simple tasks that involve attention and psychomotor skills was significantly reduced. However, no significant improvement in the performance of complex memory or attentional tasks was found. To summarize, stress has an important role in the pathophysiology of AD. The RR can contradict the stress response, but more research regarding the use of RR on AD and MCI populations is needed in order to recommend this mode of treatment for patients.

Physical Exercise

When compared with various anti-aging products and programs, physical exercise can be relatively inexpensive and is typically more accessible. In a recent review, Kramer and colleagues (2007) noted that several prospective studies found that individuals who are more physically active have a reduced chance of developing dementia. Additionally, the results of several meta-analyses based on randomized clinical trials (e.g. Ethnier et al., 2006, Heyn et al., 2004) indicate that aerobic exercise has a strong positive influence on cognition. These recent meta-analyses also concluded that normal and cognitively impaired older adults can equally benefit from physical exercise. Research has also found that the improvement in cognition was most prominent in the functions involving executive control. Interestingly, studies with fewer female participants showed smaller effects of physical exercise on cognition than studies with more female participants, suggesting that this finding may be explained by the synergistic effect of estrogen and exercise.

Other studies have tried to examine the effects of exercise on the structure and function of the human brain. Pereira and colleagues (2007) used MRI measurements of cerebral blood volume in the hippocampus of middle-aged subjects who participated in a physical exercise intervention. Findings indicated an increase in verbal memory tasks and volume associated with improvement in physical fitness. Another study using MRI with older adults ages 60-79 found an increase in gray and white matter volume in brain areas associated with learning and memory after six months of regular aerobic exercise (Colombe et al., 2006).

Sleep

Many studies have demonstrated the importance of sleep for memory consolidation (Smith, 2001; Maquet et al., 2003). Sleep following a learning period has been shown to enhance both declarative and non-declarative memories (Fischer et al. 2002; Walker et al. 2002). Notably, both types of memory can benefit from different stages of sleep. For example, it was found that pairing early sleep (stage 1) with high amounts of slow wave sleep supports consolidation in paired associate tasks, a typical form of declarative memory, whereas the late part of sleep, which is predominantly characterized by rapid eye movement (REM) sleep, seems particularly effective in consolidating procedural memory (Plihal and Born, 1997).

After the age of 30, the amount of slow wave sleep (stages 3 and 4) is declining, while the lighter non-REM sleep (stages 1 and 2) are increasing. This decline in slow wave or delta sleep, which is the deepest and most restful sleep, continues to decline with age, resulting in older adults having less overall sleep and more sleep disorders (Van Cauter et al., 2000; Wolkove et al., 2007). Advancing age and declining slow wave sleep may be associated with more memory difficulties, particularly in declarative memory (Backhaus et al., 2007; Hedden et al., 2004). Declines in declarative memory performance are often accompanied by structural and functional changes in the hippocampus, prefrontal cortex, and frontal white matter (Daselaar et al., 2003; Driscoll et al., 2003), which are areas of the brain that are implicated in the progression of AD.

Summary of Lifestyle Interventions

Overall, previous research suggests that lifestyle may have a significant effect on cognitive functioning and may even be neuroprotective and preventative against MCI. Some of the main factors that have been found to be involved in protecting against dementia include anti-oxidants, a balanced and healthy diet, physical exercise, reduced stress, and adequate sleep. Furthermore, these factors are highly interrelated. For example, maintaining a balanced diet may enhance physical exercise, which in turn, may improve sleep and reduce stress. In addition, there is emerging evidence regarding the efficacy of alternative supplements, such as curcumin, in protecting against dementia and possibly MCI.

COGNITIVE INTERVENTIONS

In recent years, geriatric researchers and healthcare providers have begun to look beyond the limits of traditional pharmacological interventions in the treatment of cognitive impairment secondary to pathological aging. Specifically, the use of non-pharmacological interventions, such as cognitive training and rehabilitation, began to emerge as viable options in promoting longevity, enhancing existing cognitive capacities, and prolonging independence in functional activities for older adults. The remainder of the current discussion presents an overview of cognitive interventions that have been utilized in MCI groups, as well as those used in healthy and demented groups as they are relevant. The majority of research in this area is focused on memory systems, just as MCI conceptually emerged from concerns related to Alzheimer's type dementia. The definition of MCI now encompasses deficits in non-amnestic domains that can potentially lead to varying dementias in addition to AD. As conceptualizations of MCI have expanded, it is assumed that cognitive interventions will likely encompass other domains affected by dementia above and beyond memory (e.g., executive, language domains). Thus, the overview will include memory systems targeted by cognitive interventions, types of interventions, distinctions between intervention populations, current efficacy research and techniques, and limitations of cognitive interventions with older adults.

Memory Systems

Understanding the nuances of the memory systems is critical to evaluating the appropriateness of the cognitive intervention. Interventions developed for individuals with memory impairments are typically focused on targeting encoding and retrieval processes of two content areas: non-declarative and declarative memory (Clare, 2008; DeVreese, 2001). Nondeclarative memory, also called implicit or procedural memory, implies execution of tasks without conscious awareness and does not rely on declarative memory, such as tying one's shoes (Sohlberg and Mateer, 2001). Declarative memory, also referred to as explicit memory, is comprised of an individual's knowledge base and implies conscious awareness and the ability to explicitly report something (Sohlberg and Mateer, 2001). The declarative memory system is further broken down into two subsystems: semantic and episodic memory. Semantic memory refers to acquired knowledge and storage of factual information, whereas episodic memory is made up of memories of personally relevant events in life.

The pathological process of MCI and AD initially impacts declarative memory, but does not typically impact procedural memory until cognitive decline advances. In particular, it has been demonstrated that individuals with amnestic MCI and early AD present with deficits in semantic and episodic memory (Cummings, 2003; Perri et al., 2005), making it difficult to encode and retrieve information from the explicit memory system. For example, individuals with AD may have trouble learning a list of new words on a neuropsychological evaluation, or have difficulty recalling the dates for significant events in their own life. In contrast, the implicit memory system has been observed to be relatively well preserved until the later stages of AD (Bozoki et al., 2006; DeVreese, 2001). Examples of preserved implicit memory in people with early to moderate AD might include playing bridge, cooking, or personal hygiene. As such, identification of the degree and type of memory impairment is critical when considering cognitive intervention.

The Role of Metamemory

Metamemory is a term used to describe a person's subjective understanding of their memory functioning. Most people hold some awareness and understanding of their strengths and weaknesses in regard to their memory and ability to learn new information. Often this awareness is what guides subsequent behaviors (Sohlberg and Mateer, 2001). For example, an individual who knows she has some difficulty with prospective memory, or memory for carrying out future tasks, may compensate by leaving a message on the answering machine at home as a cue or reminder. While individuals with severe memory impairment also typically demonstrate limited insight or awareness, the literature on metamemory in MCI is not well-developed. Some studies have observed older adults with memory impairment to demonstrate compromised awareness of their memory difficulties (Collie et al., 2002; Feher et al., 1994; Perrotin et al., 2007; Vogel et al., 2004), whereas others have found a greater sense of awareness of memory dysfunction (Correa et al., 1996; Small et al., 1995). Therefore, it is difficult to determine the "typical" degree of metamemory in MCI, and as such, each individual should be treated uniquely, and interventions should be developed in consideration of both cognitive impairment and awareness. Generally, insight toward understanding one's own strengths and weaknesses is advantageous, as the more insight one possesses about his or her memory impairments, the better position they are in to remediate these functions (Clare et al, 2004).

Types of Cognitive Interventions

Clare et al. (2005) noted three primary approaches to cognitive intervention depending on the degree and nature of deficit: *cognitive stimulation, cognitive rehabilitation*, and *cognitive training*. First, general *cognitive stimulation* and reality orientation approaches typically involve participation in group activities and/or discussions that are aimed at general enhancement of cognitive and social functioning (Boylin et al., 1976; Taulbee and Folsom, 1966). These types of interventions are non-specific to a cognitive domain, and include such activities as group discussions of current events, supervised recreational activities, and group reminiscence therapies. Cognitive stimulation is typically utilized in demented populations with limited learning abilities, and thus has not been as applicable to individuals with MCI.

Second, *cognitive rehabilitation* is a more individualized approach in which healthcare providers work collaboratively with patients and their families or caregivers in order to identify personally-relevant goals in day-to-day living and to develop strategies for addressing these goals (Clare et al., 2005). According to Wilson (2002), "cognitive rehabilitation should focus on real-life, functional problems" (p. 99). In short, the practical focus of cognitive rehabilitation involves the use of any strategy or technique that will enhance functional tasks and activities of daily living, rather than increasing performance on a specific cognitive task (Clare, 2008). Two distinct goals in cognitive rehabilitation have been suggested in the literature: (1) capitalize on remaining memory functions (e.g. implicit memory systems), and (2) find additional ways of compensating for functional difficulties (e.g. retrieval cues) (Clare et al., 2005). A review of memory rehabilitation in early AD provides evidence supporting the clinical effectiveness and pragmatic use of rehabilitation strategies. These have the potential of moderate to long term performance gains and functional applicability from training session to in-vivo environment (De Vreese et al., 2001). Originally designed for patients with non-progressive neurological disorders, such as brain injury (Wilson, 1998) and commonly used in AD populations, cognitive rehabilitation may be utilized in MCI populations for the purpose of preserving complex functional abilities. The primary goal of cognitive interventions with AD patients, similar to those with MCI, is to optimize existing cognitive and functional skills for as long as possible (Acevedo and Lowenstein, 2007), and tasks are structured and presented in a way that reflects this goal.

Whereas the focus of *cognitive stimulation* is on exercising preserved abilities and *cognitive rehabilitation* is focused on improving functional activities, *cognitive training* targets improvement of specific cognitive domains (Belleville, 2007; Cipriani et al., 2006). According to Clare and colleagues (2005), "cognitive training involves guided practice on a set of tasks that reflect particular cognitive functions, such as memory, attention, or problem-solving, which can be done in a variety of settings and formats" (p. 2). The assumption in using cognitive training with MCI individuals is that practicing the use of structured strategies to enhance encoding and retrieval has the potential to improve, or at the very least, maintain cognitive functioning, and that with intensive training, the learned strategies will generalize beyond the training sessions. Cognitive training typically involves teaching theoretically-based skills and strategies in a standardized and structured fashion on an individual basis or to a small group of individuals (Belleville, 2007). Tasks vary in difficulty level and can be traditional paper-pencil tasks, computerized activities, and/or involve activities of daily living (Clare et al., 2005). One of the primary goals of cognitive training is to improve existing cognitive functions or to compensate for impaired capacities. This often requires baseline identification of compromised domains through neuropsychological testing, which, for example, can help determine specific faulty memory processes (i.e. encoding, retrieval, or recognition) and subsequently inform treatment planning.

Heterogeneity of Techniques and Applications

The success of the efficacy research on the use of cognitive interventions with healthy older adults paved a path for its potential clinical utility in pathological aging. However, clinical and pathophysiological considerations for individuals with MCI and dementia differ considerably from healthy older adults. First, some of the typical cognitive techniques utilized with healthy older adults are complex and require multiple steps, which may pose a challenge to individuals with impaired memory and other cognitive skills (i.e. executive functioning) (Clare et al., 2000). Additionally, cognitive interventions for individuals with dementia or pre-dementia often have appropriately different goals (i.e. functional tasks and ADLs) and may require regular support from caregivers (McKitrick and Camp, 1992), as compared to interventions designed for healthy older adults (Troyer et al., 2007). Furthermore, it is critical that cognitive techniques utilized with a memory-impaired population consider the availability of intact memory systems (e.g. implicit vs. residual explicit) in order to take the greatest advantage of the possibility of new learning, as learning processes can be resistant in memory impaired individuals (Perri et al., 2005). Recent research suggests that when dual cognitive support is provided, both at encoding and retrieval, new learning may be successful in AD (Clare, 2008); however, thus far the efficacy literature on cognitive interventions in pathological aging has been inconsistent, and the majority of studies have been completed with small samples and/or no controls, thereby limiting the power of the results (Belleville, 2007).

Meta-analytic studies of pre- and post-treatment gains using mnemonic strategies in healthy adult populations have revealed inconsistent results with relatively small (Floyd and Scogin, 1997) to large (Verhaeghen et al., 1992) effect sizes when compared with controls and placebo groups. Consistent with previous research (Brooks et al., 1998), both studies reported a positive relationship between pre-training (introducing cognitive techniques) and memory improvement. Conditions that contributed to memory improvement included younger age, more intact gross cognitive functioning (higher MMSE), group training sessions (versus individual training), shorter duration of sessions, and the inclusion of a memory-related interventions, such as education about memory and aging (Verhaeghen et al., 1992). In addition, Floyd and Scogin (1997) revealed that optimal efficacy in a cognitive training program should include an integration of memory skill enhancement and expectancy modification, including the development of more adaptive attitudes towards memory and aging. Interestingly, some studies have noted that type of technique (e.g. mnemonic) did not render any differences in treatment gain (Verhaeghen et al., 1992), although a vast majority of studies combine various cognitive techniques, making it difficult to evaluate the effectiveness of each on it own merit.

The use of cognitive interventions for disorders related to pathological aging was initially met with uncertainty in regard to the efficacy of the interventions (APA, 1997) and spawned much debate until psychometrically sound research revealed promising effects (Sitzer et al., 2006; Verhaeghen et al., 1992). Now, the debate about the efficacy of cognitive interventions with older adults has shifted from *"Does it work?"* to *"How and why does it work, and for how long?"* While some authors have suggested that cognitive techniques are meant to target implicit memory systems (Baddeley and Wilson, 1994), others have made the argument that these interventions result in the activation of residual explicit memory systems (Hunkin et al., 1998). Still others have suggested that the most efficacious interventions tap into both implicit and explicit memory systems (Clare et al., 2000), or that the process of new learning may depend on the severity of the memory impairment in relation to available memory systems (Tailby and Haslam, 2003). For example, some authors have hypothesized that new learning in severely memory-impaired individuals relies primarily on implicit processes, while those with mild memory impairment utilize more explicit processes (Tailby and Haslam, 2003). Studies illustrating this point conceptualized categories of interventions based primarily upon the learning processes involved. For example, as De Vreese and colleagues (2001) outlined, stage one consists of interventions that target explicit memory systems, such as mnemonics and semantic cueing, and the second stage focuses more on interventions that utilize implicit systems, such as errorless learning and spaced retrieval (Landauer and Bjork, 1978) or expanded rehearsal. The interventions at both stages serve to cultivate more efficient processes for encoding and retrieval, and therefore have frequently been combined and proven efficacious in a number of studies for AD (Clare et al., 2001, 2002, 2003). In addition, it has been suggested that cognitive training in AD takes advantage of a cognitive reserve capacity (Farina et al., 2006), and the goal in MCI would be to extend this reserve as long as possible.

Long-Term Outcomes

Few studies have evaluated the long-term effects of cognitive interventions in older adults. In the largest clinical trial to date (ACTIVE, n = 2832), Ball and colleagues (2002) evaluated the effectiveness and durability of cognitive interventions using neuropsychological tests and measures of cognitively demanding IADLs (e.g. financial management, driving). Participants were taught mnemonic strategies in order to complete laboratory-like tasks of verbal episodic memory (e.g. recall of a word list or paragraph), as well as memory tasks that were relevant to daily life (e.g. recall of a shopping list and recall of a prescription label). Follow-up results from two (Ball et al., 2002) and five years (Willis et al., 2005) revealed that the cognitive interventions in each group helped increase performance on objective measures of cognitive ability for which they were trained; however, the interventions were not generalized to everyday tasks. Similarly, Brooks and colleagues (1999) evaluated the efficacy of mnemonic training for word list recall and face-name association. In general, their findings suggest that older age (70+) had a greater positive relationship, with benefit from pre-training and subsequent training. Furthermore, almost half of the subjects who originally employed the mnemonic strategy immediately after training reported continued use of the mnemonic five years later, suggesting that those who benefited from the initial mnemonic training actually sustained long-term benefits and may have avoided further cognitive decline (O'Hara et al., 2007). These studies are consistent with previous research suggesting that healthy older adults trained to use more efficient encoding strategies, such as mnemonics, can demonstrate long-term gains (Neely and Backman, 1993). It is important to note that even when outcomes are positive, the lifespan of these interventions still largely lies with the individual. Future research in this area may consider factors such as motivation and maintenance in order to preserve treatment gains.

Cognitive Interventions in MCI

Relative to the amount of research on the efficacy of cognitive training with healthy older adults and those with dementia, research utilizing these techniques in MCI still appears to be in its infancy, with only nine published articles to date. Nonetheless, cognitive training interventions for individuals with MCI present with a number of important benefits, as well as some limitations. Perhaps of most importance, because memory problems are often less severe in MCI than dementia, there is greater opportunity to utilize residual memory and non-memory skills, such as executive functioning, to help compensate. Additionally, goals seem to have a clearer boundary for distinguishing effectiveness – that is, cognitive techniques are typically employed with the goal of maintaining a distinct level of functional independence (Troyer et al., 2007), since this is critical in the conceptualization of MCI versus AD (Petersen, 2004). As noted by Belleville (2007), individuals with MCI are also typically more motivated for treatment and can learn new strategies, which may help alleviate some anxiety about further memory decline and improve overall quality of life. In contrast, some of the limitations of cognitive training with individuals with MCI may include the lack of techniques that have demonstrated adequate ecological validity and the noted tendency for individuals to discontinue use of the strategies after training has been terminated (Rapp et al., 2002). Despite these limitations, preliminary research has revealed encouraging findings.

Pre-Training

Meta-analytic studies on episodic memory tasks have found a significant relationship between pre-training and memory enhancement (Floyd and Scogin, 1997; Verhaeghen et al., 1992). Pre-training was first introduced to cognitive training in the early 1980's, and refers to training of various memory-related processes (e.g. visual imagery and semantic processing) before introducing visually-based mnemonic techniques (Stigsdotter Neely, 2000). According to the initial research (Yesavage et al., 1989), pre-training was primarily introduced to decrease anxiety about learning mnemonics, which was believed to subsequently facilitate encoding and enhance memory performance (Stigsdotter Neely, 2000). For example, Brooks and colleagues (1999) asked subjects in their study to compare the work of two artists by forming images, noting similarities and differences, verbally elaborating on the images by making mental comments about the images, and incorporating progressive muscle relaxation (Rimm and Masters, 1974). Pre-training builds upon the levels of processing theory (Craik and Lockhart, 1972), which suggests that information encoded at deeper levels will be easier to recall than information processed at shallow levels. Combining methods of pre-training has been found to enhance learning and long-term gains (Sheikh, Hill, and Yesavage, 1986).

Mnemonic Strategies

Mnemonic strategies were perhaps the first memory interventions utilized within clinical settings. Generally, mnemonic strategies include verbal organization (i.e. formation of acronyms), semantic clustering and elaboration (i.e. categorizing lists of words into semantic clusters or creating a story linking all target words on a list), and visual imagery (i.e. method of loci, face-name association, creating a mental picture of a target) (Sohlberg and Mateer, 2001). While semantic clustering has been found to be one of the most efficient strategies for memory enhancement (Delis et al., 1988), recent studies have revealed that individuals with MCI and AD demonstrate less semantic clustering and supportive encoding strategies than controls (Perri et al., 2005; Ribeiro et al., 2007). However, by providing additional support via categorical cueing at the encoding stage, individuals with memory impairments are able to recall and recognize names and categories upon recall (Bozoki et al., 2006; Lipinksa and Backman, 1997; Ribeiro et al., 2007).

One of the most popular mnemonic strategies is the method of loci technique. This was used by ancient orators and integrates visual association, visual imagery, and organization (Stigsdotter Neely, 2000). The key in using this technique is to use visual imagery to imagine a familiar path one can walk through, including homes, offices, etc. where landmarks can be quickly identified. Once the path has been identified and imagined, an individual can begin to associate various target items (e.g. word lists) with each landmark (or loci) along the imagined path. This technique relies primarily on explicit memory and has been proven efficacious with older adults (e.g. Brooks et al., 1999), especially on tasks that may be generalized to various settings and daily tasks, such as grocery shopping (Anschutz et al., 1985). Additionally, the method of loci can be self-taught in healthy older adults and has been reported to improve subjective feelings of memory functioning six months after training (Scogin and Prochaska, 1992). There is limited research using the method of loci technique to enhance memory in MCI and AD; perhaps this is because this technique requires additional executive skills, such as planning and organization, which may be compromised in individuals with progressive neurodegenerative disease (Canellopoulou and Richardson, 1998).

Another commonly studied visually-based mnemonic strategy is Face-Name Association (McCarty, 1980). The face-name association strategy involves three steps for encoding and three subsequent steps for recall. In encoding, or learning, new information, the individual must, (1) choose a prominent feature of the person's face, (2) develop a concrete and highly imaginative transformation of the person's name, and (3) develop a visual image integrating the prominent facial feature with the transformed name. For example, if one was attempting to remember an older woman named Mercedes with striking red hair, one might develop a visual image of her prominent facial feature (e.g. her red hair) with her name (a visual image of an old-fashioned convertible Mercedes), and then imagine the old-fashioned red convertible Mercedes parked on her head. In order to recall her name at a later time, the individual would use the three steps for efficient recall; (1) recognize the prominent facial feature (e.g. red hair), (2) use the facial feature as a retrieval cue for the image association (e.g. an old-fashioned red convertible Mercedes parked on her head), and (3) recall the name from the image (e.g. Mercedes). Belleville and colleagues (2006) employed the face-name association technique as part of a multi-factorial intervention with MCI individuals and found significant improvements post-intervention in delayed memory for people's names, evidencing the clinical utility and possible generalizability of such interventions with this population. The benefit of this technique is the relative simplicity for learning it; however, it has been suggested that even three steps and the necessity to organize various loci and target items may be challenging for those with cognitive impairments related to aging (Yesavage et al., 1990).

Overall, improving episodic memory systems involves integrating strategies that provide unique and substantial encoding that can subsequently enhance recall, such as use of mnemonics. Because individuals with MCI are still able to learn some new information and generalize strategies across tasks and settings, using mnemonic strategies with this population may warrant more successful outcomes (Sohlberg and Mateer, 2001). Not only do these studies indicate that encoding is possible, but offers encouraging prospects about the role of semantic-based and mnemonic strategies in memory enhancement programs for individuals with MCI.

Errorless Learning

Another technique, errorless learning (EL), is based upon the notion that remembering new information will be more efficient if errors during the acquisition, or encoding, phase, are minimized and/or immediately corrected. To this regard, only accurate information will be supported during encoding and subsequent recall. One author summarized the use of errorless learning in memory impaired populations by stating, "The old adage that the best way to learn is from your mistakes may be true if you have a good memory with which to remember your mistakes" (Evans et al., 2000, p. 68). Therefore, avoiding errors during the initial encoding process will theoretically result in more efficient learning (Evans et al., 2004). Considering the nature of memory impairment in pathological aging, the principle of EL is meant to target the implicit memory system since it is believed to remain spared until later stages of disease (Baddeley and Wilson, 1994 DeVreese et al., 2001), although some studies reveal that errorless learning may also activate some residual systems involved in explicit memory (Clare et al., 2003; Hunkin et al., 1998)

Akhtar, Moulin, and Bowie (2006) were interested in observing whether learning in an errorless learning paradigm was of benefit to individuals with MCI for an explicit memory task of rote word recall, and if the subjects in the study were subsequently aware of the benefits of EL. Similar to the strategy used in Baddeley and Wilson (1994), Akhtar et al. (2006) provided errorless and errorful learning conditions, but included an additional component where the subject was instructed to make a judgment of learning. Judgments of learning evaluate memory monitoring by asking participants to predict future recall performance (Akhtar et al., 2006). For example, first participants were provided with the cue and target word (i.e., "I am thinking of a word beginning with WA and the word is WATER"), they were then instructed to write the word down on a piece of paper containing the first two letters of each word (a semantic cue). Participants were then asked to make judgments of learning for each word (i.e. "How likely do you think you will be able to remember the word you have just written down?" on a scale of 0-100%, where 0% is not likely and 100% is very likely). The authors reported greater levels of cued immediate and delayed recall in the EL condition, with some participants increasing their recall by as much as 200 percent. In addition, their findings are consistent with previous research suggesting that people with MCI have some awareness of their declining memory (Correa et al., 1996; Small et al., 1995) and of the benefits of EL learning, as noted by higher predictions of subsequent recall on items learned in the EL condition (Akhtar et al., 2006). Unfortunately, there were no outcome measures for delayed recall and no long-term follow-up (as of yet) in order to gauge the true benefits of EL over a length of time.

Researchers studying the effectiveness of errorless learning in AD have used it in combination with other cognitive techniques (i.e. mnemonics, repeated practice, vanishing cues etc.) in order to evaluate functional skills, such as face-name association (Clare et al., 2000, 2002, 2003; McCarty, 1980), and to tap into both implicit and residual explicit memory systems. Even when used alone, EL has proven to be a more effective learning strategy than errorful conditions in early AD (Metzler-Baddeley and Snowden, 2005). Single case studies using these combinations have reported relatively successful results in individuals with AD in very brief periods of time (Clare et al., 2000; Winter and Hunkin, 1999), with mnemonic and expanded rehearsal (Landauer and Bjork, 1978) conditions observed as most efficient (Clare et al., 2000). Even after initial training was completed, improvements were maintained at a level above baseline (Clare et al., 2003). Similar findings have been reported in larger standardized and controlled research (Clare et al., 2002), with significant long-term gains and applicability to functional tasks (Clare et al., 2000). Even in severely memory-impaired individuals, enhanced EL conditions via the use of elaboration (e.g. providing semantic context) and self-generation have proven to improve accuracy and recall (Tailby and Haslam, 2003). These studies suggest that, with regular practice, contextual learning, active participation, and dual support in encoding and recall, it is possible for individuals with AD to benefit from a combination of cognitive techniques within an errorless learning paradigm.

Spaced Retrieval

Another well-examined strategy used in the cognitive training of individuals with AD is spaced retrieval (Landauer and Bjork, 1978), also known as expanded rehearsal (Moffat, 1989). Spaced retrieval involves learning and retaining new information by recalling the information over increasingly longer periods of time, and has been referred to as a shaping paradigm (Bjork, 1988; Camp et al., 1995). If retrieval is successful, the time interval between recall trials is increased; however, if recall is unsuccessful, the individual is told the correct response and asked to repeat it, and the following interval for recall returns to the last interval at which success was observed. Camp and colleagues (2000) suggested that successful retrieval after intervals of 15-60 minutes typically indicates adequate long-term storage of the targeted information. Additionally, this method appears to require little outlay of cognitive effort, and while the exact locus of the method remains unclear, it is believed that priming is the essential ingredient for its effectiveness (De Vreese et al., 2001). Moreover, this method has been utilized with success in both residential and outpatient settings, and can be further enhanced by extending training to family and caregivers in few training sessions (McKitrick and Camp, 1992), which ultimately allows continuous learning at lower costs (Farina et al., 2002). The research utilizing this strategy to remediate impaired memory functions secondary to AD has demonstrated positive learning and recall of small, but important, pieces of information, including face-name associations (Camp and Foss, 1997; Hawley and Cherry, 2004), calendar training (Camp et al., 1996), external memory aids (Bourgeois et al., 2003), prospective memory tasks (e.g. redeeming coupons for money; McKitrick et al., 1992), and object naming (Camp et al., 2000). It has also been observed to have a positive impact on behavioral disturbances associated with dementia (Bird and Kinsella, 1996). To date, only one single-case study of an individual with early AD has demonstrated self-training and generalization of the method (Riley, 1992), and no studies were found that were able to demonstrate generalizability to non-trained target material. Utilization of this technique in MCI individuals remains unknown but would be beneficial to consider in future research.

Conflicting Evidence

Not all research has supported cognitive training in memory impaired older adults. Farina and colleagues (2002) argued that cognitive training of residual cognitive functions is not as effective or useful for individuals with AD as rehabilitation targeted towards functional activities, such as improving ADL, which is supported by implicit memory. Additionally, some authors have reported no significant effect of cognitive training in AD (Clare and Woods, 2005; Davis et al., 2001), and in fact, some studies have stated concern that these complex techniques may actually have a negative impact on mood (Small et al., 1997) and well-being. Other studies have continued to evaluate the efficacy of cognitive techniques, and some have additionally examined the true benefit of errorless versus errorful conditions in the dementia population (Dunn and Clare, 2007). For example, Haslam, Gilroy, Black and Beesley (2006) did not find overwhelming evidence for the advantage of the errorless learning principle in their study with individuals with early AD and vascular dementia. Additionally, Dunn and Clare (2007) compared the effects of four different learning techniques under errorless, errorful, effortless, and effortful conditions for learning previously known and novel face-name associations in individuals with AD, mixed, and vascular dementia. Results indicated that all four techniques resulted in significant learning of both familiar and novel faces. However, there was no significant difference between the four learning methods, suggesting that errorful methods are at least equally efficacious as errorless methods for learning name-face associations.

Comprehensive Interventions

In addition to cognitive training programs, there is recent evidence that the role of lifestyle and environmental factors can be neuroprotective against the development of Alzheimer's disease (Kramer et al., 2004). As such, some researchers have developed comprehensive healthy lifestyle programs that incorporate aspects of diet, physical exercise, relaxation strategies, and mental exercise (Small et al., 2006). Small and colleagues (2006) developed a lifestyle program designed for older adults with age-related memory complaints. Individuals in the experimental group received a manual that detailed a 14-day program, consisting of memory mnemonics, mind-teasers, solving puzzles, mazes, and other specific strategies (e.g. Look-Snap-Connect). In addition to memory techniques, the healthy lifestyle program focuses on daily cardiovascular exercises, diet and recipe suggestions, education regarding alternative supplements, and brief relaxation strategies. The intervention group demonstrated significant improvement on objective measures of verbal fluency, and FDG-PET imaging revealed a 5% decrease in activity in the left dorsolateral prefrontal cortex, an area associated with working memory, semantic organization skills, anxiety, and verbal fluency. This decrease in activity was interpreted as greater cognitive efficiency (Small et al., 2006).

Researchers have developed similar programs for individuals with amnestic MCI (Rapp et al., 2002; Troyer et al., 2007). These studies are typically comprised of multi-faceted group training sessions that include relaxation techniques, education regarding memory and aging, memory skills training, cognitive restructuring of memory-related beliefs, information regarding appropriate diet and recreational activities, and availability of community resources (Troyer et al., 2007). Previous studies with healthy older adults had the general goal of overall longevity, memory enhancement, and healthy living, but intervention programs for individuals with MCI have typically focused on improving memory for daily tasks and maintaining a level of functional independence, since this is a key factor in distinguishing MCI from AD (Petersen, 2004). Troyer et al. (2007) reported successful findings for a multidisciplinary memory intervention program, including the use of external memory aids, to alter daily behavioral memory immediately after the intervention and upon three-month follow-up. Participants in their study reported incorporating the memory strategies appropriately into their daily lives and indicated adequate generalizability and maintenance of the strategies, which in turn was believed to aid in the maintenance of functional independence and reduce the rate of decline. They demonstrated that, despite the fact that new behaviors are often difficult to incorporate into daily living, individuals with MCI who are appropriately trained can learn and effectively utilize these techniques over the course of time. In contrast, an earlier multi-faceted study did not find a significant difference in the recall of word lists between experimental and control groups, but did observe significantly better appraisals of memory function in subjects who had received cognitive restructuring (Rapp et al., 2002). This suggests that perhaps it is important to teach older adults with MCI new ways to perceive control of their memory and overall memory functioning, and then aim to gradually integrate relevant memory strategies (e.g. memory for daily tasks versus rote word recall) and external memory aids over time.

Computer-Assisted Cognitive Interventions

With the advancement of technology, researchers have also begun to publish preliminary studies investigating the effect of the computer-assisted training interventions for healthy older adults and those with memory impairments. Gunther and colleagues (2003) investigated the long- and short-term effects of a computer-assisted cognitive training program in a group of 19 older adults diagnosed with age associated memory impairment (Crook, Bartus and Ferris, 1986). Results from this original study revealed significant improvements in the majority of cognitive functions, including verbal and visual working memory and episodic memory, information processing speed, verbal learning, and ability to block out interference. Moreover, the authors reported significant improvements in verbal learning and memory upon five month follow-up, suggesting that the computer-assisted training program may improve minor age-associated cognitive deficits, and that the effects may be relatively long-lasting. While these findings are impressive, the small sample size and lack of a control group poses a threat to some of the psychometric features of the study.

Computer-based software technology has also recently been introduced in the rehabilitative and training efforts in MCI. Initial studies have demonstrated that computer-based cognitive training has increased learning efficiency in healthy older adults (Hickman et al., 2007) and supported cognitive and functional improvements in AD populations (Schreiber et al., 1999). To date, only three articles have been published on the use and efficacy of these interventions specific to individuals with MCI. Two of these combined computer-assisted and pharmacological intervention (Requena et al., 2004; Rozzini et al., 2007). Talassi et al. (2007) integrated computer-based cognitive training with other multidisciplinary therapies (i.e. occupational therapy and behavioral therapy) and observed improvements in cognitive and affective status in the MCI group when compared to a mildly demented group. Similarly, after only 3-months of cognitive training, Cipriani and colleagues (2006) revealed significant improvements in behavioral memory (i.e. memory for skills related to daily situations) in their MCI group, as well as improvements in language and executive functioning in their AD group. Moreover, they suggested that the same or similar rehabilitative strategies could result in different outcomes according to patient diagnosis (e.g. MCI vs. mild AD vs. moderate AD), making the case that computer-based training programs may be more advantageous given their ability to rapidly tailor individual interventions based upon available memory functions.

Another study examined the effectiveness of an interactive computer-based memory training program for individuals with mild to moderate Alzheimer's disease and vascular dementia (Schreiber et al., 1999). Ten 30-minute training sessions were developed to improve immediate and delayed recall of objects and routes in a virtual apartment made up of several familiar rooms (e.g. living room, kitchen, bedroom, bathroom, etc.). The authors reported significant improvements upon post-tests in the areas of immediate recall of meaningful visual information and delayed retention of topographical information. Still other authors have combined treatment interventions in order to evaluate the efficacy of a multi-modal intervention. Mate-Kole and colleagues (2007) used a combination of an interactive group cognitive training program and individually-based computer-assisted training program with six elderly individuals with a diagnosis of moderate to severe dementia. The two interventions consisted of Mind Aerobics (paper/pencil and hands-on activities focused on memory, attention, cognitive flexibility, manual dexterity, and problem solving) and a series of computerized tasks that were conducted individually for 30 minutes, four times per week during the intervention period of six weeks. Results revealed that participants demonstrated significant improvement on measures of global cognitive functioning and short-term memory (via a selective reminding task), as well as behavioral and social improvements after completion of both interventions. Four weeks after the initial training ended, cognitive and behavioral decline was observed and noted by caregivers, thus providing evidence in support of the immediate effects of the training program in maintaining level of cognitive functioning, but suggesting the absence of longer-term effects.

As our older generation becomes more technologically savvy, it seems only natural that cognitive interventions for memory disorders should move in the same direction. These newer computer-based cognitive training interventions have presented with some significant advantages and some limitations to consider before accepting them as reliable and efficacious methods of intervention. First, the majority of the studies published on computer-assisted cognitive interventions were completed with small sample sizes and some lack controls, making comparisons to other modes of intervention difficult. In addition, many of the tasks included in these interventions are laboratory-based and likely lack ecological validity for functional activities. On a more functional level, many older adults have not had regular exposure to modern technology and thus may be hesitant or cautious in using them. However, some of the advantages to using computer-assisted cognitive training programs are their flexibility and ability to tailor interventions to specific aspects of cognitive impairments (Gunther et al., 2003; Talassi et al., 2007), as well as the ability of the computer to provide immediate and specific feedback regarding performance (Gunther et al., 2003). Computers are also ideal for simulating real-life environments and integrating goal-directed behaviors in order to increase ecological validity (Schreiber et al., 1999). In sum, while the efficacy of computer-assisted cognitive interventions is far from perfect, recent research has provided encouraging evidence for its usefulness.

Combined Approaches

Researchers have also evaluated the efficacy of combining medication with a computer-based cognitive training program. Rozzini and colleagues (2007) evaluated the efficacy of a cognitive training program in MCI patients treated with acetylcholinesterase inhibitors (AChEI), compared with MCI patients treated only with AChEIs and patients not treated at all over a one-year follow-up study. Findings suggested that a combination of pharmacological and non-pharmacological treatment in MCI may maximize the effects of the AChEIs and delay memory deterioration and conversion to AD. It is unclear, however, whether treatment gains were attributable to the cognitive training alone, or whether a positive relationship exists between cognitive training and pharmacological treatment, as observed in previous research in healthy aging (Yesavage et al., 2007) and AD (Olazaran et al., 2004; Requena et al., 2004).

Requena and colleagues (2004 and 2006) completed a similar study using individuals with mild AD. At one year follow-up, Requena et al. (2004) reported significant gains in cognition in those receiving a combination of donepezil and computerized cognitive stimulation, relative to those with no treatment or either treatment alone. After two years, however, the authors (Requena et al., 2006) reported gradual deterioration in all groups and concluded that cognitive deterioration is inevitable after two years of treatment in people with mild dementia. Similarly, after a one-year, 103-session training period, Olazaran and colleagues (2004) reported that those with MCI and mild and moderate AD maintained cognitive status after 6 months of receiving cognitive-motor, psychosocial, and ACHEI intervention, with significant cognitive declines among those receiving psychosocial interventions alone. After 12 months, a significant improvement was observed in behavior and affective status, which was not attributable to the pharmacological intervention alone. These findings suggest a complementary relationship between cognitive and drug therapy for both cognitive and psychosocial disturbances; however, there is some indication that improvements subside after the first year. In sum, the evidence in support of combining cognitive training and pharmacological treatment in MCI and mild dementia is exciting; however, additional studies should be completed before assuming the reliability of these findings.

Limitations to Cognitive Interventions

The development of cognitive interventions designed for older adults has come a long way since initial research in this area over a decade ago, but these interventions still present with some significant limitations. Along with generally small and homogenous samples, and absence of appropriate controls (Belleville, 2007), one of the chief concerns regarding the use of cognitive techniques in memory enhancement is the overwhelming lack of evidence for its ecological validity, or generalizability. Many tasks used in research studies rely on laboratory-based tasks (e.g. word list recall), which are highly specific to the mnemonic ability being trained (Ball et al., 2002) and therefore result in more efficient recall for tasks that are congruent with training (Neely and Backman, 1993). This makes it more challenging for older adults to transfer the training toward application to functional situations, and leads to the conclusion that training on tasks that simulate real-life situations may be more useful.

One factor that appears to weigh heavily in the success of the long-term studies is the adherence of cognitive strategies after initial training ends. Cognitive gains in healthy older adults resulting from these strategies have been observed immediately post intervention (Anschutz, 1985), and at subsequent one year, three year (Anschutz, 1987; Neely and Backman, 1993), and even five year follow-up (O'Hara et al., 2007; Willis et al., 2005). Conversely, subjects who discontinued use of the cognitive strategies, or reverted back to faulty methods of learning, did not demonstrate significant long-term gain (O'Hara et al., 2007). At the same time, it is important to note that individuals with AD have been found to lose the benefit of cognitive training only three months after initial training (Farina et al., 2002). Perhaps issues of noncompliance partially account for the lack of generalization and maintenance of the strategies. There is some long-term benefit for individuals who utilize cognitive techniques on a regular basis or with more frequent follow-up. Thus, the results from these studies suggest that continued "booster" sessions (Ball et al., 2002) applied regularly and indefinitely after the initial training may further help individuals utilize and employ techniques with greater consistency and in more generalized situations (e.g. daily "to-do" lists).

Despite these limitations, there are some distinct characteristics that have contributed to the success of cognitive interventions with older adults. For example, interventions that were multidisciplinary in nature and gradually introduced the memory strategies with pre-training, distributed practice, regular homework assignments, booster sessions, and components of cognitive restructuring demonstrated the most enduring effects for healthy older adults and those with MCI. Because of the high vulnerability to interference that exists for people with MCI (Della Sala et al., 2005), regular maintenance and application of the strategies to daily tasks is a critical component of cognitive intervention. In addition, interventions which provide support at both encoding and recall for material that is relevant to daily functioning appear to be more successful. Comprehensive and multimodal intervention programs that utilize both traditional and computer-assisted training have also provided evidence that individuals with MCI who are trained appropriately can learn and effectively utilize these techniques over the course of time. Even without long-term data, this research has revealed the importance of considering each individual's unique strengths and weaknesses in order to best develop multimodal interventions that can maintain functional independence and improve overall quality of life.

In sum, the limited research published on the use of cognitive training techniques and programs with individuals with MCI has been encouraging, but presents clinicians with a number of factors to consider before implementing treatment. At the most general level, these issues include the lack of standardized criteria for MCI diagnosis, which has an impact on the reliability of the studies published thus far. Additionally, because this area of research is still in its infancy, there is no long-term data to support the efficacy of cognitive interventions in MCI over a long period of time, and/or the subsequent rate of conversion to AD (Belleville, 2007). At a more functional level, most of the research was not able to demonstrate an adequate transfer of training to everyday tasks, making it highly specific to the trained task. Moreover, techniques used among AD populations cannot be automatically generalized to MCI individuals without further investigation. Overall, it is apparent that while cognitive training techniques can be beneficial to individuals with MCI, more research is necessary before any definitive decisions can be made about its effectiveness with this population.

CONCLUSIONS

With the continued growth and longevity of the aging population, the detection, diagnosis, and treatment of MCI has increasing importance in clinical practice. To date, no standardized diagnostic criteria exist; however, clinicians and researchers alike have operationalized MCI as a representation of progressive cognitive decline in the absence of dementia. In addition to clinically accepted criteria, there is increasing agreement that informant data, multiple evaluations of cognition over time, and impairment of complex functional activities must be considered. A multimodal approach combining data from neuropsychological testing and neuroimaging is highly recommended for confirmation of diagnosis. While no pharmacological treatment has been approved specifically for the treatment of MCI, off-label use of medications for dementia is currently being utilized. There is also a growing body of supportive research regarding the use of lifestyle and cognitive intervention techniques for preserving cognition. For example, a balanced diet, adequate sleep, and reduced stress have been positively associated with prevention of cognitive decline, and cognitive training interventions such as mnemonics and errorless learning have proven efficacious in the process of learning new information for individuals with MCI. Overall, however, the most efficacious interventions are those that combine education about aging and memory, biological and lifestyle interventions, and cognitive training.

MCI is a relatively new diagnostic construct, fraught with heterogeneity in terms of etiology, diagnosis, progression, prognosis, and intervention efficacy. This increases the complexity of application and relevance of current information to MCI, especially in a population with intermediate changes in neuropathology and minimal functional impairment. This also makes additional research necessary for all aspects of MCI. Specifically, future research using sensitive and specific neuropsychological tests and advanced neuroimaging, such as FDDNP-PET, may enhance diagnostic confidence and aid in addressing the extent and subtype of MCI. Investigation is also needed to determine the diagnostic utility of biomarkers such as genetic and CSF testing. Medications that are differentiated from dementia treatment and specific to MCI have yet to be determined. Many of the studies published on the neuroprotective characteristics and clinical utility of lifestyle and cognitive interventions have been done in healthy aging and/or AD populations, but very few have been completed with MCI groups. More studies demonstrating adequate ecological validity and transfer of training to daily tasks, as well as meaningful exercises to maintain independence in functional activities, are necessary. The concept of MCI is also being increasingly used to inform impairment in domains other than memory (and AD), allowing for a better understanding of diseases such as frontotemporal or vascular dementia. Additional research is needed to establish a base of knowledge about the many conditions that MCI may indicate. Hopefully, data demonstrating the long-term benefits of interventions and their role in slowing the rate of conversion to dementia may provide clinicians with additional tools for improving the quality of life and longevity in our burgeoning aging population.

REFERENCES

Acevedo A and Lowestein DA (2007). Nonpharmacological interventions in aging and dementia. *Journal of Geriatric Psychiatry and Neurology, 20,* 239-249.

Adabag AS, Nelson DB, and Bloomfield HE (2007). Effects of statin therapy on preventing atrial fibrillation in coronary disease and heart failure. *American Heart Journal, 154*(6), 1140-5.

Adak S, Illouz K, Gorman W, Tandon R, Zimmerman EA, Guariglia R, Moore MM, and Kaye, JA (2004). Predicting the rate of cognitive decline in aging and early Alzheimer disease. *Neurology, 63,* 108-114.

ADAPT Research Group (2006). Cardiovascular and cerebrovascular events in the randomized, controlled Alzheimer's Disease Anti-inflammatory Prevention Trial (ADAPT). *Public Library of Science Clinical Trials, 1*(7), e33. Retrieved on December 15 2007, at http://clinicaltrials.ploshubs.org/article/info:doi/10.1371/journal.pctr.0010033

ADAPT Research Group; Lyketsos CG, Breitner JC, Green RC, Martin BK, Meinert C, Piantadosi S, Sabbagh M (2007). Naproxen and celecoxib do not prevent AD in early results from a randomized controlled trial. *Neurology, 68*(21), 1800-8.

Aenlle KK, Kumar A, Cui L, Jackson TC, and Foster TC (in press). Estrogen effects on cognition and hippocampal transcription in middle-aged mice. *Neurobiology of Aging..*

Aggarwal NT, Wilson RS, Beck TL, Bienias JL, and Bennett DA (2005). Mild cognitive impairment in different functional domains and incident Alzheimer's disease. *Journal of Neurology, Neurosurgery, and Psychiatry, 76*(11), 1479-84.

Akhtar S, Moulin CJ and Bowie, PC (2006). Are people with mild cognitive impairment aware of the benefits of errorless learning? *Neuropsychological Rehabilitation, 16*(3), 329-46.

Albert M, Blacker D, Moss MB, Tanzi R and McArdle, JJ (2007). Longitudinal change in cognitive performance among individuals with mild cognitive impairment. *Neuropsychology, 21*, 158-169.

Alexander DM, Williams LM, Gatt JM, Dobson-Stone C, Kuan SA, Todd EG, Schofield PR, Cooper NJ, and Gordon, E (2007). The contribution of apolipoprotein E alleles on cognitive performance and dynamic neural activity over six decades. *Biological Psychology, 75*, 229-238.

Almkvist O, and Winblad B (1999). Early diagnosis of Alzheimer dementia based on clinical and biological factors. *European Archives of Psychiatry and Clinical Neuroscience,249*(Suppl. 3), 3-9.

Allain H, Bentué-Ferrer D and Akwa Y (2007). Treatment of mild cognitive impairment (MCI). *Human Psychopharmacology, 22*, 189-97.

Almeida OP, Lautenschlager NT, Vasikaran S, Leedman P, Gelavis A and Flicker, L (2006). A 20-week randomized controlled trial of estradiol replacement therapy for women aged 70 years and older: Effect on mood, cognition, and quality of life. *Neurobiology of Aging, 27*, 141-9.

American Psychiatric Association (1994). *Diagnostic and Statistical Manual of Mental Disorders* (4th ed.). Arlington, VA: American Psychiatric Publishing, Inc.

American Psychiatric Association; Workgroup on Alzheimer's disease and related disorders (1997). *APA Practice guidelines. Practice Guideline for the Treatment of Patients with Alzheimer's Disease and Other Dementias of Late Life.* Retrieved on December 15, 2007, at http://www.psych.org/psych_pract/treatg/pg/AlzPG101007.pdf

Ames D, Peterson RC, Knopman DS, Visser PJ, Brodaty H, Gauthier S (2006). For debate: Is mild cognitive impairment a clinically useful concept? *International Psychogeriatrics, 18*(3), 393-414.

Amieva H, Jacqmin-Gadda H, Orgogozo JM, Le Carret N, Helmer C, Letenneur L, et al. (2005). The 9 year cognitive decline before dementia of the Alzheimer type: A prospective population-based study. *Brain, 128*, 1093-1101.

Andel R, Hughes TF and Crowe, M (2005). Strategies to reduce the risk of cognitive decline and dementia. *Aging Health, 1*(1), 107-116.

Anderer P, Saletu B, Saletu-Zyhlarz G, Gruber D, Metka M, Huber J, and Pascual-Marqui RD (2004). Brain regions activated during an auditory discrimination task in insomniac postmenopausal patients before and after hormone replacement therapy: Low-resolution brain electromagnetic tomography applied to event-related potentials. *Neuropsychobiology, 49*(3), 134-53.

Andreasen N, Minthon L, Davidsson P, Vanmechelen E, Vanderstichele H, Winblad B, Blennow K (2001). Evaluation of CSF-tau and CSF-Abeta42 as diagnostic markers for Alzheimer disease in clinical practice. *Archives of Neurology, 58*(3), 373-9.

Andreasen N, Vanmechelen E, Van de Voorde A, Davidsson P, Hesse C, Tarvonen S, et al. (1998). Cerebrospinal fluid tau protein as a biochemical marker for Alzheimer's disease:

a community based follow up study. *Journal of Neurology, Neurosurgery, and Psychiatry, 64*(3), 298-305.

Anschutz L., Camp CJ, Markley RP and Kramer JJ. (1985). Maintenance and generalization of mnemonics for grocery shopping by older adults. *Experimental Aging Research* 11(3): 157-160.

Anschutz L, Camp CJ, Markley RP and Kramer JJ. (1987). Remembering mnemonics: A three-year follow-up on the effects of mnemonics training in the elderly. *Experimental Aging Research* 13(3): 141-143.

Anstey KJ, and Low LF (2004). Normal cognitive changes in aging. *Australian Family Physician, 33,* 783-787.

Apostolova LG and Cummings JL (2008). Neuropsychiatric manifestations in mild cognitive impairment: A systematic review of the literature. *Dementia and Geriatric Cognitive Disorders, 25,* 115-126.

Arai H, Morikawa Y, Higuchi M, Matsui T, Clark CM, Miura M, et al. (1997). Cerebrospinal fluid tau levels in neurodegenerative diseases with distinct tau-related pathology. *Biochemical and Biophysical Research Communication, 236*(2), 262-4.

Arca M and Gaspardone, A (2007). Atorvastatin efficacy in the primary and secondary prevention of cardiovascular events. *Drugs, 67*(Suppl. 1), 29-42.

Ardila A, Ostrosky-Solis F, Rosselli M and Gomez, C (2000). Age-related cognitive decline during normal aging: The complex effect of education. *Archives of Clinical Neuropsychology, 15*(6), 495-513.

Arnaiz E, Almkvist O (2003). Neuropsychological features of mild cognitive impairment and preclinical Alzheimer's disease. *Acta Neurologica Scandinavica, 107*(Suppl. 179), 34-41.

Artero S, Petersen R, Touchon J and Ritchie, K (2006). Revised criteria for mild cognitive impairment: Validation within a longitudinal population study. *Dementia and Geriatric Cognitive Disorders, 22*(5-6), 465-70.

Babiloni C, Benussi L, Binetti G, Cassetta E, Dal Forno G, Del Percio C, et al. (2006). Apolipoprotein E and alpha brain rhythms in mild cognitive impairment: A multicentric electroencephalogram study. *Annals of Neurology, 59,* 323-334.

Babiloni C, Binetti G, Cassarino A, et al. (2006). Sources of cortical rhythms in adults during physiological aging: A multicentric EEG study. *Human Brain Mapping, 27*(2), 152-72.

Backhaus J, Born J, Hoeckesfeld R, Fokuhl S, Hohagen F and Junghanns, K (2007). Midlife decline in declarative memory consolidation is correlated with a decline in slow wave sleep. *Learning and Memory, 14*(5), 336-41.

Backman L, Jon es S, Berger AK, Laukka EJ, and Small BJ (2004). Multiple cognitive deficits during the transition to Alzheimer's disease. *Journal of Internal Medicine, 256,* 195-204.

Backman L, Jones S, Berger AK, Laukka EJ, and Small BJ (2005). Cognitive impairment in preclinical Alzheimer's disease: A meta-analysis. *Neuropsychology, 19,* 520-531.

Backman L, Jones S, Small BJ, Aguero-Torres H and Fratiglioni L (2003). Rate of cognitive decline in preclinical Alzheimer's disease: The role of comorbidity. *Journal of Gerontology:Psychological Sciences, 58B,* 228-236.

Baddeley AD and Wilson BA (1994). When implicit learning fails: Amnesia and the problem of error elimination. *Neuropsychologia, 32,* 53-68.

Ball K, Berch DB, Helmers KF, Jobe JB, Leveck MD, Marsiske E, Morris JM, Rebok GW, Smith DM, Tennstedt SL, Unverzagt FW and Willis SL (2002). Effects of cognitive training interventions with older adults: A randomized controlled trial. *Journal of the American Medical Association* 288: 2271-2281.

Balthazar ML, Martinelli JE, Cendes F and Damasceno BP (2007). Lexical semantic memory in amnestic mild cognitive impairment and mild Alzheimer's disease. *Arquivos de neuro-psiquiatria, 65*(3A), 619-22.

Barnes DE, Alexopoulos GS, Lopez OL, Williamson JD, Yaffe K (2006). Depressive symptoms, vascular disease, and mild cognitive impairment: Findings from the Cardiovascular Health Study. *Archives of General Psychiatry, 63*(3), 273-9.

Bassuk SS, Berkman LF, Wypij D (1998). Depressive symptomatology and incident cognitive decline in an elderly community sample. *Archives of General Psychiatry, 55*(12), 1073-81.

Bell-McGinty S, Lopez OL, Meltzer CC, Scanlon JM, Whyte EM, Dekosky ST and Becker, JT (2005). Differential cortical atrophy in subgroups of mild cognitive impairment. *Archives of Neurology, 62*(9), 1393-7.

Belleville S (2007). Cognitive training for persons with mild cognitive impairment. *International Psychogeriatrics, 20*(1), 57-66.

Belleville S, Chertkow H and Gauthier S (2007). Working memory and control of attention in persons with Alzheimer's disease and mild cognitive impairment. *Neuropsychology, 21*, 458-469.

Belleville S, Gilbert B, Fontaine F, Gagnon L, Menard E and Gauthier S (2006). Improvement of episodic memory in persons with mild cognitive impairment and healthy older adults: Evidence from a cognitive intervention program. *Dementia and Geriatric Cognitive Disorder*s, 22, 486-99.

Bennett DA, Wilson RS, Schneider JA, Evans DA, Beckett LA, Aggarwal NT, Barnes LL, Fox JH and Bach J (2002). Natural history of mild cognitive impairment in older persons, *Neurology, 59*(2), 198-205.

Benson H, Beary IF and Carol MP (1974). The relaxation response. *Psychiatry, 37*, 37-45.

Biessels GJ, van der Heide LP, Kamal A, Bleys RL and Gispen EH (2002). Ageing and diabetes: Implications for brain function. *European Journal of Pharmacology, 441*(1-2), 1-14.

Bigler ED, Tate DF, Miller MJ, Rice SA, Hessel CD, Earl HD, et al. (2002). Dementia, asymmetry of temporal lobe structures, and Apolipoprotein E genotype: Relationships to cerebral atrophy and neuropsychological impairment. *Journal of the International Neuropsychological Society, 8*, 925-933.

Bird M and Kinsella G (1996). Long-term cued recall of tasks in senile dementia. *Psychology and Aging* 11: 45-56.

Blackford RC and La Rue A (1989). Criteria for diagnosing age associated memory impairment: Proposed improvements in the field. *Developmental Neuropsychoogyl, 5*, 295-306.

Blackwell AD, Sahakian BJ, Vesey R, Semple JM, Robbins TW, and Hodges JR (2004). Detecting dementia: Novel neuropsychological markers of preclinical Alzheimer's disease. *Dementia and Geriatric Cognitive Disorders, 17*, 42-48.

Bondi MW, Salmon DP, Galasko D, Thomas RG and Thal LJ (1999). Neuropsychological function and apolipoprotein E genotype in the preclinical detection of Alzheimer's disease. *Psychology and Aging, 14*, 295-303.

Bourgeois MS, Camp C, Rose M, White B, Malone M, Carr J and Rovine M (2003). A comparison of training strategies to enhance use of external aids by persons with dementia. *Journal of Communication Disorders, 36*, 361-78.

Bouwman FH, Schoonenboom SN, van der Flier WM, van Elk EJ, Kok A, Barkhof F, et al. (2007). CSF biomarkers and medial temporal lobe atrophy predict dementia in mild cognitive impairment. *Neurobiology of Aging, 28*(7), 1070-4.

Boylin W, Gordon S and Nehrke M (1976). Reminiscence and ego integrity in institutionalized elderly. *Gerontologist, 16*, 118-24.

Bozoki A, Grossman M and Smith EE (2006). Can patients with Alzheimer's disease learn a category implicitly? *Neuropsychologia, 44*, 816-27.

Brooks JO, Friedman L, Pearman AM, Gray C and Yesavage JA (1999). Mnemonic training in older adults: Effects of age, length of training, and type of cognitive pretraining. *International Psychogeriatrics* 11(1): 75-84.

Brusoli M and Lovestone S (2004). Is MCI really just early dementia? A systematic review of conversion studies. *International Psychogeriatrics, 16*(2), 129-40.

Bugiani O, Constantinidis B, Ghetti B, Bouras C and Tagliavini F (1991). Asymmetrical cerebral atrophy in Alzheimer's disease. *Clinical Neuropathology, 10*, 55–60.

Burns A and Zaudig M (2002). Mild cognitive impairment in older people *Lancet, 360*(9349), 1963-5.

Buschke H and Fuld PA (1974). Evaluating storage, retention, and retrieval in disordered memory and learning. *Neurology, 24*, 1019-25.

Busse A, Hensel A, Gühne U, Angermeyer MC and Riedel-Heller SG (2006). Mild cognitive impairment: Long-term course of four clinical subtypes. *Neurology, 67*(12), 2176-85.

Camp CJ (2001). From efficacy to effectiveness to diffusion: Making the transitions in dementia intervention research. *Neuropsychological Rehabilitation* 11: 495-517.

Camp CJ and Foss JW (1997). Designing ecologically valid intervention for persons with dementia. In DG Payne and FG Conrad (Eds.), *Intersections in Basic and Applied Memory Research* (311-5). New York: Springer.

Camp CJ, Foss JW, O'Hanlon AM and Stevens AB (1996). Memory interventions for persons with dementia. *Applied Cognitive Psychology* 10: 193-210.

Camp CJ, Bird MJ and Cherry KE (2000). Retreival strategies as a rehabilitation aid for cognitive loss in pathological aging. In RD Hill, L Backman, and A Stigsdotter-Neely (Eds.), *Cognitive Rehabilitation in Old Age* (224-8). Oxford: Oxford University Press.

Camp CJ, Foss JW, O'Hanlon A and Stevens AB (1996). Memory intervention for persons with dementia. *Applied Cognitive Psychology, 10*, 193-210.

Canellopoulou M and Richardson JT (1998). The role of executive functioning in imagery mnemonics: Evidence from multiple sclerosis. *Neuropsychologia, 36*(11), 1181-8.

Canon WB (1914). The emergency function of the adrenal medulla in pain and major emotions. *American Journal of Physiology, 33*(2), 356-72.

Caretti B, Borella E and De Beni R (2007). Does strategic memory training improve the working memory performance of younger and older adults? *Experimental Psychology* 54(4): 311-320.

Caselli RJ, Reiman EM, Osborne D, Hentz JG, Baxter LC, Hernandez JL and Alexander GG (2004). Longitudinal changes in cognition and behavior in asymptomatic carriers of the APOE e4 allele. *Neurology, 62*, 1990-1995.

Casserly I and Topol E (2004). Convergence of atherosclerosis and Alzheimer's disease: Inflammation, cholesterol, and misfolded proteins. *Lancet, 363*(9415), 1139-46.

Catani M, Cherubini A, Howard R, Tarducci R, Pelliccioli GP, Piccirilli M, Gobbi G, Senin U, Mecocci P (2001). (1)H-MR spectroscopy differentiates mild cognitive impairment from normal brain aging. *Neuroreport, 12*(11), 2315-7.

Cerhan JH, Ivnik RJ, Smith GE, Machulda MM, Boeve BF, Knopman DS, Petersen RC and Tangalos EG (2007). Alzheimer's disease patients' cognitive status and course years prior to symptom recognition. *Aging, Neuropsychology, and Cognition, 14*, 227-235.

Chan DC, Kasper JD, Black BS, Rabins PV (2003). Prevalence and correlates of behavioral and psychiatric symptoms in community-dwelling elders with dementia or mild cognitive impairment: The Memory and Medical Care Study. *International Journal of Geriatric Psychiatry, 18*(2), 174-82.

Chantal S, Braun CM, Bouchard RW, Labelle M, Boulanger Y (2004). Similar 1H magnetic resonance spectroscopic metabolic pattern in the medial temporal lobes of patients with mild cognitive impairment and Alzheimer disease. *Brain Research, 1003*(1-2), 26-35.

Chen P, Ratcliff G, Belle SH, Cauley JA, DeKosky ST and Ganguli M (2000). Cognitive tests that best discriminate between presymptomatic AD and those who remain nondemented. *Neurology, 55*, 1847-1853.

Chen P, Ratcliff G, Belle SH, Cauley JA, DeKosky ST and Ganguli M (2001). Patterns of cognitive decline in presymptomatic Alzheimer disease. *Archives of General Psychiatry, 58*, 853-858.

Cherrier MM, Matsumoto AM, Amory JK, Asthana S, Bremmer W, Peskind ER, Raskind MA and Craft S (2005). Testosterone improves spatial memory in men with Alzheimer's disease and mild cognitive impairment. *Neurology, 64*, 2063-8.

Chong MS and Sahadevan S (2005). Preclinical Alzheimer's disease: Diagnosis and prediction of progression. *The Lancet Neurology, 4*, 576-579.

Christensen H (2001). What cognitive changes can be expected with normal aging? *New Zealand Journal of Psychiatry, 35*, 768-775.

Christensen H, Mackinnon AJ, Korten AE, Jorm AF, Henderson AS, Jacomb P and Rodgers B (1999). An analysis of diversity in the cognitive performance of elderly community dwellers: Individual differences in change scores as a function of age. *Psychology and Aging, 14*, 365-379.

Cipriani G, Bianchetti A and Trabucchi M (2006). Outcomes of a computer-based cognitive rehabilitation program on Alzheimer's disease patients compared with those on patients affected by mild cognitive impairment. *Archives of Gerontology and Geriatrics, 43*, 327-35.

Clare L (2007). Dementia, disability and rehabilitation. In *Neuropsychological Rehabilitation: A Modular Handbook, Neuropsychological Rehabilitation and People with Dementia* (5-22). New York: Psychology Press.

Clare L and Wilson BA (2006). Longitudinal assessment of awareness in early-stage Alzheimer's disease using comparable questionnaire-based and performance-based measures: A prospective one-year follow-up study. *Aging and Mental Health* 10: 156-165.

Clare L, Roth I, Wilson BA, Carter G and Hodges JR (2002). Relearning face-name associations in early Alzheimer's disease. *Neuropsychology, 16*(4), 538-47.

Clare L, Wilson BA, Carter G, Roth I and Hodges JR (2004). Awareness in early-stage Alzheimer's disease: Relationship to outcome of cognitive rehabilitation. *Journal of Clinical and Experimental Neuropsychology, 36*(2), 215-26.

Clare L, Wilson BA, Breen K and Hodges JR (1999). Errorless learning of face-name associations in early Alzheimer's disease. *Neurocase, 5,* 37-46.

Clare L, Wilson BA, Carter G, Breen K, Gosses A and Hodges JR (2000). Intervening with everyday memory problems in dementia of Alzheimer type: An errorless learning approach. *Journal of Clinical and Experimental Neuropsychology, 22*(1), 132-46.

Clare L, Wilson BA, Carter G and Hodges JR (2003). Cognitive rehabilitation as a component of early intervention in Alzheimer's disease: a single case study. *Aging and Mental Health* 7: 15-21.

Clare L, Wilson BA, Carter G, Hodges JR and Adams M (2001). Long-term maintenance of treatment gains following a cognitive rehabilitation intervention in early dementia of Alzheimer type: A single case study. *Neuropsychological Rehabilitation, 11*(3/4), 477-94.

Clare L, Woods RT, Moniz Cook ED, Orrell M and Spector A (2003). Cognitive rehabilitation and cognitive training for the early-stage Alzheimer's disease and vascular dementia. *Cochrane Database of Systemic Reviews, Issue 4*(CD003260). Retrieved December 15, 2007, from http://mrw.interscience.wiley.com/cochrane/clsysrev/articles/CD003260/frame.html

Cohen M (1997). *Children's Memory Scale Manual.* Lutz, FL: Psychological Assessment Resources.

Colcombe SJ, Erickson KI, Scalf PE, Kim JS, Prakash R, McAuley E, Elavsky S, Marquez DX, Hu L and Kramer AF (2006). Aerobic exercise training increases brain volume in aging humans. *Journal of Gerontology. Series A, Biological Sciences and Medical Sciences 61*(11), 1166-70.

Collie A, Maruff P and Currie J (2002). Behavioral characterization of mild cognitive impairment. *Journal of Clinical and Experimental Neuropsychology, 24,* 720-33.

Colombe S and Kramer AF (2003). Fitness effects on the cognitive function of older adults: A meta-analytic study. *Psychological Science, 14*(2), 125-30.

Convit A, de Leon MJ, Tarshish C, de Santi S, Tsui W, Rusinek H and George A (1997). Specific hippocampal volume reductions in individuals at risk for Alzheimer's disease. *Neurobiology of Aging, 18,* 131-138.

Convit, A Wolf OT, Tarshish C, and de Leon MJ (2003). Reduced glucose tolerance is associated with poor memory performance and hippocampal atrophy among normal elderly. *Proceedings of the National Academy of Sciences of the United States of America, 100*(4), 2019-22.

Cook TH, Bartus RT, Ferris SH, Whitehouse P, Cohen GD and Gershon S (1986). Age-associated memory impairment: Proposed diagnostic criteria and measures of clinical change; Report of a National Institute of Mental Health Work Group. *Developmental Neuropsychology, 2,* 261-76.

Corral M, Rodriguez M and Amenedo E (2006). Cognitive reserve, age, and neuropsychological performance in healthy participants. *Developmental Neuropsychology, 29*(3), 479-91.

Correa DD, Graves RE and Costa L (1996). Awareness of memory deficit in Alzheimer's disease patients and memory-impaired older adults. *Aging Neuropsychology and Cognition, 3*, 215-28.

Craig MC, Maki PM and Murphy DGM (2005). The Women's Health Initiative Memory Study: Findings and implications for treatment. *The Lancet Neurology, 4*(3), 190-4.

Craik F and Lockhart RS (1972). Levels of processing: A framework for memory research. *Journal of Verbal Learning and Verbal* Behavior, 11, 671-84.

Crook TH, Bartus R and Ferris SH (1986). Age-associated memory impairment: Proposed diagnostic criteria and measures of change. *Developmental Neuropsychology, 2*, 261-76.

Cucchiara B and Kasner SE (2001). Use of statins in CNS disorders. *Journal of Neurological Sciences, 187*(1-2), 81-9.

Cummings JL (2003). The neuropsychiatry of Alzheimer's disease and related dementias. Kentucky, Taylor Francis Group.

Dai Q, Borenstein AR, Wu Y, Jackson JC and Larson EB (2006). Fruit and vegetable juices and Alzheimer's disease: The Kame Project. *The American Journal of Medicine, 119*, 751-9.

Darvesh S, Martin E, Walsh R and Rockford K (2004). Differential effects of lipid-lowering agents on human cholinesterases. *Clinical Biochemistry, 37*(1), 42-9.

Davis RN, Massman PJ and Doody RS (2001). Cognitive intervention in Alzheimer disease: A randomized placebo-controlled study. *Alzheimer's Disease and Associated Disorders, 15*(1), 1-9.

de Leon MJ, Convit A, Wolf OT, Tarshish CY, DeSanti S, Rusinek H, et al. (2001). Prediction of cognitive decline in normal elderly subjects with 2-[(18)F]fluoro-2-deoxy-D-glucose/poitron-emission tomography (FDG/PET). *Proceedings of the National Academy of Sciences USA, 98*(19), 10966-71.

de Leon MJ, DeSanti S, Zinkowski R, Mehta PD, Pratico D, Segal S, Clark C, Kerkman D, DeBernardis J, Li J, Lair L, Reisberg B, Tsui W, Rusinek H (2004). MRI and CSF studies in the early diagnosis of Alzheimer's disease. *Journal of Internal Medicine, 256*(3), 205-23.

De Ronchi D, Berardi M, Menchetti M, Ferrari G, Serretti A, Dalmonte E and Fratiglioni L (2005). *Dementia and Geriatric Cognitive Disorders, 19*, 97-105.

De Santi S, de Leon MJ, Rusinek H, Convit A, Tarshish CY, Roche A, Tsui WH, Kandil E, Boppana M, Daisley K, Wang GJ, Schlyer D and Fowler J (2001). Hippocampal formation glucose metabolism and volume losses in MCI and AD. *Neurobiological Aging, 22*, 529-539.

De Vreese LP, Mirco N, Fioravanti M, Belloi L and Zanetti O (2001). Memory rehabilitation in Alzheimer's disease: A review of progress. *International Journal of Geriatric Psychiatry, 16*, 794-809.

Deaselaar SM, Veltman DJ, Rombouts SA, Raaijmakers JG and Jonker C (2003). Neuroanatomical correlates of episodic encoding and retrieval in young and elderly subjects. *Brain, 126*(1), 43-56.

DeCarli C (2003). Mild cognitive impairment: Prevalence, prognosis, aetiology, and treatment. *Lancet Neurology, 2*(1), 15-21.

Delis DC, Kaplan E, Kramer JH and Ober BA (1988). Integrating clinical assessment with cognitive neuroscience: Construct validation of the California Verbal Learning Test. *Journal of Consulting and Clinical Psychology, 56*, 123-30.

Della Sala S, Cowan N, Beschin N and Perini M. (2005). Just lying there, remembering: Improving recall of prose in amnesic patients with mild cognitive impairment by minimizing interference. *Memory* 13: 435-440.

Devanand DP, Pradhaban G, Liu X, Khandji A, De Santi S, Segal S, Rusinek H, Pelton GH, Honig LS, Mayeux R, Stern Y, Tabert MH and de Leon MJ (2007). Hippocampal and entorhinal atrophy in mild cognitive impairment: Prediction of Alzheimer disease. *Neurology, 68*(11), 828-36.

Di Carlo A, Lamassa M, Baldereschi M, Inzitari M, Scafato E, Farchi G and Inzitari D (2007). CIND and MCI in the Italian elderly: Frequency, vascular risk factors, progression to dementia. *Neurology, 68*(22), 1909-16.

Dierckx E, Engelborghs S, De Raedt R, De Deyn PP and Ponjaert-Kristoffersen I (2007). Mild cognitive impairment: What's in a name? *Gerontology, 53*(1), 28-35.

Dixit A, Vaney N and Tandon OP (2006). Evaluation of cognitive brain functions in caffeine users: A P3 evoked potential study. *Indian Journal of Physiology and Pharmacology, 50*(2), 175-80.

Doody RS, Stevens JC, Beck C, Dubinsky RM, Kaye JA, Gwyther L, Mohs RC, Thal LJ, Whitehouse PJ, DeKosky ST and Cummings JL (2001). Practice parameter: Management of dementia (an evidence-based review). Report of the Quality Standards Subcommittee of the American Academy of Neurology. *Neurology, 56*(9), 1154-66.

Drachman DA (2006). Aging of the brain, entropy, and Alzheimer disease. *Neurology, 67*, 1340-52.

Driscoll I, Hamilton DA, Petropoulos H, Yeo RA, Brooks WM, Baumgartner RN and Sutherland RJ (2003). The aging hippocampus: Cognitive, biochemical and structural findings. *Cerebral Cortex, 13*, 1344-51.

Driscoll I, McDaniel MA and Guynn MJ (2005). Apolipoprotein E and prospective memory in normally aging adults. *Neuropsychology, 19*, 28-34.

Dunn J and Clare L (2007). Learning face-name associations in early-stage dementia: Comparing the effects of errorless learning and effortful processing. *Neuropsychological Rehabilitation, 17*(6), 735-54.

Engelhart MJ, Geerinlings MI, Ruitenberg A, van Swieten JC, Hofman A, Witteman JC and Breteler MM (2002). Dietary intake of antioxidants and risk of Alzheimer disease. *The Journal of the American Medical Association, 287*(24), 3223-9.

Esch T, Fricchione GL and Stefano GB (2003). The therapeutic use of the relaxation response in stress-related diseases. *Medical Science Monitor, 9*(2), RA23-34.

Esch T, Stefano GB, Fricchione GL and Benson H (2002). The role of stress in neurodegenerative diseases and mental disorders. *Neuroendocrinology Letters, 23*, 199-208.

Etnier JL, Nowell PM, Landers DM and Sibley BA (2006). A meta-regression to examine the relationship between aerobic fitness and cognitive performance. *Brain ResearchRreviews, 52*(1), 119-30.

Evans J, Levine B and Bateman A (2004). Errorless learning. *Neuropsychological Rehabilitation, 14*(4), 467-76.

Evans JJ, Wilson BA, Schuri U, Andrade J, Baddeley A, Bruna O, Canavan T, Della Sala S, Green R, Laaksonen R, Lorenzi L and Taussik I (2000). A comparison of "errorless" and "trial-and-error" learning methods for teaching individuals with acquired memory deficits. *Neuropsychological Rehabilitation* 10: 67-101.

Fabrigoule C, Rouch I, Taberly A, Letenneur L, Commenges D, Mazaux J, Orgogozo JM and Dartigues JF (1998). Cognitive process in preclinical phase of dementia. *Brain, 121*, 135-141.

Farina E, Fioravanti R, Chiavari L, Imbornone E, Alberoni M, Pomati S, Pinardi G, Pignatti R and Mariani C (2002). Comparing two programs of cognitive training in Alzheimer's disease: A pilot study. *Acta Neurologica Scandanivica, 105*, 365-71.

Farina E, Mantovani F, Fioravanti R, Pignatti R, Chiavari L, Imbornone E, Olivotto F, Alberoni M, Mariani C and Nemni R (2006). Evaluating two group programmes of cognitive training in mild-to-moderate AD: Is there any difference between a 'global' stimulation and a 'cognitive-specific' one? *Aging and Mental Health* 10: 211-218.

Feher EP, Larrabee GJ, Sudilovsky A and Crook TH (1994). Memory self-report in Alzheimer's disease and in age-associated memory impairment. *Journal of Geriatric Psychiatry and Neurology*, 7: 58-65.

Feldman H, Scheltens P, Scarpini E, Hermann N, Mesenbrink P, Mancione L, Tekin S, Lane R, Ferris S (2004). Behavioral symptoms in mild cognitive impairment. *Neurology, 62*(7), 1199-201.

Fillit HM, Butler RN, O'Connell AW, Albert MS, Birret JE, Cotman CW, et al. (2002). Achieving and maintaining cognitive vitality with aging. *Mayo Clinic Proceedings, 77*, 681-696.

Fischer P, Jungwirth S, Zehetmayer S, Weissgram S, Hoenigschnabl S, Gelpi E, Krampla W and Tragl KH (2007). Conversion from subtypes of mild cognitive impairment to Alzheimer dementia. *Neurology, 68*(4), 288-91.

Fischer S, Hallschmid M, Elsner AL and Born J (2002). Sleep forms memory for finger skills. *Proceedings of the National Academy of Sciences of the United States of America, 99*(18), 11987-91.

Fisk JD, Merry HR and Rockwood K (2003). Variations in case definition affect prevalence but not outcomes of mild cognitive impairment. *Neurology, 61*(9), 1179-84.

Fleisher AS, Sowell BB, Taylor C, Gamst AC, Peterson RC and Thal LJ (2007). Alzheimer's Disease Cooperative Study. Clinical predictors of progression to Alzheimer disease in amnestic mild cognitive impairment. *Neurology, 68*(19), 1588-95.

Floyd M and Scogin F (1997). Effects of memory training on the subjective memory functioning and mental health of older adults: A meta-analysis. *Psychology and Aging* 12: 150-161.

Folstein MF, Folstein SE and McHugh PR (1975). "Mini-mental state". A practical method for grading the cognitive state of patients for the clinician. *Journal of Psychiatric Research, 12*(3), 189-98.

Forsell Y, Palmer K, Fratiglioni L (2003). Psychiatric symptoms/syndromes in elderly persons with mild cognitive impairment. Data from a cross-sectional study. *Acta neurologica Scandinavica. Supplementum, 179*, 25-8.

Fox NC, Warrington EK, Seiffer AL, Agnew SK and Rossor MN (1998). Presymptomatic cognitive deficits in individuals at risk of familial Alzheimer's disease: A longitudinal prospective study. *Brain, 121*, 1631-1639.

Frank B and Gupta S (2005). A review of antioxidants and Alzheimer's disease. *Annals of Clinical Psychiatry, 17*(4), 269-86.

Fredholm BB, Bättig K, Holmén J, Nehlig A and Zuartau EE (1999). Actions of caffeine in the brain with special reference to factors that contribute to its widespread use. *Pharmacological Reviews, 51*(1), 83-133.

Galvin JA, Benson H, Deckro GR, Fricchione GL and Dusek JA (2006). The relaxation response: Reducing stress and improving cognition in healthy aging adults. *Complementary Therapies in Clinical Practice, 12*(3), 186-91.

Galvin JE, Powlishta KK, Wilkins K, McKeel DW, Jr Xiong C, Grant E, Storandt M and Morris JC (2005). Predictors of preclinical Alzheimer disease and dementia. *Archives of Neurology, 62*, 758-765.

Ganguli M (2006). Mild cognitive impairment and the 7 uses of epidemiology. *Alzheimer Disease and Associated Disorders, 20*, S52-S7.

Gauthier S, Resiberg B, Zaudig M, Peterson RC, Ritchie K, Broich K, Belleville S, Brodaty H, Bennett D, Chertkow H, Cummings JL, de Leon M, Feldman H, Ganguli M, Hampel H, Scheltens P, Tierney MC, Whitehouse P and Winblad B (2006). Mild cognitive impairment. *Lancet, 367*, 1262-70.

Geda YE, Smith GE, Knopman DS, Boeve BF, Tangalos EG, Ivnik RJ, Mrazek DA, Edland SD, Petersen RC (2004). De novo genesis of neuropsychiatric symptoms in mild cognitive impairment (MCI). *International Psychogeriatrics, 16*(1), 51-60.

Glisky EL, Schacter DL and Tulving E (1986). Learning and retention of computer-related vocabulary in memory impaired patients: Method of vanishing cues. *Journal of Clinical and Experimental Neuropsychology, 8*, 292-312.

Gouras GK, Xu H, Gross RS, Greenfield JP, Hai B, Wang R and Greengard P (2000). Testosterone reduces neuronal secretion of Alzheimer's beta-amyloid peptides. *Proceedings of the National Academy of Sciences, 97*(3), 1202-5.

Graham JE, Rockwood K, Eattie BL, Eastwood R, Gauthier S, Tuokko H and McDowell I (1997). Prevalence and severity of cognitive impairment with and without dementia in an elderly population, *Lancet, 349*, 1793-6.

Greene RA and Dixon W (2002). The role of reproductive hormones in maintaining cognition. *Obstetrics and Gynecology Clinics of North America, 29*, 437–53.

Grundman M, Peterson RC, Ferris SH, Thomas RG, Aisen PS, Bennett DA, et al. for the Alzheimer's Disease Cooperative Study (2004). Mild cognitive impairment can be distinguished from Alzheimer disease and normal aging for clinical trials. *Archives of Neurology, 61*, 59-66.

Gunstad J, Paul RH, Brickman AM, Cohen RA, Arns M Roe D, Lawrence JJ and Gordon E (2006). Patterns of cognitive performance in middle-aged and older adults: A cluster analytic examination. *Journal of Geriatric Psychiatry and Neurology, 19*, 59-64.

Gunther VK, Schafer P, Holzner BJ and Kemmler GW (2003). Long-term improvements in cognitive performance through computer-assisted cognitive training: A pilot study in a residential home for older people. *Aging and Mental Health, 7*(3), 200-6.

Gurland BJ, Dean LL, Copeland J, Gurland R and Golden R (1982). Criteria for the diagnosis of dementia in the community elderly. *Gerontologist, 22*(2), 180-6.

Guttman CR, Joesz FA and Kikinis R (1998). White matter changes with normal aging. *Neurology, 50*(4), 972-8.

Hall CB, Lipton RB, Sliwinski M and Stewart WF (2000). A change point model for estimating the onset of cognitive decline in preclinical Alzheimer's disease. *Statistics in Medicine, 19*, 1555-66.

Haslam C, Gilroy D, Black S and Beesley T (2006). How successful is errorless learning in supporting memory for high and low-level knowledge in dementia? *Neuropsychologica Rehabilitation, 16,* 505-36.

Hawley KS and Cherry KE (2004). Spaced-retrieval effects on name-face recognition in older adults with probable Alzheimer's disease. *Behavior Modification, 28*(2), 276-96.

Hayden KM, Zandi PP, Khachaturian AS, Szekely CA, Fotuhi M, Norton MC, Tschanz Pieper CF, Corcoran C, Lyketos CG, Breitner JCS and Welsh-Bohmer KA; for the Cache County Investigators (2007). *Neurology, 69,* 275-82.

Hedden T and Gabrieli JDE (2004). Insights into the ageing mind: A view from cognitive neuroscience. *Nature Reviews. Neuroscience, 5*(2), 87-96.

Herholz K, Salmon E, Perani D, Baron JC, Holthoff V, Frölich L, et al. (2002). Discrimination between Alzheimer dementia and controls by automated analysis of multicenter FDG PET. *Neuroimage, 17*(1), 302-16.

Heun R, Kolsch H and Jessen F (2006). Risk factors and early signs of Alzheimer's disease in a family study sample: Risk of AD. *European Archives of Psychiatry and Clinical Neuroscience, 256,* 28-36.

Heyn P, Abreu BC and Ottenbacher KJ (2004). The effects of exercise training on elderly persons with cognitive impairment and dementia: A meta-analysis. *Archives of Physical Medicine and Rehabilitation, 85*(10), 1694-704.

Hickman JM, Rogers W and Fisk A (2007). Training older adults to use new technology. *Journals of Gerontology, Series B, 62B,* 77-84.

Higdon JV and Frei E (2006). Coffee and health: A review of recent human research. *Critical Reviews in Food Science and Nutrition, 46,* 101-23.

Hogervorst E and Bandelow S (2007). Should surgical menopausal women be treated with estrogens to decrease the risk of dementia? *Neurology, 69*(11).

Hogervorst E, De Jager C, Budge M and Smith AD (2004). Serum levels of estradiol and testosterone and performance in different cognitive domains in healthy elderly men and women. *Psychoneuroendocrinology, 29,* 405-21.

Höschl C and Hajek T (2001). Hippocampal damage mediated by corticosteroids-A neuropsychiatric research challenge. *European Archives of Psychiatry and Clinical Neuroscience, 251*(Suppl 2), II81-8.

Hu L, Yue Y, Zuo PP, Jin ZY, Feng F, You H, Li ML and Ge QS (2006). Evaluation of neuroprotective effects of long-term low dose hormone replacement therapy on postmenopausal women brain hippocampus using magnetic resonance scanner. *Chin Med Sci J, 21*(4), 214-8.

Hull M, Strauss S, Berger M, Volk B, and Bauer J (1996). The participation of interleukin-6, a stress-inducible cytokine, in the pathogenesis of Alzheimer's disease. Behavioural Brain Research, 78(1), 37-41.

Hunkin NM, Squire EJ, Parkin AJ and Tidy JA (1998). Are the benefits of errorless learning dependent on implicit memory? Neuropsychologia, 36, 25-36.

Hwang TJ, Masterman DL, Ortiz F, Fairbanks LA and Cummings JL (2004). Mild cognitive impairment is associated with characteristic neuropsychiatric symptoms. *Alzheimer Disease and Associated Disorders, 18*(1), 17-21.

Janowsky JS, Oviatt SK and Orwoll ES (1994). Testosterone influences spatial cognition in older men. Behavioral Neuroscience, 108, 325-32.

Jarvik GP, Wusman EM, Kukull WA, Schellenberg GD, Yu C and Larson EB (1995). Interactions of apolipoprotein e genotype, total cholesterol level, age, sex in prediction of Alzheimer's disease: A case-control study. Neurology, 45, 1092-6.

Jernigan TL, Archibald SL, Berhow MT, Sowell ER, Foster DS and Hesselink JR (1991). Cerebral structure on MRI, part I: Localization of age-related changes. *Biological Psychiatry, 29*(1), 55-67.

Jicha GA, Parisi JE, Dickson DW, Johnson K, Cha R, Ivnik RJ, Tangalos EG, Boeve BF, Knopman DS, Braak H and Petersen RC (2006). Neuropathologic outcome of mild cognitive impairment following progression to clinical dementia. *Archives of Neurology, 63*(5), 674-81.

Johansson B and Zarit SH (1997). Early cognitive markers of the incidence of dementia and mortality: A longitudinal population-based study of the oldest old. *International Journal of Geriatric Psychiatry, 12*, 53-9.

Jones RS and Eayrs CB (1992). The use of errorless learning procedures in teaching people with learning disability: A critical review. *Mental Handicap Research, 5*, 204-12.

Jonker C, Geerlings MI and Schmand B (2000). Are memory complaints predictive for dementia? A review of clinical and population-based studies. *International Journal of Geriatric Psychiatry, 15*(11), 983-91.

Kantarci K, Jack CR Jr, Xu YC, Campeau NG, O'Brien PC, Smith GE, Ivnik RJ, Boeve BF, Kokmen E, Tangalos EG and Petersen RC (2000). Regional metabolic patterns in mild cognitive impairment and Alzheimer's disease: A 1H MRS study. *Neurology, 55*(2), 210-7.

Kavé G and Heinik J (2005). Issues to consider when using the new diagnosis of mild cognitive impairment. *The Israel Medical Association Journal, 7*, 732-5.

Kelley BJ and Petersen RC (2007). Alzheimer's disease and mild cognitive impairment. *Neurologic Clinics, 25*, 577-609.

Kendler KS and Prescott CA (1999). Caffeine intake, tolerance, and withdrawal in women: A population-based twin study. *The American journal of psychiatry, 156*(2), 223-8.

Kendler KS, Myers J and Gardner CO (2006). Caffeine intake, toxicity and dependence and liftime risk for psychiatric and substance use disorders: An epidemioilogic and co-twin control analysis. *Psychological medicine, 36*(12), 1717-25.

Kenny AM, Fabregas G, Song C, Biskup B and Bellantonio S (2004). Effects of testosterone on behavior, depression, and cognitive function in older men with mild cognitive loss. *The Journals of Gerontology. Series A, Biological Sciences and Medical Sciences, 59*(1), 75-8.

Kerr JE, Allore RJ, Beck SG and Handa RJ (1995). Distribution and hormonal regulation of androgen receptor (AR) and AR messenger ribonucleic acid in the rat hippocampus. *Endocrinology, 136*(8), 3213-21.

Keys A, Aravanis C and Sdrin H (1968). The diets of middle-aged men in two rural areas of Greece. In C Den Hartog, K Buzina, F Fidanza, A Keys and P Roine (Eds.), *Dietary Studies and Epidemiology of Heart Diseases* (57-68). The Hague: The Stichting.

Kirk A (2007). Target symptoms and outcome measures: Cognition. *Canadian Journal of Neurological Sciences, 34*(Suppl 1), S42-6.

Kivipelto M, Soloman A and Winblad B (2005). Statin therapy in Alzheimer's disease. *The Lancet Neurology, 4*(9), 521-2.

Knopman DS and Ryberg S (1989). A verbal memory test with high predictive accuracy for dementia of the Alzheimer type. *Archives of Neurology, 46*(2), 141-5.

Kokmen E, Naessens JM and Offord KP (1987). A short test of mental status: Description and preliminary results. *Mayo Clinic Proceedings, 62*(4), 281-8.

Koontz J and Baskys A (2005). Effects of galantamine on working memory and global functioning in patients with mild cognitive impairment: A double-blind placebo-controlled study. *American Journal of Alzheimer's Disease and Other Dementias, 20*(5), 295-302.

Kral VA (1962). Senescent forgetfulness: Benign and malignant. *Canadian Medical Association Journal, 86*, 257-60.

Kramer AF and Erickson KI (2007). Capitalizing on cortical plasticity: Influence of physical activity on cognition and brain function. *Trends in Cognitive Sciences, 11*(8), 342-8.

Kramer AF, Bherer L, Colcombe SJ, Dong W and Greenough WT (2004). Environmental influences on cognitive and brain plasticity during aging. *Journal of Gerontology: Medical Sciences, 59*, 940-57.

Krausz Y, Bonne O, Gorfine M, Karger H, Lerer B and Chisin R (1998). Age-related changes in brain perfusion of normal subjects detected by 99mTc-HMPAO SPECT. *Neuroradiology, 40*(7), 428-34.

Kugaya A, Epperson CN, Zoghbi S, van Dyck CH, Hou Y, Fujita M, Staley JK, Garg PK, Seibyl JP and Innis RB (2003). Increase in prefrontal cortex serotonin 2A receptors following estrogen treatment in postmenopausal women. *American Journal of Psychiatry, 160*, 1522-4.

Landauer TK and Bjork RA (1978). Optimal rehearsal patterns and name learning. In MM Gruneberg, PE Harris and RN Sykes (Eds.), *Practical aspects of memory* (pp. 625-632). New York: Academic Press.

Lazar SW, Bush G, Gollub RL, Fricchione GL, Khalsa G and Benson H (2000). Functional brain mapping of the relaxation response and meditation. *Neuroreport, 11*(7), 1581-5.

Le Blanc ES, Janowsky J, Chan BKS and Nelson HD (2001). Hormone replacement therapy and cognition: Systematic review and meta-analysis. *Journal of the American Medical Association, 285*, 1489–99.

Levey A, Lah J, Goldstein F, Steenland K and Bliwise D (2006). Mild cognitive impairment: An opportunity to identify patients at high risk for progression to Alzheimer's disease. *Clinical Therapeutics, 28*(7), 991-1001.

Levy R (1994). Aging-associated cognitive decline; Working Party of the International Psychogeriatric Association in collaboration with the World Health Organization., *International Psychogeriatrics, 6*, 63-8.

Lezak MD, Howieson DB and Loring DW (2004). *Neuropsychological Assessment* (4th ed.). New York: Oxford University Press.

Li L, Cao D, Kim H, Lester R and Fukuchi K (2006). Simvastatin enhances learning and memory independent of amyloid load in mice. *Annals of Neurology, 60*, 729-39.

Liddell BJ, Paul RH, Arns M, Gordon N, Kukla M, Rowe D, Cooper N, Moyle J and Williams LM (2007). Rates of decline distinguish Alzheimer's disease and mild cognitive impairment relative to normal aging: Integrating cognition and brain function. *Journal Integrative Neuroscience, 6*(1), 141-74.

Lim GP, Calon F, Morihara T, Yang F, Teter B, Ubeda O, Salem N, Frautschy SA and Cole GM (2005). A diet enriched with the omega-3 fatty acid docosahexaenoic acid reduces amyloid burden in an aged Alzheimer mouse model. *The Journal of Neuroscience, 25*(12), 3032-40.

Lim GP, Chu T, Yang F, Beech W, Frautschy SA and Cole GM (2001). The curry spice curcumin reduces oxidative damage and amyloid pathology in an Alzheimer transgenic mouse. *The Journal of Neuroscience, 21*(21), 8370-7.

Lind J, Larsson A, Persson J, Ingvar M, Nilsson L, Backman L, et al. (2006). Reduced hippocampal volume in non-demented carriers of the apolipoprotein E e4: Relation to chronological age and recognition memory. *Neuroscience Letters, 396*, 23-27.

Lipinska G and Backman L (1997). Encoding-retreival interactions in mild Alzheimer's disease: The role of access to categorical information. *Brain and Cognition, 34*, 274-86.

Luis CA, Loewenstein DA, Acevedo A, Barker WW and Duara R (2003). Mild cognitive impairment: Directions for future research. *Neurology, 61*, 438-44.

Lyketsos CG, Lopez O, Jones B, Fitzpatrick AL, Breitner J, DeKosky S (2002). Prevalence of neuropsychiatric symptoms in dementia and mild cognitive impairment: Results from the cardiovascular health study. *The Journal of the American Medical Association, 288*(12), 1475-83.

Machens K and Schmidt-Gollwitzer K (2003). Issues to debate on the Women's Health Initiative WHI study. Hormone replacement therapy: An epidemiological dilemma? *Human Reproduction, 1810*, 1992-9.

Maioli F, Cover, M, Pagni P, Chiandetti C, Marchetti C, Ciarrocchi R, Ruggero C, Nativio V, Onesti A, D'Anastasio C and Pedone V (2007). Conversion of mild cognitive impairment to dementia in elderly subjects: A preliminary study in a memory and cognitive disorder unit. *Archives of Gerontology and Geriatrics, 44*(Suppl. 1), 233-41.

Manach C, Scalbert A, Morand C, Remesy C and Jimenez L (2004). Polyphenols: Food sources and bioavailability. *American Journal of Clinical Nutrition, 79*, 727-47.

Maquet P, Smith C and Stickgold R (2003). *Sleep and brain plasticity.* Oxford: Oxford University Press.

Mariani E, Monastero R and Mecocci P (2007). Mild cognitive impairment: A systematic review. *Journal of Alzheimer's Disease, 12*(1), 23-35.

Mate-Kole CC, Fellows RP, Said PC, McDougal K, Catayong K, Dang V and Gianesini J (2007). Use of computer assisted and interactive cognitive training programmes with moderate to severely demented individuals: A preliminary study. *Aging and Mental Health, 11*(5), 485-95.

Mayeux R, Small SA, Tang M, Tycko B and Stern Y (2001). Memory performance in healthy elderly without Alzheimer's disease: Effects of time and apolipoprotein-E. *Neurobiology of Aging, 22*, 683-689.

McCarty DL (1980). Investigation of a visual imagery mnemonic device for acquiring face-name associations. *Journal of Experimental Psychology: Human Learning and Memory, 6*, 145-55.

McConnell LM, Sanders GD, Owens DK (1999). Evaluation of genetic tests: APOE genotyping for the diagnosis of Alzheimer disease. *Genetic Testing, 3*(1), 47-53.

McDougall GJ, Vaughan PW, Acee TW and Becker H (2007). Memory performance and mild cognitive impairment in black and white community elders. *Ethnicity and Disease, 17*(2), 381-8.

McEwen B (2002). Estrogen actions throughout the brain. *Recent Progress in Hormone Research, 57*, 357-84.

McKitrick LA and Camp CJ (1993). Relearning the names of things: The spaced-retrieval intervention implemented by a caregiver. *Clinical Gerontologist, 14,* 60-2.

McKitrick LA, Camp CJ and William-Black F (1992). Prospective memory intervention in Alzheimer's disease. *Journal of Gerontology: Series B Psychological Sciences, 47*(5), 337-43.

Mecocci, P (2004). Oxidative stress in mild cognitive impairment and Alzheimer disease: A continuum. *Journal of Alzheimer's Disease, 6*(2), 159-63.

Messier C (2005). Impact of impaired glucose tolerance and type 2 diabetes on cognitive aging. *Neurobiology of aging, 26*(1), 26-30.

Messier C, Tsiakas M, Gagnon M, Desrochers A and Awad N (2003). Effect of age and glucoregulation on cognitive performance. *Neurobiology of aging, 24*(7), 985-1003.

Metzler-Baddeley C and Snowden, JS (2005). Brief report: Errorless versus errorful learning as a memory rehabilitation approach in Alzheimer's disease. *Journal of Clinical and Experimental Neuropsychology, 27,* 1070-9.

Miller KJ and Rogers SA (2007). *The estrogen-depression connection.* Oakland, CA: New Harbinger Publications.

Minkeviciene R, Banerjee P and Tanila H (2004). Memantine improves spatial learning in a transgenic mouse model of Alzheimer's disease. *Journal of Pharmacology and Experimental Therapeutics, 311*(2), 677-82.

Mizoguchi K, Kunishita T, Chui DH and Tabira T (1992). Stress induces neuronal death in the hippocampus of castrated rats. *Neuroscience Letters, 138*(1), 157-60.

Modrego PJ and Ferrández J (2004). Depression in patients with mild cognitive impairment increases the risk of developing dementia of Alzheimer type: A prospective cohort study. *Archives of Neurology, 61*(8), 1290-3.

Moffat NJ (1989). Home-based cognitive rehabilitation with the elderly. In LW Poon, DC Rubin, and BA Wilson (Eds.), *Everyday Cognition in Adulthood and Late Life* (659-80). New York: Cambridge University Press.

Moffat SD, Zonderman AB, Metter EJ, Kawas C, Blackman MR, Harman SM, and Resnick SM (2004). Free testosterone and risk for Alzheimer disease in older men. *Neurology, 62*(2), 188-93.

Monastero R, Palmer K, Qiu C, Winblad B and Fratiglioni L (2007). Heterogeneity in risk factors for cognitive impairment, no dementia: Population-based longitudinal study from the Kungsholmen Project. *American Journal of Geriatric Psychiatry, 15*(1), 60-9.

Morris JC (1993). The Clinical Dementia Rating Scale (CDR): Current version and scoring rules, *Neurology, 43,* 2412-4.

Morris JC, Mohs RC, Rogers H, Fillenbaum G and Heyman A; Consortium to Establish a Registry for Alzheimer's Disease (CERAD) (1988). Clinical and neuropsychological assessment of Alzheimer's disease. *Psychopharmacology Bulletin, 24,* 641–52.

Morris JC, Storandt M, Miller JP, McKeel DW, Price JL, Rubin EH and Berg L (2001). Mild cognitive impairment represents early-stage Alzheimer disease. *Archives of Neurology, 58*(3), 397-405.

Morris MC, Evans DA, Bienias JL, Tngney CC, Bennet DA, Wilson RS, Aggarwal N and Schneider J (2003). Consumption of fish and n-3 fatty acids and risk of incident Alzheimer disease. *Archives of Neurology, 60*(7), 940-6.

Mosconi L (2005). Brain glucose metabolism in the early and specific diagnosis of Alzheimer's disease. FDG-PET studies in MCI and AD. *European Journal of Nuclear Medicine and Molecular Imaging, 32*(4), 486-510.

Mosconi L, Brys M, Glodzik-Sobanska L, De Santi S, Rusinek H and de Leon MJ (2007). Early detection of Alzheimer's disease using neuroimaging. *Experimental Gerontology, 42*, 129-138.

Mosconi L, De Santi S, Li Y, Li J, Zhan J, Tsui WH, et al. (2006). Visual rating of medial temporal lobe metabolism in mild cognitive impairment and Alzheimer's disease using FDG-PET. *European Journal of Nuclear Medicine and Molecular Imaging, 33*(2), 210-21.

Mueller SG, Weiner MW, Thal LJ, Peterson RC, Jack CR, Jagust W, Trojanowski JQ, Toga AW and Beckett L (2005). Ways toward an early diagnosis in Alzheimer's disease: The Alzheimer's Disease Neuroimaging Initiative (ADNI). *Alzheimer's and Dementia, 1*(1), 55-66.

Mulnard RA, Cotman CW, Kawas C, van Dyck CH, Sano M, Doody R, Koss E, Pfeiffer E, Jin S, Gamst A, Grundman M, Thomas R and Thal LJ (2000). Estrogen replacement therapy for treatment of mild to moderate Alzheimer disease: A randomized controlled trial. Alzheimer's Disease Cooperative Study. *The Journal of the American Medical Association, 283*(8), 1007-15.

Nasreddine ZS, Phillips NA, Bedirian V, Charbonneau S, Whitehead V, Collin I, Cummings JL, and Chertkow H. (2005). The Montreal Cognitive Assessment (MoCA): A brief screening tool for mild cognitive impairment. *Journal of American Geriatrics Society, 53*, 695-9.

Neely AS and Backman L (1993). Long-term maintenance of gains from memory training in older adults: Two 3 ½ year follow-up studies. *Journal of Gerontology, 48*(5) 233-7.

Negrao AB, Deuster PA, Gold PW, Singh A and Chrousos GP (2000). Individual reactivity and physiology of the stress response. *Biomedicine and Pharmacotherapy, 54*(3), 122-8.

Newcomer JW, Selke G, Melson AK, Hershey T, Craft S, Richards K and Alderson AL (1999). Decreased memory performance in healthy humans induced by stress-level cortisol treatment. *Archives of General Psychiatry, 56*(6), 527-33.

Ng T, Chiam P, Lee T, Chua H, Lim L and Kua E (2006). Curry consumption and cognitive function in the elderly. *American Journal of Epidemiology, 164*(9), 898-906.

Ng T, Graham DI, Adams JH and Ford I (1989). Canges in the hippocampus and the cerebellum resulting from hypoxic insults: Frequency and distribution. *Acta Neuropathologica, 78*(4), 438-43.

Nilsen J, Shuhua C, Irwin RW, Iwamoto S and Brinton RD (2006). Estrogen protects neuronal cells from amyloid beta-induced apoptosis via regulation of mitochondrial proteins and function. *BMC Neuroscience, 7*(74). Retrieved on December 15, 2007, at http://www.biomedcentral.com/1471-2202/7/74

O'Hara R, Brooks JO, Friedman L, Schroder CM, Morgan K and Kraemer HC (2007). Long-term effects of mnemonic training in community-dwelling older adults. *Journal of Psychiatric Research* 41: 585-590.

Okamura N, Arai H, Maruyama M, Higuchi M, Matsui T, Tanji H, et al. (2002). Combined analysis of CSF tau levels and [(123)I]Iodoamphetamine SPECT in mild cognitive impairment: Implications for a novel predictor of Alzheimer's disease. *American Journal of Psychiatry, 159*(3), 474-6.

Olazaran J, Muniz R, Reisberg B, Pena-Casanova J, der Ser T, Cruz-Jentoft AJ, Serrano P, Navarro E, Garcia de la Rocha ML, Frank A, Galiano M, Fernandez-Bullido Y, Serra JA, Gonzalez-Salvador MT and Seville C (2004). Benefits of cognitive-motor intervention in MCI and mild to moderate Alzheimers disease. *Neurology, 63,* 2348-53.

Panza F, D'Introno A, Colacicco AM, Capurso C, Del Parigi A, Caselli RJ, Pilotto A, Argentieri G, Scapicchio PL, Scafato E, Capurso A and Solfrizzi V (2005). Current epidemiology of mild cognitive impairment and other predementia syndromes. *American Journal of Geriatric Psychiatry, 13*(8), 633-44.

Parasuraman R, Greenwood PM and Sunderland T (2002). The apolipoprotein E gene, attention, and brain function. *Neuropsychology, 16,* 254-274.

Pereira AC, Huddleston DE, Brickman AM, Sosunov AA, Hen R, McKhann GM, Sloan R, Gage FH, Brown TR and Small SA (2007). An in vivo correlate of exercise-induced neurogenesis in the adult dentate gyrus. *Proceedings of the National Academy of Sciences of the United States of America, 104*(13), 5638-43.

Perneczky R, Pohl C, Sorg C, Hartmann J, Komossa K, Alexopoulos P, Wagenpfeil S and Kurz A (2006). Complex activities of daily living in mild cognitive impairment: Conceptual and diagnostic issues. *Age Ageing, 35*(3), 240-5.

Perri R, Carlesimo GA, Serra L, Caltagirone C, and the early diagnosis group of the Italian interdisciplinary network on Alzheimer's disease. (2005). Characterization of a memory profile in subjects with amnestic mild cognitive impairment. *Journal of Clinical and Experimental Neuropsychology* 27: 1033-1055.

Perrotin A, Belleville S and Isingrini M (2007). Metamemory monitoring in mild cognitive impairment: Evidence of a less accurate episodic feeling-of-knowing. *Neuropsychologia, 45,* 2811-26.

Peskind ER, Potkin SG, Pomara N, Ott BR, Graham SM, Olin JT and McDonald S; for the Memantine MEM-MD-10 Study Group (2006). Memantine treatment in mild to moderate Alzheimer disease: A 24-week randomized, controlled trial. *American Journal of Geriatric Psychiatry, 14,* 704-15.

Petersen RC (2004). Mild cognitive impairment as a diagnostic entity. *Journal of Internal Medicine, 256,* 183-94.

Peterson RC (2006). Conversion. *Neurology, 67*(Suppl 3), S12-S3.

Peterson RC (2007). Mild cognitive impairment: Current research and clinical implications. *Seminars in Neurology, 27,* 22-31.

Petersen RC, Doody R, Kurz A, Mohs RC, Morris JC, Rabins PV, Ritchie K, Rossor M, Thal L and Winblad B (2001). Current concepts in mild cogntive impairment, *Archives of Neurology, 58,* 1985-92.

Peterson RC and O'Brien J (2006). Mild cognitive impairment should be considered for DSM-V. *Journal of Geriatric Psychiatry and Neurology, 19,* 147-54.

Peterson RC, Smith GE, Waring SC, Ivnik RJ, Kokmen E and Tangelos EG (1997). Aging, memory, and mild cognitive impairment. *International Psychogeriatrics, 9*(Suppl.1), 65-9.

Peterson RC, Smith GE, Waring SC, Ivnik RJ, Kokmen E and Tangelos EG (1999). Mild cognitive impairment clinical characterization and outcome. *Archives of Neurology, 56,* 303-8.

Petersen RC, Thomas RG, Grundman M, Bennet D, Doody R, Ferris S, Galasko D, Jin S, Kaye J, Levey A, Pfeiffer E, Sano M, vanDyck CH and Thal LJ; Alzheimer's Disease

Cooperative Study Group (2005). Vitamin E and donepezil for the treatment of mild cognitive impairment. *The New England Journal of Medicine, 352*(23), 2379-88.

Philal W and Born J (1997). Effects of early and late nocturnal sleep on declarative and procedural memory. *The Journal of Cognitive Neuroscience, 9*(4), 534-47.

Poirier J, Nalbantoglu J, Buillaume D and Bertrand P (1995). Apolipoprotein E and Alzheimer's disease. In A Goate and F Ashall (Eds), *Pathobiology of Alzheimer's Disease* (pp. 225-246). New York: Academic.

Pomara N, Ott BR, Peskind E and Resnick EM; for the Memantine MEM-MD-10 Study Group (2007). Memantine treatment of cognitive symptoms in mild to moderate Alzheimer disease: Secondary analyses from a placebo-controlled randomized trial. *Alzheimer Disease and Associated Disorders, 21*, 60-4.

Portet F, Ousset PJ, Visser PJ, Frisoni GB, Nobili F, Scheltens PH, Vellas B and Touchon J; the MCI Working Group of the European Consortium on Alzheimer's Disease (EADC) (2006). Mild cognitive impairment (MCI) in medical practice: A critical review of the concept and new diagnostic procedure. Report of the MCI Working Group of the European Consortium on Alzheimer's disease. *Journal of Neurology, Neurosurgery, and Psychiatry, 77*, 714-8.

Rapp S, Brenes G and Marsh AP (2002). Memory enhancement training for older adults with mild cognitive impairment: A preliminary study. *Aging and Mental Health, 6*(1), 5-11.

Rasgon NL, Silverman D, Siddarth P, Miller K, Ercoli LM, Bookheimer SY, Lavretsky H, Huang SC, Barrio JR, and Phelps ME (2005). Estrogen use and brain metabolic change in postmenopausal women. *Neurobiology of Aging, 26*(2), 229-35.

Rasgon NL, Small GW, Siddarth P, Miller K Ercoli LM, Bookheimer SY, Lavretsky H, Huang SC, Barrio JR, and Phelps ME (2001). Estrogen use and brain metabolic change in older adults. A preliminary report. *Psychiatric Research, 107*, 11-8.

Raz N and Rodrigue KM (2006). Differential aging of the brain: Patterns, cognitive correlates and modifiers. *Neuroscience and Biobehavioral Reviews, 30*, 730-748.

Reiman EM, Caselli RJ, Yun LS, Chen K, Bandy D, Minoshima S, et al. (1996). Preclinical evidence of Alzheimer's disease in persons homozygous for the _4 allele for apolipoprotein E. *New England Journal of Medicine, 334*, 752–758.

Reisberg, B (2007). Global measures: Utility in defining and measuring treatment response in dementia. *International Psychogeriatrics, 19*(3), 421-56.

Reisberg B, Doody R, Stöffler A, Schmitt F, Ferris S and Möbius HJ; Memantine Study Group (2003). Memantine in moderate-to-severe Alzheimer's disease. *The New England Journal of Medicine, 348*(14), 1333-41.

Reisberg B, Ferris SH, de Leon MJ, Crook T (1982). The Global Deterioration Scale for assessment of primary degenerative dementia. *American Journal of Psychiatry, 139*(9), 1136-9.

Requena C, Lopez Ibor MI, Maestu F, Campo P, Lopez Ibor JJ and Ortiz T (2004). Effects of cholinergic drugs and cognitive training on dementia. *Dementia and Geriatric Cognitive Disorders, 18*, 50-4.

Requena C, Maestu F, Campo P, Fernandez A and Ortiz T (2006). Effects of cholinergic drugs and cognitive training on dementia: 2-year follow-up. *Dementia and Geriatric Cognitive Disorders, 22*, 339-45.

Resnick SM, Coker LH, Maki PM, Rapp SR, Espeland MA and Shumaker SA (2004). The Women's Health Initiative Study of Cognitive Aging (WHISCA): A randomized clinical trail of the effects of hormone therapy on age-associated cognitive decline. *Clinical Trials, 1*, 440-50.

Ribeiro F, Guerreiro M and De Mendonca A (2007). Verbal learning and memory deficits in mild cognitive impairment. *Journal of Clinial and Experimental Neuropsychology, 29*(2), 187-97.

Rich JB, Rasmusson DX, Folstein MF, Carson KA, Kawas C and Brandt J (1995). Nonsteroidal anti-inflammatory drugs in Alzheimer's disease. *Neurology, 45*(1), 51-5.

Riley KP (1992). Bridging the gap between researchers and clinicians: Methodological perspectives and choices. In RL West and JD Sinnicott (Eds.), *Everyday Memory and Aging: Current Research and Methodology* (182-9). New York: Springer-Verlag.

Rimm DC and Masters JC (1974). *Behavior therapy: Techniques and empirical findings.* New York: Academic Press.

Rinaldi P, Polidori MC, Metastasio A, Mariana E, Mattiolo P, Cherubini A, Catani M, Cecchetti R, Senin U and Mecocci P (2003). Plasma antioxidants are similarly depleted in mild cognitive impairment and in Alzheimer's disease. *Neurobiology of Aging, 24*(7), 915-9.

Ritchie K, Artero S and Touchon J (2001). Classification criteria for mild cognitive impairment. *Neurology, 56*, 37-42.

Ritchie K, Carrière de Mendoça A , Portet F, Dartigues JF, Rouaud O, Barberger-Gateau P and Ancelin ML (2007). The neuroprotective effects of caffeine: A prospective population study (the Three City Study). *Neurology, 69*(6), 536-45.

Ritchie K, Ledesert B and Touchon J (2000). Subclinical cognitive impairment: Epidemiology and clinal characteristics. *Comprehensive Psychiatry, 41*, 61-5.

Robert PH, Berr C, Volteau M, Bertogliati C, Benoit M, Sarazin M, Legrain S, Dubois B; the PréAL study (2006). Apathy in patients with mild cognitive impairment and the risk of developing dementia of Alzheimer's disease: A one-year follow-up study. *Clinical Neurology and Neurosurgery, 108*(8), 733-6.

Rocca WA, Bower JH, Maraganore DM, Ahlskog JE, Grossardt BR, de Andrade M and Melton LJ (2007). Increased risk of cognitive impairment or dementia in women who underwent oophorectomy before menopause. *Neurology, 69*(11), 1074-83.

Rogers PJ, Smith JE, Heatherley SV and Pleydell-Pearce CW (2008). Time for tea: Mood, blood, pressure and cognitive performance effects of caffeine and theanine administered alone and together. *Psychopharmacology, 195*(4), 569-77.

Rogers SA, Kang CH and Miller KJ (2007). Cognitive profiles of aging and aging-related conditions. *Aging Health, 3*(4), 457-70.

Rogers SA, Miller KJ, Ercoli LM, Siddarth P and Small GW (2005 August). *Verbal memory deficits as a preclinical risk factor for Alzheimer's disease.* Proceedings of the American Psychological Association Annual Meeting, Washington, D.C.

Rosen VM, Bergenson JL, Putnam K, Harwell A and Sunderland T (2002). Working memory and apolipoprotein E: What's the connection? *Neuropsychologia, 40*, 2226-2233.

Rosenberg PB, Johnston D and Lyketsos CG (2006). A clinical approach to mild cognitive impairment. *American Journal of Psychiatry, 163*(11), 1884-90.

Rossini PM, Rossi S, Babiloni C and Polich J (2007). Clinical neurophysiology of aging brain: From normal aging to neurodegeneration. *Progress in Neurobiology, 83*(6), 375-400.

Roth M, Tym E, Mountjoy CQ, Huppert FA, Hendrie H, Verma S and Goddard R (1986). CAMDEX: A standardised instrument for the diagnosis of mental disorder in the elderly with special reference to the early detection of dementia. *British Journal of Psychiatry*, 149, 698-709.

Rozzini L, Costardi D, Chilovi BV, Franzoni S, Trabucchi M and Padovani A (2007). Efficacy of cognitive rehabilitation in patients with mild cognitive impairment treated with cholinesterase inhibitors. *International Journal of Geriatric Psychiatry, 22,* 356-60.

Rozzini L, Vicini Chilovi B, Conti M, Delrio I, Borroni B, Trabucchi M and Padovani A (2007). Neuropsychiatric symptoms in amnestic and nonamnestic mild cognitive impairment. *Dementia and Geriatric Cognitive Disorders, 25,* 32-36.

Royall DR, Palmer R, Chiodo LK and Polk MJ (2005). Normal rates of cognitive change in successful aging: The Freedom House study. *Journal of the International Neuropsychological Society, 11*, 899-909.

Rusinek H, De Santi S, Frid D, Tsui WH, Tarshish CY, Convit A and de Leon MJ (2003). Regional brain atrophy rate predicts future cognitive decline: 6-year longitudinal MR imaging study of normal aging. *Radiology, 229*(3), 691-6.

Sair HI, Doraiswamy PM and Petrella JR (2004). In vivo amyloid imaging in Alzheimer's disease. *Neuroradiology, 46*(2), 93-104.

Saletu B (2003). Sleep, vigilance and cognition in postmenopausal women: Placebo-controlled studies with 2mg estradiol valerate, with and without 3mg dienogest. *Climacteric 6*(Suppl 2), 37-45.

Salloway S, Ferris S, Kluger A, Goldman R, Griesing T, Kumar D and Richardson S; Donepezil 401 Study Group (2004). Efficacy of donepezil in mild cognitive impairment: A randomized placebo-controlled trial. *Neurology, 63*(4), 651-7.

Salthouse TA and Babock RA (1991). Decomposing adult age differences in working memory. *Developmental Psychology, 27*(5), 763-77.

Saxton J, Lopez OL, Ratcliff G, Dulberg C, Fried LP, Carlson MC, Newman AB, and Kuller L (2004). Preclinical Alzheimer disease: Neuropsychological test performance 1.5 to 8 years prior to onset. *Neurology, 63*, 2341-2347.

Saunders AM, Strittmatter WJ, Schmechel D, George-Hyslop PH, Pericak-Vance MA, Joo SH, et al. (1993). Association of apolipoprotein E allele epsilon 4 with late-onset familial and sporadic Alzheimer's disease. *Neurology, 43*(8), 1467-72.

Scalbert A, Johnson IT and Saltmarsh M (2005). Dietary polyphenols and health: Proceedings of the 1st international conference on polyphenols and health. *American Journal of Clinical Nutrition, 81*(1), 215S-7S.

Scarmeas N, Stern Y, Ming-Xin T, Mayeux R and Luchsinger JA (2006). Mediterranean diet and risk for Alzheimer's disease. *Annals of Neurology, 59*(6), 912-21.

Schaie KW (1994). The course of adult intellectual development. *The American Psychologist, 49*(4), 304-13.

Scharf JM and Daffner KR (2007). NSAIDs in the prevention of dementia: A Cache-22? *Neurology, 69*, 235-6.

Schiff R, Bulpitt CJ, Wesnes KA and Rajkumar C (2005). Short-term transdermal estradiol therapy, cognition and depressive symptoms in healthy older women. A randomized placebo controlled pilot cross-over study. *Psychoneuroendocrinology, 30*, 309-15.

Schott JM, Kennedy J and Fox NC (2006). New developments in mild cognitive impairment and Alzheimer's disease. *Current Opinion in Neurology, 19*(6),552-8.

Schreiber M, Schweizer A, Lutz K, Kalveram KT and Jancke L (1999). Potential of an interactive computer-based training in the rehabilitation of dementia: An initial study. *Neuropsychological Rehabilitation, 9*(2), 155-67.

Schumaker SA, Legault C, Kuller L, Rapp SR, Thal L, Lane DS, Fillit H, Stefanick ML, Hendrix SL, Lewis CE, Masaki K and Coker LH; Women's Health Initiative Memory Study (2004). Conjugated equine estrogens and incidence of probable dementia and mild cognitive impairment in postmenopausal women. *The Journal of the American Medical Association, 291*(24), 2947-58.

Scogin F and Prochaska M (1992). The efficacy of self-taught memory training for community-dwelling adults. *Educational Gerontology, 18*(8), 751-66.

Sherwin BB (2005). Estrogen and memory in women: How can we reconcile the findings? *Hormones and Behavior, 47*, 371-5.

Sherwin BB (2006). The clinical relevance of the relationship between estrogen and cognition in women. *The Journal of Steroid Biochemistry and Molecular Biology, 106* (1-5), 151-6.

Shiekh JI, Hill RD and Yesavage JA (1986). Long-term efficacy of cognitive training for age-associated memory impairment: A six-month follow-up study. *Developmental Neuropsychology, 2*, 413-21.

Silveri MC, Reali G, Jenner C and Puopolo M (2007). Attention and memory in the preclinical stage of dementia. *Journal of Geriatric Psychiatry and Neurology, 20*, 67-75.

Silverman I, Kastuk D, Choi J and Phillips K (1999). Testosterone levels and spatial ability in men. *Psychoneuroendocrinology, 24*, 813-22.

Simard M and van Reekum R (1999). Memory assessment in studies of cognition-enhancing drugs for Alzheimer's disease. *Drugs Aging, 14*(3), 197-230.

Simons M, Schwarzler F, Lutjohann D, von Bergmann K, Beyreuther K, Dichgans J, Wormstall H, Hartmann T and Schulz JB (2002). Treatment with simvastatin in normocholesterolemic patients with Alzheimer's disease: A 26-week randomized, placebo-controlled, double-blind trial. *Annals of Neurology, 52*(3), 346-50.

Sitzer DI, Twamley EW and Jeste DV (2006). Cognitive training in Alzheimer's disease: A meta-analysis of the literature. *Acta Psychiatrica Scandinavica, 114*, 75-90.

Sliwinski M and Buschke H (1999). Cross-sectional and longitudinal relationships among age, cognition, and processing speed. *Psychology and Aging, 14*(1), 18-33.

Small BJ, Fratiglioni L, Viitanen M, Winblad B and Backman L (2000). The course of cognitive impairment in preclinical Alzheimer disease. *Archives of Neurology, 57*, 839-844.

Small BJ, Gagnon E and Robinson B (2007). Early identification of cognitive deficits: Preclinical Alzheimer's disease and mild cognitive impairment. *Geriatrics, 62*(4), 19-23.

Small BJ, Rosnick CB, Fratiglioni L and Backman L (2004). Apolipoprotein E and cognitive performance: A meta-analysis. *Psychology and Aging, 19*, 592-600.

Small GW and Vorgan G (2004). *The Memory Prescription*. New York: Hyperion.

Small GW (2002). *The Memory Bible*. New York: Hyperion.

Small GW, La Rue A, Komo S, Kaplan A and Mandelkern MA (1995). Predictors of cognitive change in middle-aged and older adults with memory loss. *American Journal of Psychiatry, 152*, 1757-64.

Small GW, Rabins PV, Barry PP, Buckholtz NS, DeKosky ST and Ferris SH (1997). Diagnosis and treatment of Alzheimer disease and related disorders: Consensus statement of the American Association for Geriatric Psychiatry, the Alzheimer's Association and the American Geriatric Society. *Journal of the American Medical Association, 278,* 1363-71.

Small GW, Silverman DHS, Siddarth P, Ercoli LM, Miller KJ, Lavretsky H, Wright BC, Bookheimer SY, Barrio JR and Phelps ME (2006). Effects of a 14-day healthy longevity lifestyle program on cognitive and brain function. *American Journal of Geriatric Psychiatry, 14*(6), 538-45.

Small GW, Kepe V, Ercoli, LM, Siddarth P, Bookheimer SY, Miller KJ, et al. (2006). PET of brain amyloid and tau in mild cognitive impairment. *New England Journal of Medicine, 355*(25), 2652-63.

Smith C (2001). Sleep states and memory processes in humans: Procedural versus declarative memory systems. *Sleep Medicine Reviews, 5*(6), 491-506.

Smith CD, Chebrolo H, Wekstein DR, Schmitt FA, Jicha GA, Cooper G and Markesbery WR (2007). Brain structural alterations before mild cognitive impairment. *Neurology, 68*(16), 1268-73.

Smith GE, Pankratz VS, Negash S, Machulda MM, Petersen RC, Boeve BF, et al. (2007). A plateau in pre-Alzheimer memory decline: Evidence for compensatory mechanisms? *Neurology, 69,* 133-139.

Smith T, Gildeh N and Holmes C (2007). The Montreal Cognitive Assessment: Validity and utility in a memory clinic setting. *Canadian Journal of Psychiatry, 52*(5), 329-32.

Snowden JS, Stopford CL, Julien CL, Thompson JC, Davidson Y, Gibbons L, et al. (2007). Cognitive phenotypes in Alzheimer's disease and genetic risk. *Cortex, 43,* 835-845.

Sohlbert MM and Mateer CA (2001). *Cognitive rehabilitation: An integrative neuropsychological approach.* New York: Guilford Press.

Sparks DL, Connor DJ, Wasser DR, Lopez JE and Sabbagh MN (2000). The Alzheimer's disease atorvastatin treatment trial: Scientific basis and position on the use of HMG-CoA reductase inhibitors (statins) that do or do not cross the blood-brain barrier. In HM Fillet and AW O'Connell (Eds.), *Advances in drug discovery and drug development for cognitive aging and Alzheimer's disease* (244-52). NY: Springer Publishing Company.

Sparks DL, Sabbagh M, Connor D, Soares H, Lopez J, Stankovic G, Johnson-Traver S, Ziolkowski C and Browne P (2006). Statin therapy in Alzheimer's disease. *Acta Neurology Scandinavian, 114* (Suppl. 185), 78-86.

Sparks DL, Scheff SW, Hunsaker JC III, Liu H, Landers T and Gross DR (1994). Induction of Alzheimer-like β-amyloid immunoreactivity in the brain of rabbits with dietary cholesterol. *Experimental Neurology, 126,* 88-94.

Stephan BC, Matthews FE, McKeith IG, Bond J and Brayne C; Medical Research Council Cognitive Function and Aging Study (2007). Early cognitive change in the general population: How do different definitions work? *Journal of the American Geriatrics Society, 55,* 1534-40.

Stigsdotter-Neely A and Backman L (1993). Long-term maintenance of gains from memory training in older adults: Two 31/2-year-follow-up studies. *Journal of Gerontology* 48: 233-237.

Stoub TR, deToledo-Morrell L, Stebbins GT, Leurgans S, Bennett DA and Shah RC (2006). Hippocampal disconnection contributes to memory dysfunction in individuals at risk for Alzheimer's disease. *Proceedings of the National Academy of Sciences of the United States of America, 103*(26), 10041-5.

Szekely CA, Town T and Zandi PP (2007). NSAIDs for the chemoprevention of Alzheimer's disease. *Subcellular Biochemistry, 42,* 229-48.

Tabert MH, Manly JJ, Liu X, Pelton GH, Rosenblum S, Jacobs M, Zamora D, Goodkind M, Bell K, Stern Y and Devanand DP (2006). Neuropsychological prediction of conversion to Alzheimer disease in patients with mild cognitive impairment. *Archives of General Psychiatry, 63*(8), 916-24.

Tailby R and Haslam C (2003). An investigation of errorless learning in memory-impaired patients: improving the technique and clarifying theory. *Neuropsychologia* 41: 1230-1240.

Talassi E, Guerreschi M, Feriani M, Fedi V, Bianchetti A, and Trabucchi M (2007). Effectiveness of a cognitive rehabilitation program in mild dementia (MD) and mild cognitive impairment (MCI): A case control study. *Archives of Gerontology and Geriatrics, 44*(Suppl. 1), 391-9.

Tariot PN, Farlow MR, Grossberg GT, Graham SM, McDonald S and Gergel I; Memantine Study Group (2004). Memantine treatment in patients with moderate to severe Alzheimer's disease already receiving donepezil: A randomized controlled trial. *Journal of the American Medical Assocation, 291*(3), 317-24.

Taulbee LR and Folsom JC (1966). Reality orientation for geriatric patients. *Hospital Community Psychiatry, 17,* 133-5.

Teng EL and Chui HC (1987). The Modified Mini-Mental State (3MS) Examination. *Journal of Clinical Psychiatry, 48,* 314–8.

Teng E, Lu PH and Cummings JL (2007). Neuropsychiatric symptoms are associated with progression from mild cognitive impairment to Alzheimer's disease. *Dementia and Geriatric Cognitive Disorders, 24*(4), 253-9.

Tschanz JT, Welsh-Bohmer KA, Lyketsos CG, Corcoran C, Green RC, Hayden K, Norton MC, Zandi PP, Toone L, West NA and Breitner JC; Cache County Investigators (2006). Conversion to dementia from mild cognitive disorder: The Cache County Study. *Neurology, 67*(2), 229-34.

Troyer AK, Murphy KJ, Anderson ND, Moscovitch M and Craik FI (2008). Changing everyday memory behaviour in amnestic mild cognitive impairment: A randomized controlled trial. *Neuropsychological Rehabilitation, 18*(1), 65-88.

Twamley EW, Legendre Ropacki SA and Bondi MW (2006). Neuropsychological and neuroimaging changes in preclinical Alzheimer's disease. *Journal of the International Neuropsychological Society, 12,* 707-735.

Van Cauter E, Leproult R and Plat L (2000). Age-related changes in slow wave sleep and REM sleep and relationship with growth hormone and cortisol levels in healthy men. *Journal of the American Medical Association, 284*(7), 861-8.

Van de Pol LA, Korf ES, Van der Flier WM, Brashear HR, Fox NC, Barkhof F, and Scheltens P (2007). Magnetic resonance imaging predictors of cognition in mild cognitive impairment. *Archives of Neurology, 64*(7), 1023-8.

Vaughan C, Goldstein FC and Tenover JL (2007). Exogenous testosterone alone or with finasteride does not improve measurements of cognition in healthy older men with low serum testosterone. *Journal of Andrology, 28*(6), 875-82.

Verhaeghen P, Borchelt M, and Smith J (2003). Relation between cardiovascular and metabolic disease and cognition in very old age: Cross-sectional and longitudinal findings from the Berlin aging study. *Health Psychology, 22(*6), 559-569.

Verhaeghen P, Marcoen A and Goossens L (1992). Improving memory performance in the aged through mnemonic training: A meta-analytic study. *Psychology and Aging, 7,* 242-251.

Visser PJ, Scheltens P and Verhey FR (2005). Do MCI criteria in drug trials accurately identify subjects with predementia Alzheimer's disease? *Journal of Neurology, Neurosurgery, and Psychiatry, 76*(10), 1348-54.

Vogel A, Stokholm J, Gade A, Anderson BB, Hejl AM and Waldemar G (2004). Awareness of deficits in mild cognitive impairment and Alzheimer's disease: Do MCI patients have impaired insight? *Dementia and Geriatric Cognitive Disorders, 17,* 181-7.

Walker MP, Brakefield T, Morgan A, Hobson JA and Stickgold R (2002). Practice with sleep makes perfect: Sleep-dependent motor skill learning. *Neuron, 35*(1), 205-11.

Wang JY, Zhou DH, Li J, Deng J, Tang M, Gao C, et al. (2006). Leisure activity and risk of cognitive impairment: The Chongqing aging study. *Neurology, 66,* 911-913.

Weaver JC, Maruff P, Collie A and Masters C (2006). Mild memory impairment in healthy older adults is distinct from normal aging. *Brain and Cognition, 60*(2), 146-55.

Weggen S, Eriksen JL, Das P, Sagi SA, Wang R, Pietrzik CU, Findlay KA, Smith TE, Murphy MP, Bulter T, Kang DE, Marquez-Sterling N, Golde TE and Koo EH (2001). A subset of NSAIDs lower amyloidogenic Abeta42 independently of cyclooxygenase activity. *Nature, 414*(6860), 212-6.

Welch R, West DC and Yassuda MS (2000). Innovative approaches to memory training for older adults. In RD Hill, L Backman, and AS Neely (Eds.), *Cognitive Rehabilitation in Old Age* (81-105). New York: Oxford University Press.

Wetter SR, Delis DC, Houston WS, Jacobson MW, Lansing A, Cobell K, Salmon DP and Bondi MW (2006). Heterogeneity in verbal memory: A marker of preclinical Alzheimer's disease? *Aging, Neuropsychology, and Cognition, 13,* 503-515.

Weycker D, Taneja C, Edelsberg J, Erder MH, Schmitt FA, Setyawan J and Oster G (2007). Cost-effectiveness of memantine in moderate-to-severe Alzheimer's disease patients receiving donepezil. *Current Medical Research and Opinion, 23*(5), 1187-97.

Willis SL, Tennstedt SL, Marsiske M, Ball K, Elias J, Mann Koepke K, Morris JN, Rebok GW, Unverzagt FW, Stoddard AM and Wright E. (2006). Long-term effects of cognitive training on everyday functional outcomes in older adults. *Journal of the American Medical Association* 296: 2805-2814.

Wilson BA (1998). Recovery of cognitive functions following non-progressive brain injury. *Current opinion in neurobiology, 8,* 281-7.

Wilson BA (2002). Towards a comprehensive model of cognitive rehabilitation. *Neuropsychological Rehabilitation, 12*(2), 97-110.

Wilson PW, Myers RH, Larson MG, Ordovas JM, Wolf PA and Schaefer EJ (1994). Apolipoprotein E alleles, dyslipidemia, and coronary heart disease: The Framingham offspring study. *The Journal of the American Medical Association, 272*(21), 339-45.

Winblad B, Palmer K, Kivipelto M, Jelic V, Fratiglioni L, Wahlund LO, et al. (2004). Mild cognitive impairment – Beyond controversies, towards a consensus: Report of the International Working Group on Mild Cognitive Impairment. *Journal of Internal Medicine, 256,* 240-6.

Winter NM and Hunkin J (1999). Re-learning in Alzheimer's disease. *International Journal of Geriatric Psychiatryi, 14,* 983-90.

Wolkove N, Elkholy O, Baltzan M and Palayew M (2007). Sleep and aging: 1. Sleep disorders commonly found in older people. *Canadian Medical Association Journal, 176*(9), 1299-304.

World Health Organization (1996). *International Statistical Classification of Diseases and Related Health Problems* (10th ed.). Geneva: WHO Press.

Writing Group for the Women's Health Initiative Investigators (2002). Risks and benefits of estrogen plus progestin in healthy postmenopausal women. *The Journal of the American Medical Association, 288*, 321-33.

Writing Group for the Women's Health Initiative Investigators (2004). Effects of conjugated equine estrogen in postmenopausal women with hysterectomy. *The Journal of the American Medical Association, 291*, 1701-12.

Xu G, Meyer JS, Huang Y, Chen G, Chowdhury M, and Quach M (2004). Cross-cultural comparison of mild cognitive impairment between China and USA. *Current Alzheimer Research, 1*(1), 55-61.

Xu H, Wang R, Zhang YW and Zhang X (2006). Estrogen, β-amyloid metabolism/trafficking, and Alzheimer's disease. *Annals of the New York Academy of Sciences, 1089*, 324-42.

Yaffe K, Barnes D, Lindquist K, Cauley EM, Simonsick EM, Penninx B, Satterfield S, Harris T, and Cummings SR; Health ABC Investigators (2007). Endogenous sex hormone levels and risk of cognitive decline in an older biracial cohort. *Neurobiology of Aging, 28*, 171-8.

Yaffe K, Blackwell T, Gore R, Sands L, Reus V, Browner WS (1999). Depressive symptoms and cognitive decline in nondemented elderly women: A prospective study. *Archives of General Psychiatry, 56*(5), 425-30.

Yaffe K, Lui LY, Zmuda J and Cauley J (2002). Sex hormones and cognitive function in older men. *Journal of the American Geriatric Society, 50*, 707-12.

Yesavage J, Hoblyn J, Friedman L, Mumenthaler M, Schneider B and O'Hara R. (2007). Should one use medication with cognitive training? If so, which ones? *Journals of Gerontology, Series B* 62B: 11-18.

Yesavage J, Sheikh JI, Friedman L and Tanke E (1990). Learning mnemonics: Roles of aging and subtle cognitive impairment. *Psychology and Aging, 5*(1), 133-7.

Ylikoski R, Ylikoski A, Keskivaara P, Tilvis R, Sulkava R, Erkinjuntti T (1999). Heterogeneity of cognitive profiles in aging: successful aging, normal aging, and individuals at risk for cognitive decline. *European Journal of Neurology, 6*, 645-652.

Zaudig M (1992). A new systematic method of measurement and diagnosis of "mild cognitive impairment" and dementia according to ICD-10 and DSM-III-R criteria. *International Psychogeriatrics*, (Suppl 2), 203-19.

In: Alzheimer's Disease in the Middle-Aged
Editor: Hyun Sil Jeong, pp. 67-96

ISBN: 978-1-60456-480-8
© 2008 Nova Science Publishers, Inc.

Chapter 2

AGE AND DISEASE EFFECTS ON WORKING MEMORY

William J. McGeown[1] and Annalena Venneri[1,2]**

[1] Clinical Neuroscience Centre, University of Hull. UK
[2] Division of Neurology, Department of Neuroscience,
University of Modena and Reggio Emilia, Italy

ABSTRACT

There is a large body of evidence which has established the neural network supporting working memory (WM). Several functional imaging studies have identified functional changes within this network in the course of physiological brain ageing. Behavioural studies have also shown that in the course of pathological cognitive decline, for example that due to Alzheimer's disease (AD), WM deficits are detectable very early and appear different from those of normal ageing. In normal ageing, WM decline may be due to slower processing, a reduced capacity for inhibition or a less highly directed attentional focus. Healthy elderly, therefore, appear to mostly use the same cognitive processes as the young, just not as effectively. In AD on the other hand, the drop in WM capacity and performance appears to be due to different causes, for example, disease related functional and anatomical impairments. WM decline also tends to be more severe in AD. These behavioural hypotheses can be tested using functional magnetic resonance imaging (fMRI) working memory paradigms.

Through fMRI, it is possible to detect abnormalities in the activation patterns of patients with AD when compared to normal ageing individuals. People that are in the preclinical stages of AD should be expected to have malformed patterns of brain activity underlying the behavioural deficits. These differences may vary from increases in activation (compensatory effects) to decreases or absences of activation in task relevant areas. Both of these effects are likely to be due to early disease related pathology and/or genetic influences. Differences should be robust in middle-aged individuals with preclinical AD, as confounds such as the physiological effects of age would not be as prominent (compared to the very elderly) and if healthy, a high level of cognitive functioning would be expected. This approach, now confined to research, might be

* Professor Annalena Venneri;Clinical Neuroscience Centre;University of Hull,Cottingham Road;Hull HU6 7RX, UK;e-mail: a.venneri@hull.ac.uk

translated into clinical application and provide a way to increase confidence in clinical diagnosis very early in the disease process.

In this chapter behavioural and functional neuroimaging studies on the effects of normal and pathological ageing on working memory will be reviewed. Original results of fMRI studies demonstrating the differences in brain activation patterns between young and elderly people and younger and older patients with AD will also be included. A prospective validation study of diagnostic techniques of this kind in individuals who experience mild cognitive impairment who have a greater risk than the normal ageing population of developing AD will also be presented.

INTRODUCTION

A number of early signs of Alzheimer's disease (AD) may originate from a compromised attentional and working memory network. For example, a reduced ability to acquire new information is recognized as one of the first signs of AD and working memory impairment may be a contributing factor (Germano and Kinsella, 2005). Calculation deficits can also be an early sign of AD (Carlomagno et al., 1999), as can difficulties in comprehension (Almor, Kempler, MacDonald, Andersen, and Tyler, 1999). Both these functions also rely heavily on working memory (WM) and can be influenced profoundly by its impairment. Cognitive tests that assess WM should, therefore, be of use when attempting to diagnose AD at an early stage. Attention and WM appear to be intrinsically linked and tasks that examine attentional processing in AD should also be important for diagnosis. Previous research has shown that impairments in WM have been detected in patients with AD, for example using digit span (Belleville, Peretz, and Malenfant, 1996; Kopelman, 1985) or word span tests (Collette, Van der Linden, Bechet, and Salmon, 1999). Deficits are also noted when patients are required to divide (Baddeley, Logie, Bressi, Della Sala, and Spinnler, 1986; MacPherson, Della Sala, Logie, and Wilcock, 2007) or shift attention (Parasuraman, Greenwood, Haxby, and Grady, 1992; Parasuraman and Haxby, 1993).

Problems in WM and attention have also been reported in normal ageing. In WM, lower capacity has been described e.g. Gregoire and Van der Linden (1997) and Foos (1989), as has the decreased ability to chunk information (Naveh-Benjamin, Cowan, Kilb, and Chen, 2007). The deficits that occur under normal ageing appear to be more readily observed during the completion of more complex tasks than for example, forward digit span (Babcock and Salthouse, 1990). Problems updating information, shifting attention (Fisk and Sharp, 2004) or inhibiting interfering stimuli (Gazzaley and D'Esposito, 2007; Hasher and Zacks, 1988; McDowd and Craik, 1988; Plude and Hoyer, 1986) can also occur with age and these attentional shortcomings can potentially influence WM functioning.

Behavioural deficits that are shared in AD and normal ageing, even if varying in severity, do not make diagnosis an easy task. The impairments that can be observed in patients with AD and normal elderly may, however, be due to different underlying functional and anatomical alterations. Neuropathological formations typical of AD can precede clinical symptoms by many years (Braak and Braak, 1991), and corresponding changes in perfusion and metabolism may be expected. Knowledge of the brain activation patterns that occur in normal and pathological ageing should be beneficial when attempting to diagnose AD at a very early stage (when clinical signs point towards, but are not sufficient for a diagnosis of AD to be made). To extend this concept further, by examining brain activation patterns it may be possible to identify a person at risk of developing AD a number of years in advance of any behavioural impairment.

WORKING MEMORY

Working memory is the memory system that utilizes input from the sensory systems, either to maintain information (temporarily) and/or to make use of the information in the present by integrating it with prior knowledge. Working memory has been likened to Short Term Memory (STM), as the information that is to be maintained is retained only as long as it is required and both of the systems are limited in capacity. The concept of working memory differs from STM, however, as working memory can also include the manipulation of information during the limited period of time it is to be maintained. The concept of STM on the other hand refers to a temporary store in which information can be maintained, but not manipulated.

Working memory includes a vital attentional component and to be successful on a working memory task, attentional abilities must be intact. The descriptions of attention tend to fractionate the ability into three types: vigilance, selective attention and executive control (Parasuraman, Greenwood, Haxby, and Grady, 1992). Vigilance refers to the state when one is paying close and continuous attention, selective attention is the preferential processing of one type of stimuli over another and executive control consists of the ability to coordinate processing by dividing resources.

THEORIES AND MODELS OF WORKING MEMORY

One of the most popular models of working memory is that of Baddeley and Hitch (1974). The model introduced two hypothetical slave components, which are now known as the phonological loop and the visuo-spatial sketch pad. The slave components are co-ordinated by a central executive system. The phonological loop is composed of a phonological store, which retains auditory information over a period of a few seconds, unless the information is renewed by a process of phonological/articulatory rehearsal (Baddeley, 2000). The visuo-spatial sketch pad is the component of working memory in which visual representations of objects and their spatial locations can be retained for a limited period of time (Baddeley, 1998). Logie (1995) describes visuo-spatial working memory as a system which incorporates a visual temporary store (visual cache) and a spatial temporary store (inner scribe). The visual cache stores visual information, but is prone to decay and interference. The inner scribe, on the other hand, is used to both plan movement and rehearse the contents of the visual cache. The central executive is the system that is in control of the perceptual slave components (Baddeley and Hitch, 1974). It is this attentional system that allocates resources, co-ordinates working memory activity and enables participants to perform two or more tasks simultaneously. The model has now been reconfigured with an additional storage site named the episodic buffer (Baddeley, 2000). The episodic buffer is a temporary storage system with a limited capacity that has the capability of integrating information from a number of sources i.e. from long term memory and/or from the slave systems. The central executive acts upon the episodic buffer by controlling the content of the storage site and by allocating attentional resources to the various sources of information available.

THE EFFECT OF NORMAL AGEING ON WORKING MEMORY

There is a large amount of evidence that forward and backward spans are reduced with age. Multiple studies demonstrate this often small but reliable decrease. For example, Gregoire et al. (1997) examined the forward and backward digit spans from the standardization sample of the French adaptation of the Wechsler Adult Intelligence Scale – Revised (WAIS-R). Both types of span decreased significantly with age. The largest reductions in span occurred in adults over the age of 65. Two meta-analyses also provide corroborating evidence that lower span lengths occur with advanced age (Babcock and Salthouse, 1990; Verhaeghen, Marcoen, and Goossens, 1993). In the Babcock and Salthouse analyses, a visual inspection of the data from thirty-eight comparisons shows that the mean digit and word spans are reduced in older individuals (on both simple and complex tasks) on all but one of the comparisons, which appears to be an anomaly. The meta-analysis by Verhaeghen et al. (1993) also demonstrated reduced span length in older adults by comparing in total 5679 elderly and 5254 young participants.

Some researchers have suggested that differences due to age are more common in tasks that require manipulation of information rather than simple maintenance. The rationale behind this is that the central executive system is impaired in normal ageing, but the slave components of the model are intact e.g. the phonological loop. If this theory holds, one might expect that backward digit spans (requiring manipulation via the central executive) will be disproportionately reduced as people grow older compared to forward digit spans (requiring maintenance through the phonological loop). The meta-analysis by Babcock and Salthouse (1990) supported this hypothesis. They found that elderly participants were more impaired on the backward digit span task compared to the forward digit span. Some studies have provided evidence to the contrary showing that forward and backward digit spans do not decrease at different rates with advancing age (Gregoire and Van der Linden, 1997; Hester, Kinsella, and Ong, 2004). Furthermore, the meta-analysis by Verhaegen et al. (1993) showed that with increasing age, backward span was no more impaired than forward span. The evidence appears to be controversial for whether backward digit span is more impaired with age than forward span. It is clear however, that reductions in both types of span occur with age.

Reduced performance of aged individuals on both forward and backward span tasks does not rule out central executive impairment, however, as even forward digit span can be influenced by this system (Baddeley, 1986). For example, the central executive can be used to chunk information in WM, therefore increasing capacity. Furthermore, both the abovementioned meta-analyses found bigger decrements in complex WM tasks, in older, rather than younger individuals, suggesting that the central executive is dysfunctioning at some level in the elderly.

Further age-related impairments to the central executive system are found when shifting attention (Fisk and Sharp, 2004; Verhaeghen and Basak, 2005), choosing strategies (Lemaire, Arnaud, and Lecacheur, 2004) and inhibiting interfering stimuli (Gazzaley and D'Esposito,

2007; Hasher and Zacks, 1988; McDowd and Craik, 1988; Plude and Hoyer, 1986). Perseverations also increase in older adults (Ridderinkhof, Span, and van der Molen, 2002) and they have a less highly peaked attentional focus (Baddeley, 1996). The above studies point towards a deficit in the central executive system of older individuals.

There is another potential cause of cognitive processing deficits in the elderly, including those of memory. Salthouse (1991; 1996) found that there is shared variance between processing speed and memory performance and the difference in memory performance between young and old individuals is less pronounced, after statistically controlling for speed of processing. General cognitive slowing related to ageing may, therefore, be accountable for part of the impairment that occurs in WM.

In summary, the evidence shows that WM spans tend to get lower as age increases. A variety of impairments can also be found due to failure of the central executive system in older individuals. Speed of processing appears to be an important factor that contributes considerably to WM decline. We will see in a later section that the impairments of WM and attention found in AD are more marked than in normal ageing.

WHY MIGHT NORMAL AGEING INFLUENCE WORKING MEMORY?

The atrophy of regions associated with working memory functioning may contribute to the differences that are observed between older and younger adults. Volumetric analyses have demonstrated that age related changes in brain matter do exist. Using Magnetic Resonance Imaging (MRI), Salat, Kaye and Janowsky (1999) investigated the differences in grey and white matter volumes between a group of young elderly (mean age 70) and a group of old elderly (mean age 90). The researchers showed that the old group had significantly less total prefrontal volume than the young group (approximately 15% less). Examining only the white matter, the old elderly group had a significantly lower volume than the young elderly (approximately 30% less). The old elderly group also had a significantly higher grey/white matter volume ratio than the young elderly group. The white matter volume appears to decrease disproportionately faster than the grey matter volume as an effect of age. A further study by Salat, Kaye and Janowsky (2001) examined the volumetric differences in prefrontal regions that exist between young elderly (mean age 71.7) and old elderly (mean age 88.9). The older group of elderly participants had less prefrontal white matter than the group of young elderly participants. The orbital frontal region was preserved in the old elderly group compared to the other prefrontal regions. An additional study to investigate the effect of ageing on the volume of white matter in the brain was carried out by Bartzokis et al. (2003). MRI was used to measure the volume of frontal lobe white matter (FLWM) in participants (n = 252) ranging from 19 to 82 years old. The volume of FLWM increased up until the age of 38 and then decreased noticeably with age. These age-related decreases in FLWM may be important for WM, as the core of the central executive system resides in the frontal lobes.

Another reason for central executive impairment in older adults might be due to changes in the levels of various neurotransmitters. Phasic and tonic changes in dopaminergic activity may be occurring (Braver and Barch, 2002). Braver and Cohen (2000) proposed that the phasic activity may trigger the updating of context information in the prefrontal cortex and Braver and Barch (2002) stated that the tonic levels of dopamine activity might be important in the maintenance of the context representation. There may be a differential time-course for the impairment of both phasic and tonic dopaminergic activity. This theory of ageing still requires further investigation.

Decreases in the resting brain glucose utilisation of elderly individuals compared to young people have also been found. By measuring glucose metabolic rate this decrease has been estimated to be approximately 6% for every 10 years (Petit-Taboue, Landeau, Desson, Desgranges, and Baron, 1998). The ongoing decreases in brain metabolism through time may also play a role in the WM problems found in older people.

The atrophy in prefrontal areas, changes in neurotransmitters and decreased metabolism that occurs in older adults, may contribute to the reduced working memory performance in this population.

THE EFFECT OF PATHOLOGICAL AGEING ON WORKING MEMORY

The working memory system generally becomes impaired early in the course of AD. Specific tasks can be used, for example, digit, letter, word and spatial location span tasks, as well as delayed response tasks, to identify which components of the working memory system are affected by the disease process.

A number of researchers have investigated the amount of information that patients with AD can hold in WM. For example, Belleville et al. (1996), Cherry et al. (1996) and Kopelman (1985) tested the capacity of WM using digit span. Belleville and colleagues compared the span of a group of patients with AD to the digit spans of young and elderly controls. The mean digit span scores of the young, elderly and patients with AD were 6.33, 6.08 and 4.85, respectively. The span of the patients with AD was significantly lower than the span of the elderly control group, but the young and elderly controls did not differ significantly. Kopelman (1985) also reported a significant decrease in the digit span of patients with AD compared to adult controls (the effect was still present after co-varying for age). Investigating letter spans, Belleville et al. (1996) found that patients with AD performed worse than young or elderly controls. The exact length of the letter spans was not included in the paper however, as the main reason behind the experiment was to test phononological similarity. The similarity effect was reduced in the AD patients, which may demonstrate limited involvement of the phonological store when engaging WM and dysfunction of the brain area associated with the store. Collette et al. (1999) examined word span and found shorter spans and a decreased phonological similarity effect in patients with AD when compared to elderly controls. The combined findings from the span studies illustrate a reduced capacity for working memory in patients with AD.

The deficits in the passive storage of information, reported in e.g. the Belleville et al. (1996) and Kopelman (1985) studies might have been found because the AD patients investigated were in the moderate to severe stages of the disease (Germano and Kinsella, 2005). Previously, Morris (1984) provided evidence that not all the components of the working memory system are impaired in early (mild) AD. In his research, Morris did not detect any specific problems with the functioning of the phonological loop.

If the severity of the disease determines working memory capacity, at what stage does impairment in storage begin and which part of the WM system is to blame? Subsequent research suggests that a breakdown of the central executive system is responsible for the problems seen in working memory. Due to the involvement of the central executive system in allocating attentional resources in WM, this component can be assessed using tasks that require the division of attention or the manipulation of information in WM.

Baddeley, Logie, Bressi, Della Sala and Spinnler (1986) used a dual task paradigm to investigate the issue of central executive dysfunction in AD. One of the tasks involved tracking, in which the participant had to follow a moving stimulus on a computer screen with a light pen, and the other, digit repetition. Patients with AD and normal participants (both young and elderly) performed the tasks. The difficulty of each of the tasks was equated for each individual (i.e. performance was recorded when the tasks were performed separately, and this was the level that was used subsequently for the dual task). When completing the tasks simultaneously, the performance of the patients with AD was substantially lower than that of the control groups. Baddeley, Bressi, Della Sala, Logie and Spinnler (1991) also carried out a follow up study on the patients with AD after a period of six months. The performance of the patients when doing each task separately remained unchanged. The scores of the patients when doing both tasks simultaneously, however, had decreased significantly. The impaired performance of the patients on this dual task demonstrates the executive dysfunction that appears to affect patients with AD. The executive impairment also seems to increase over time, as disease severity increases, even while the patient is still capable of completing the tasks adequately when performed separately. Using dual-task paradigms, Morris (1986) discovered that central executive impairments in AD could be observed even when using relatively simple distractor tasks. For example, if the patient engaged in a short term memory task while also consistently tapping the palm of their hand on a desk, a deficit in memory performance could be seen, that was not present in the controls. Morris (1986) also showed that a secondary task of adding or reversing the order of two single digit numbers was enough to cause impairment in patients with AD.

Vecchi, Saveriano and Paciaroni (1998) examined specific functions of working memory, such as passive storage and the active processing of information in patients with AD and elderly controls. Lower accuracy was observed in the AD group than the controls on all the tasks. The greatest impairment was found on tasks that involved active processing, independently of whether the task was verbal or visuo-spatial. This study and others like it show that the impairment of WM found in early AD is more evident in tasks that require the manipulation of information rather than maintenance only. A further example of this impairment is seen when the differences between forward and backward digit spans are compared. Carlesimo (1998) found the difference to be significantly larger in patients with mild AD compared to age-matched elderly controls.

Stuart-Hamilton (2000) suggested that the reduced capacity of working memory in normal healthy elderly is quantitative in nature. The deficit of working memory capacity in patients with AD, instead, appeared to be more than a simple reduction in performance. Healthy elderly participants seem to perform WM tasks in the same ways as young participants and fail in similar ways. One experiment showed that if the elderly were aided with additional memory cues (i.e. coloured stimuli), performance tended to increase (Stuart-Hamilton, Rabbitt, and Huddy, 1988). The reverse was true for patients with AD. If additional information was provided the patients still tended to perform at lower levels than usual. This different effect may have been because the patients were easily confused and the additional information interfered, hindering performance rather than increasing it (Stuart-Hamilton,

Rabbitt, and Huddy, 1988). Alternative evidence of the different alteration of WM abilities in AD can be seen in additional results of the study by Carlesimo (1998), in which a decline in forward digit span was found with increased age (comparing young, elderly and older elderly). This decreasing performance on forward digit span with age may be viewed as quantitative. A significant difference was also observed, however, which may be interpreted as qualitative. The difference between forward and backward digit spans in patients with AD in the mild and moderate stages was significantly larger than in the group of healthy age-matched controls and even the group of older-elderly participants. The forward-backward difference values between the young, elderly and older-elderly controls remained stable and did not differ with increasing age. These findings imply that impairment of a different form compared to that found in normal ageing occurs in patients that have AD.

Dysfunction of the working memory system, in addition to affecting the maintenance and/or manipulation of information over short periods, may also have an impact on new learning. Moss, Albert, Butters and Payne (1986) carried out a study which consisted of a delayed recognition span test. Disks conveying various information e.g. positions, colours, words, patterns and faces, were consecutively laid out on a board that was out of view of the participant. After the addition of each disk, the board was revealed and the participant had to point to the last disk that was added. To do well in the task the participant must remember an increasingly large amount of information. The disks are added one by one until an error is made, this reveals the participants delayed recognition span. A group of patients with AD was significantly impaired compared to the control group on the recognition of all the types of information, as were patients with Korsakoff's syndrome (KS). Patients with Huntington's disease (HD) were impaired on all information types except the verbal information. Perhaps more interestingly, however, the researchers also added a recall task to the study that was to be completed at both 15 seconds and 2 minutes after the completion of the last verbal recognition trial. All three patient groups were equally impaired compared to the control groups at the 15 second period. The AD patients recalled significantly fewer words at the 2 minute mark than either the patients with HD or KS, however. At the 2 minute interval, eleven out of twelve of the patients with AD could recall fewer than 3 of the 16 available words. Of these eleven, seven were unable to recall any of the words at the 2 minute mark. On average the patients with HD and KS appeared to lose about 10-15% of the verbal information between the 15 second and 2 minute interval. This is in contrast to the patients with AD who appeared to lose on average about 75% of the information between the two intervals. This study demonstrates the rapid rate of loss of information from verbal working memory that can be observed in patients with AD. The findings also suggest that although verbal information is lost in patients with HD, KS and AD after only a short time interval (15 seconds), if the amount of verbal information retained at this point is compared with a longer interval (i.e. 2 minutes), this may be of diagnostic significance. Only the patients with AD had a significant loss of verbal information between the two time periods. A further study by Moss and Albert (1988) investigated AD and frontotemporal dementia using the same delayed recognition span test. The difference in the recall of verbal information between the 15 second and 2 minute mark differentiated the two groups, with the patients with AD losing a great deal of information, whereas, the patients with frontotemporal dementia had near normal performance. Monitoring verbal recall between an interval of 15 seconds and 2 minutes, therefore, appears to distinguish AD patients from normal elderly, patients with

Huntington disease, patients with Korsakoff syndrome and patients with frontotemporal dementia.

The most recent addition to the WM model, the episodic buffer (Baddeley, 2000), should act as an interface between WM and long term memory. Impairment of this component may provide an additional reason for the deterioration of working memory in AD, but more research needs to be carried out on this component.

Kopelman (1985) considered that patients with AD would have accelerated forgetting on a version of the Brown-Peterson test when compared to normal elderly and patients with Korsakoff's syndrome. The task involved the presentation of three words that had to be remembered for varying amounts of time (0, 2, 5, 10 and 20 seconds). A distractor task was also used during the various delays (except for the time delay of zero), in which the participant had to count backwards from one hundred in either twos or threes (the number to subtract was determined prior to the experiment). The Brown-Peterson test requires the central executive system to coordinate the dual task activity and divide resources accordingly. There was a significant main effect of group for the period 0-20 seconds. There was also a significant interaction of group by interval. The fastest rate of forgetting appeared to be up to approximately 5 seconds (after which the AD patients appeared to be close to their 'floor'). Stringent investigation of the assumption that reduced ability to retain information contributes to the impairments of working memory in AD (in addition to encoding/retrieval deficits) presumes that the performance of the AD patients is intact at the zero delay. When only the period of 0-5 seconds was analysed, a significant interaction was observed for the three groups by delay. Over this time, there was also an interaction for the pairs of AD by control and AD by Korsakoff's syndrome. When the zero point was excluded and the 2-5 second interval analysed, a significant effect of group was observed, but the interaction effect fell just short of statistical significance. The outcome of the experiment, although by itself not providing concrete evidence of an increased rate of forgetting in AD in addition to encoding/retrieval deficits, when taken together with the results of e.g. the Moss et al. (1986) study, encourages the conclusion that patients with AD have an increased rate of information loss when compared to healthy elderly.

At a later date, Belleville et al. (1996) also used an adapted Brown-Peterson procedure to investigate working memory in AD. In this study, the participant had to remember three consonants presented auditorily. The experiment consisted of mixed design, with a between subjects factor, which was group (AD, elderly or young) and two within subjects factors which were delay (0, 10, 20 and 30 seconds) and interference (no interference, tapping and addition). A three-way interaction between the factors was significant. The analyses were broken down into each interference condition in order to attempt to explain the results. The no interference condition revealed a significant interaction between group and delay. The researchers explained this interaction to relate to the significant decline in performance due to delay in the patients with AD, which was not present in the elderly or young groups. The tapping condition also revealed a significant effect of group in which the patients with AD had lower recall compared to the normal control groups. The effect of delay and the interaction between group and delay only approached significance in this condition, however. The addition condition had a significant effect of delay as well as a significant interaction between delay and group. Delay was found to reduce performance significantly in all groups, the patients with AD, however, were those who were affected more severely. The experiment demonstrated that the patients with AD had impaired recall on the Brown-Peterson task, especially when required to carry out the addition interference task. The combination of the recall and the addition interference condition was considered by Belleville et al. (1996) to be the most demanding on attentional resources.

The above experiments show that patients with AD have a reduced WM capacity compared to controls and are only capable of storing information in WM for very short periods. The central executive system is a component of WM that is impaired early in the course of AD and tasks that require divided attention or manipulation provide convincing evidence of this early impairment. Furthermore, the addition of an attentionally demanding distractor test also impairs performance of patients with AD to a greater extent than it does controls. There is some behavioural evidence to suggest that the impairments in WM seen in AD are of different type and distinguishable from those seen in normal ageing.

In a number of the WM studies that have been mentioned above, it is entirely possible that within the AD patient groups under investigation, not all patients were impaired on all the tasks. This heterogeneity of patients with AD can complicate diagnosis. The analyses carried out are usually on groups and the mean scores can sometimes conceal subgroups of AD patients with differing impairments (all the patients, however, may be deemed to be of the same disease severity). It is possible to investigate the pathologies of patients with AD at the individual level as well as at the group level. Belleville et al. (1996) used a number of various tests to examine patients with AD not only at the group level, but also individually. The various tests used were an adapted Brown-Peterson procedure (as described above), a phonological similarity letter task, a word length span task (using two sets of words - monosyllabic words and words with four syllables), and three phonological judgement tasks (one in the auditory domain - syllable judgement, and two in the visual domain - a homophony task, and a rhyme judgement task). Belleville et al. found that the patients were impaired on some types of tasks but not others. For example, of the ten patients, three were impaired only on the adapted Brown-Peterson procedure. This finding suggests a problem with the central executive in these patients. Five other patients were also impaired on the Brown-Peterson test but also had further impairment. One of these patients was impaired on the auditory syllable discrimination task. The second of these patients was impaired on both the visual and auditory phonological tasks. The third patient revealed no phonological similarity effects for either the visual or auditory modalities, the researchers suggest that for this patient, information was not stored using a phonological code. The third patient was also impaired on the rhyme judgement task. The fourth patient did not exhibit the phonological similarity effect in either modality. The fifth patient again demonstrated a different pattern of performance, an intact phonological similarity effect in the auditory modality, but not in the visual modality, and vice versa for the word length effect. The test scores of the final two of the ten patients fell within the normal range for all the tasks.

These findings appear to show that various sub-types of AD pathology produced differing deficits. Although the patients in the Belleville et al. (1996) study were all classified as having approximately the same disease severity, the various tests revealed that most of the patients were impaired on the central executive component, but only some of the patients had a phonological deficiency. Of those patients that were impaired phonologically there appeared to be a range of observed deficits, which further demonstrates the variability in the progression of AD pathology. As for the central executive, as demonstrated by the Brown-Peterson procedure revealed that eight out of ten AD patients were impaired on this task. As in the group studies, executive dysfunction, therefore, appears to present a means of distinguishing normal ageing from reduced performance due to AD pathology. It should be noted that the normal aged participants in the Belleville et al. (1996) study did not present any impairment in performance on the Brown Peterson procedure, in relation to the normal young participants. An alternative study by Puckett and Lawson (1989) using the Brown-Peterson task, showed that age differences in performance were minimal to non-existent. Belleville et al. (1996) suggest that any executive impairment that is observed in normal elderly individuals (if at all present) is likely to be less severe than that found in AD, and the adapted Brown-Peterson procedure may not be sensitive enough to illustrate any such impairment.

In summary, patients with AD can be seen to have severe problems retaining information, even for very limited periods of time. Many explanations for working memory deficits in AD have referred to the central executive component of the working memory model by Baddeley (1974). This is not surprising as a multitude of evidence points towards central executive dysfunction in AD. Studying individuals with AD, as opposed to groups, has also revealed that central executive processes are often impaired, but there may be additional impairments in phonological processing and storage in some instances.

THE EFFECT OF PRECLINICAL AD ON WORKING MEMORY

The evidence above shows that normal physiological ageing can affect WM; the effects of AD, however, appear to be much more severe. WM impairments have been identified in patients with minimal to mild AD, but is it possible to detect WM dysfunction preclinically in AD? A number of studies have attempted to do this, some of which will be described in this chapter. A higher proportion of people with Mild Cognitive Impairment (MCI) convert to AD, than in the normal population (Petersen et al., 1999), suggesting that this cognitive state might be a preclinical phase of the disease. MCI people are, therefore, an informative population to study when attempting to identify markers of pathological ageing. Economou et al. (2007) found that individuals with MCI were more impaired than normal elderly on the Working Memory Index, which is the sum of the spatial span and letter-number sequencing subtest scores in the WMS-III (Wechsler, 1997). WM impairment was also significantly greater in an AD group than in the clinically derived MCI group. The results show that WM impairments are present in a population of people that are at high risk of converting to AD. The cross sectional design of the study unfortunately does not permit a subdivision of the MCI group into converters to AD and non-converters.

Belleville et al. (2007) assessed divided attention, manipulation capacities and inhibition in individuals with MCI and patients with mild AD. Divided attention was investigated using the Brown-Peterson procedure (with an addition task as the interference condition), manipulation using immediate serial recall of words compared to alphabetical reordering before recall, and inhibition using the Hayling procedure (which requires the participant to complete sentences using irrelevant words that do not fit with the context). The patients with AD were impaired on all three attentional tasks compared to normal elderly, whereas the individuals with MCI had significantly lower performance on only the Brown-Peterson task. Examining the results on the three tests for each person individually showed frequent impairment on the Brown-Peterson procedure (75% of MCI and 62% of AD). Only the participants that performed all three of the tasks were included in the individual analysis, those that could not finish all three tasks due to severe dysfunction or fatigue were excluded, which might explain the lower rate of impairment in the patients with AD, i.e. the most impaired may have been dropped from the analysis. On the manipulation task, 30% of MCI were impaired compared to 62% of AD and on the Hayling test, 35% of MCI showed a deficit, in comparison to 54% of AD. Individuals with MCI showed impairment on one (50%) or two tasks (30%), with few having a deficit on all three (10%). The patients with AD were impaired across more of the tasks, with only 8% showing impairment on a single task, 38% on two of the tasks and 31% on all three of the tests. The results of the group and individual analyses show that impairment of attentional control is common in patients with AD, despite the heterogeneity in the early stages of the disease (Belleville, Chertkow, and Gauthier, 2007). Further small group analyses revealed that the individuals with MCI that declined further (monitored with reassessment) were impaired on both the Brown-Peterson task and the alphabetical recall task at baseline when compared to controls. This suggests that as impairment begins to spread across the attentional components tapped by these tests (moving beyond divided attention to include manipulation), the prediction of further deterioration in MCI or conversion to AD may be possible.

Parasuraman et al. (2002) studied 75 healthy participants whose genetic profile differed in ApoE ε4 status (homozygotes, heterozygotes and non-carriers). They showed that attentional cueing enhanced spatial working memory in young and middle-aged adults, but those people that were homozygous for ApoE ε4 did not receive this benefit. The lower accuracy found for this group also suggests problems in forming and retaining memories for restricted regions in space.

Caselli et al. (1999) also studied cognitively intact individuals that were either homozygous for ApoE ε4, heterozygous or non-carriers. They found no significant differences between the groups on any neuropsychological measures. A correlation with age was found in the group heterozygous for ApoE ε4 on only the WAIS similarities (in which score increased with age) and no significant correlations with age were found on any neuropsychological measure for the non-carrier group. Interestingly, the group homozygous for ApoE ε4 had a negative correlation on several memory scores (which included digit span, the Auditory Visual Learning Test and the Benton Visual Retention Test) with age. Although using a cross-sectional design, the study provides evidence that ApoE ε4 homozygotes are subject to age-related memory decline earlier than heterozygotes or non-carriers. Longitudinal study of the groups may be enlightening and Caselli and colleagues had plans to do this in the future, in addition to replicating the results on another matched sample.

Estevez-Gonzalez et al. (2004) split a group of preclinical AD patients at least 2 years prior to diagnosis (mean 27.7 ± 4 months) into those that carried the APOE ε4 allele and those that did not. All participants were diagnosed with MCI at the time of neuropsychological testing. The study revealed no differences between the groups on tests of WM that evaluated digit span, visuospatial, visuoperceptive and processing speed, or any other type of memory (verbal learning, semantic, procedural and priming) for that matter. This study showed that in preclinical AD, carriers of the APOE ε4 allele did not differ on various memory tasks from non-carriers. The study may have been limited by the sensitivity of the tests used i.e. there was no task to investigate the central executive component of WM. Assessing individuals with MCI only two years prior to the diagnosis of AD may also have been too late to detect any very early changes associated with the APOE ε4 allele, i.e. any impairment may have reached the same level in non-carriers by this stage. By the time that

AD can be diagnosed, the presence of an ApoE ε4 allele does not appear to strongly influence the rate of cognitive decline (e.g. Dal Forno et al., 1996; Gomez-Isla et al., 1996; Growdon, Locascio, Corkin, Gomez-Isla, and Hyman, 1996).

The next study reviewed, that of Rapp and Reischies (2005), investigates a period earlier than 2 years prior to diagnosis. A sample of normal elderly was studied and their progression to AD charted. To investigate AD in the earliest stages possible, and to ensure that nobody was borderline AD, after two years from baseline testing a screening was carried out and any people that had converted were excluded from the study. The people that met the criteria for AD when tested 4 years on from baseline defined the converter group. This method meant that the individuals studied converted between 2 and 4 years after baseline testing (and no sooner). Using receiver operating characteristics to investigate the diagnostic accuracy of the neuropsychological tests used, those which tapped attention and executive function were reliable predictors of conversion to AD. The study shows that a detailed assessment of attentional abilities may be informative when trying to determine at an early stage, individuals that will go on to develop AD. The participants in the study were generally very old (mean age 79.63), which although hampering the transference of the results directly to younger elderly, may strengthen the theory for assessing attention, as the effects of normal ageing would be expected to be reduced in younger elderly populations, making it easier to detect pathological impairments.

To summarize, the research on at risk groups, whether it be people with MCI or carriers of the ApoE ε4 allele, has been informative in identifying tests that are sensitive to AD in its earliest stages. The evidence shows that the central executive component of working memory is affected early in the disease process and tests that evaluate these functions may have the potential of flagging up further cognitive decline. People homozygous for ApoE ε4 may undergo earlier cognitive decline than heterozygotes or non-carriers, but further research needs to be carried out in this area. A selection of tasks most sensitive to the early changes in AD may be suitable for this purpose. Research also showed that normal elderly individuals that converted to AD between 2 to 4 years after initial baseline testing could be reliably predicted using tests of attention and executive functioning.

WHY MIGHT AD INFLUENCE WORKING MEMORY?

Extensive damage of the cholinergic system is found in the brains of patients with AD. Impairment of cholinergic production is thought to occur because of damage to the nucleus basalis of Meynert (Mesulam, 2000). Neurofibrillary tangle formation can be observed extensively in the nucleus basalis of patients with AD, as well as the depletion of cholinergic axons in the cerebral cortex (Geula and Mesulam, 1994). The cholinergic deficit found in the brains of patients with AD does not appear to be generalised throughout the cortex but seems to be selective, targeting the cholinergic axons of the pathway that connects the nucleus basalis to the cerebral cortex (Mesulam, 2000). Cholinergic inhibition can interfere with performance on sustained attention (Mesulam, 2000) and, as the cholinergic pathways innervate the prefrontal cortex, impairments are likely to occur in the central executive system of working memory.

Atrophic changes in the AD brain may contribute to the impairments in working memory that can be observed in AD patients. Salat et al. (1999) investigated the differences in grey and white matter volumes between young elderly (mean age 70), old elderly (mean age 90) and patients with AD (mean age 70). The results showed that the AD patients had reduced white matter when compared to the age matched controls, but a similar decrease in white matter was also observed as an effect of ageing. The white matter declined disproportionately compared to grey matter in the old elderly group, however, and this difference did not exist in the AD patients. This result suggested that in the AD group both grey and white matter decline contributed to the decreases in prefrontal volume, whereas in the older elderly disproportionate white matter decline was the cause of the loss in prefrontal volume. In a later study, Salat et al. (2001) performed a further volumetric analysis to investigate the differences in brain volume between a group of elderly participants (mean age 72.4) and a group of patients with AD (mean age 69.8). As expected, the results confirmed that the AD group had less total prefrontal grey matter than the age-matched controls. The differences in volume were significantly lower in the inferior prefrontal cortex region alone. Bartzokis et al. (2003) also revealed structural differences between a group of patients with AD and a group of participants ageing normally. The AD group who was studied consisted of 34 participants between the ages of 59 and 85. The frontal lobe white matter volume in the AD group was significantly lower than in a group of age and gender matched control participants. The researchers claim that this greater reduction in frontal lobe white matter in patients with AD reflects more extensive myelin breakdown than that which is observed due to the effects of normal ageing.

Further reasons for impaired attention and working memory function in AD may be due to the decreased perfusion and metabolism of the temporo-parietal regions that is common amongst patients with AD. Using a longitudinal and cross-sectional design, Smith et al. (1992) reported glucose metabolism deficits in both the temporal and parietal association areas of patients with AD. In a later study, using Single Photon Emission Computed Tomography (SPECT), Hashikawa et al. (1995) showed that perfusion abnormalities also exist in the temporo-parietal regions of the patients with AD.

In summary, various deficits occur in AD that could contribute to working memory dysfunction. The working memory network is thought to consist of a fronto-parietal network and disease related changes have been reported in these brain regions. A loss of prefrontal grey and white matter has been identified in patients with AD, in addition to decreased perfusion and metabolism in the parietal regions. A cholinergic deficit has also been described that can create problems with attention and memory. Any of these impairments may affect the working memory system in patients with AD.

NEUROIMAGING THE EFFECTS OF NORMAL AGEING

Neuroimaging effects attributable to the ageing process are under-activation, non-selective over-activation and the activation of different regions, a decrease in laterality, compensatory activations and the effect of dedifferentiation. Under-activation is seen when older adults activate regions at lower levels to those activated by younger adults, or when older adults fail to activate the areas at all. The effect of non-selective over-activation is the result of older adults activating areas that the young do not and these activations may be detrimental to the functioning of cognitive mechanisms. This type of activation may be due to a breakdown in inhibitory processes, which in turn no longer prevent the activation of irrelevant areas. The activation of different regions may occur due to compensation, different strategies, or differing neural networks. Compensatory activation by the elderly might occur to offset the effects of atrophy, decreased blood flow, and changes in neural architecture that can occur with advanced age. Dedifferentiation is the term used when older adults lose the ability to activate specialised functional mechanisms that are available to the young.

An example of under-activation in older adults can be seen in a study by Jonides et al. (2000). The experiment consisted of a verbal working memory task that involved high and low conflicting response tendencies. In the young adult group during the higher conflicting response condition, activation increased in the left inferior frontal gyrus. The older adults did not recruit this region, however, and performed more poorly than the younger group. In concordance with the lesion model (in which neuropsychological patient populations are used in order to attempt to explain deficits that are thought to be the consequence of "normal" ageing), neuroimaging has revealed that the prefrontal cortex appears to be a common site which is under-activated in aged participants (Reuter-Lorenz, 2002).

In an experiment carried out in our own laboratory to investigate the effect of normal ageing on the WM network, young and elderly participants were tested on an n-back fMRI paradigm. The participants had to observe a string of letters that were presented one at a time and had to push a response button every time the same letter appeared consecutively (1-back). The task was used to produce a light working memory load.

On this low demand working memory task, the young and elderly controls activated broadly similar areas (see figure 1).

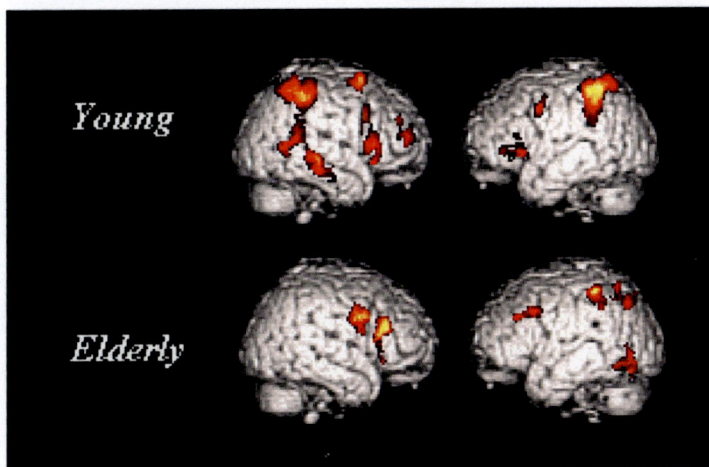

Figure 1. Areas activated on the WM task by young and elderly controls (p<0.01).

Activation was seen in the right prefrontal cortex and the left parietal lobule in both groups. These are areas that are often activated in working memory tasks (e.g. Braver et al., 1997; Veltman, Rombouts, and Dolan, 2003; Jonides et al., 1997). The right dorsolateral prefrontal cortex is part of the attentional network and the left parietal area is thought to be the anatomical correlate of the phonological store. The young also had activation in the right parietal lobule (also part of the attentional network), but the elderly lacked significant activation in this area. On the other hand, the elderly recruited the left fusiform area, unlike the young who did not have significant activation in this area. The fusiform area is activated in tasks requiring visual discrimination (e.g. Polk and Farah, 1998; Polk et al., 2002). In summary, the results showed that the patterns of activation found in the young and elderly groups were for the most part similar. No evidence of Hemispheric Asymmetry Reduction in Older Adults (HAROLD) (see below for a detailed description) (Cabeza, 2002) was seen with this particular task i.e. frontal activation did not appear any more bilateral in the elderly than the young. Certain age related differences did exist, however, and there was evidence of under-activation in the elderly group and the recruitment of an area not activated by the young. Despite the differences in activation patterns, both the young and elderly groups performed at a very high level on this WM task (100% and 98.86%, respectively). The age-related differences in activation may have been due to the utilization of different neural networks, compensatory mechanisms or alternative strategy usage.

Evidence of compensation by the elderly is provided by Reuter-Lorenz et al. (2000). A verbal WM task was used with Positron Emission Tomography (PET) to investigate the effects of age. The elderly group activated similar regions to the young, but also recruited a homologous region in the frontal lobe. Reuter-Lorenz and colleagues also carried out a spatial working memory experiment. In addition to the right hemisphere frontal regions used by the young, the older group activated the homologous frontal regions on the left. These results fit well with one of the theories of age-related decline, the HAROLD model (Cabeza, 2002). This model states that frontal cortex activity tends to be less lateralised in the elderly than in the young. Evidence for this model has been reported in other domains as well, including episodic and semantic memory.

In working memory tasks, elderly brains often recruit similar structures to younger brains and this can be seen with neuroimaging techniques. The activation in the elderly is sometimes at a lower level (under-activation) and/or in a more widespread manner (possibly resulting in bilateral activation). The patterns of activation in patients with AD can be substantially different from both young and elderly brains, however.

NEUROIMAGING THE EFFECTS OF AD

Patients with very early AD, although possibly having the capability of performing within normal limits on certain pencil and paper neuropsychological tests, may have different functional networks than those of normal participants. The changes in activation patterns may exist due to the functional and structural changes that are taking place within the brains of patients with AD. The altered activation patterns observed in the AD brains in response to certain cognitive tasks provide a visual analogue of the brain at work and, in addition to cognitive behavioural data and a clinical interview, may increase the likelihood of an accurate diagnosis.

In a review of studies that used fMRI, PET, SPECT, and electroencephalography (EEG) in conjunction with cognitive paradigms, a number of differences were found between patients with AD and normal elderly (Almkvist, 2000). Examples of these differences were a failure to activate certain brain regions, reduced levels of activation possibly due to neuronal degeneration and the spread of activation to new regions possibly due to compensation. The pattern of activation is generally dependant on the stage of the dementia, the level of atrophy in the brain, the task difficulty and the specific neuronal circuits that are required for task completion (Almkvist, 2000).

The spread of activation to new regions is exemplified in a study by Becker et al. (1996). Becker and colleagues investigated the components of auditory-verbal short term memory. The AD patients that were studied had a more extensive field of activation in those areas normally associated with working memory than normal controls. In addition, the patients with AD also activated various cortical regions that were not activated by the controls.

Another study demonstrating the spread of activation and recruitment of additional brain regions in patients with AD is that of Yetkin et al. (2006). While carrying out a visual working memory paradigm under fMRI, patients with AD had significantly higher levels of activation in the right superior frontal gyrus and the middle frontal, anterior cingulate, middle temporal and fusiform gyri, bilaterally, when compared to a group of controls. The patients were all on cholinesterase inhibitor treatment, however, which may have affected the results. Cholinesterase inhibitors have been reported to increase cerebral blood flow in responding patients (Venneri et al., 2002). In the study by Yetkin et al., under-activation was also seen in the patients with AD, and significantly lower activation was present when compared to the controls in e.g. the precuneus bilaterally.

Rombouts, Barkhof, Van Meel and Scheltens (2002) carried out an fMRI study on a group of patients with AD that was undergoing drug therapy. Assessing treatment response with an n-back task showed that increased activation occurred in the areas associated with working memory. The focus of this study was to investigate the effects of the drug therapy rivastigmine, however; the finding that certain task relevant areas increased in activation after treatment implies that these areas were underactivated before treatment. The researchers did not include an aged control group, however, so no comparisons could be made directly to investigate the effects of pathological ageing compared to normal ageing.

The n-back task might be useful for investigating the differences between normal and pathological ageing because in addition to storage (visual and/or phonological), the n-back task requires the involvement of the central executive system, which is particularly impaired in AD. The task involves manipulation of information in WM, i.e. frequent updating of the target letter and inhibition of responses to non-target letters. Impairment to either storage or executive functioning (or both) should lead to altered patterns of activation. For these reasons, substantial differences in functional brain activations were expected to exist between normal elderly individuals and patients with Alzheimer's disease. A number of previous neuroimaging studies have used versions of the n-back task to examine the working memory networks of normal controls (e.g. Braver et al., 1997; Veltman, Rombouts, and Dolan, 2003; Jonides et al., 1997; Awh et al., 1996; Schumacher et al., 1996). The tasks used previously tended to include higher working memory load conditions (e.g. the participant remembering 2 or 3 letters back in the sequence) and patients with AD are unlikely to be able to perform such complex tasks. The previous studies on normal controls document the brain areas used in phonological storage and central executive function, which is useful information when investigating patterns of pathological activation. The studies also reveal what happens in the brain when increments are made to the WM load that must be remembered.

A study was carried out in our own laboratory in order to examine the effects of AD on younger and older individuals. The AD group included a large age range (from 56 to 95 years). It was, therefore, divided into a younger group of patients (who did not differ significantly in age from the elderly controls, age range 56-76) and an older AD group (who was significantly older than both the younger AD group and the elderly control group, age range 77-95). To examine early changes to the brains of the patients only those of minimal to mild AD (MMSE $\geq$ 18) were investigated. The MMSE scores of the patient groups were significantly lower than the elderly control group, but did not differ significantly from each other.

The elderly controls, the younger AD and the older AD groups all had significant activation in the right prefrontal cortex, but the cluster of activation was smaller in the older AD group. The younger AD group had activation in the right parietal area, which was not present in the elderly controls or older AD group. This activation may reflect the activity of compensatory mechanisms and be indicative of increased effort in this group as, on average, they had a lower behavioural score than the elderly and they performed worse than the older AD group, although these differences were not significant (elderly mean 98.86%, SD 3.21; younger AD 78.79%, SD 25.95; older AD 93.94%, 10.32).

An important difference emerged that neither the younger nor older AD group had significant activation in the left parietal lobule (that was present in the young and elderly groups) (figure 2).

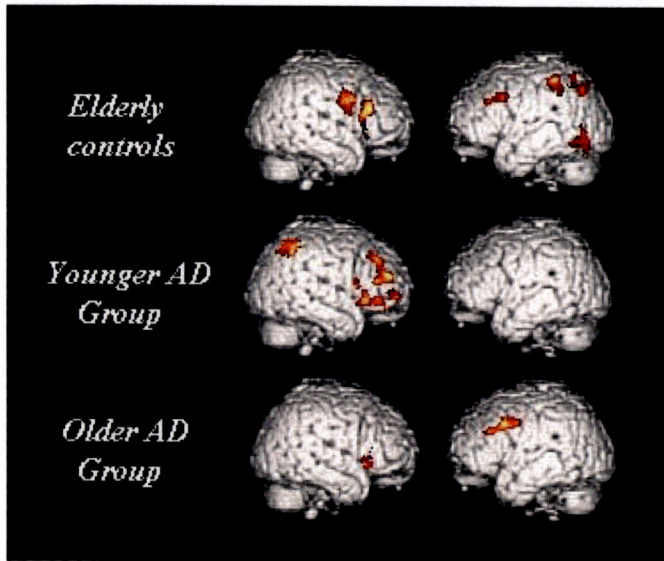

Figure 2. Areas activated on the WM task by the elderly controls, younger AD patients and older AD patients (p<0.01).

This might indicate a limited recruitment of the phonological store and the lack of activation in this area may be due to the atrophy (Fox et al., 2001) and metabolism/perfusion problems (Chase et al., 1984; Hashikawa et al., 1995; Smith et al., 1992) that commonly affect this area in AD. Atrophy of the temporoparietal areas has been reported to be greater in early onset AD than late onset AD, with more hippocampal atrophy associated with late onset (Frisoni et al., 2005). As the WM task draws upon the left inferior parietal lobule for phonological storage, this finding may help explain the trend for lower scores in the younger AD group in this study.

In summary, the elderly controls, younger patients with AD and older patients with AD all activated the right prefrontal cortex. The cluster of activation in the right frontal region was smaller in the older AD group however, and the younger AD group although activating this region seemed to compensate by recruiting the right parietal lobule. Most importantly, there appeared to be a common lack of significant activation in the left parietal lobule of both patient groups. This is in contrast to both the young and elderly controls who had significant activation in this region.

The evidence seems to show that, in some cases, patients with AD activate additional areas of the cortex and have increased fields of activation compared to normal elderly participants. This additional activation is often considered to reflect compensatory mechanisms. The study by Rombouts et al. (2002) that was described above suggests under-activation by AD patients in task relevant areas, but unfortunately it does not deal with the differences between these individuals and normal elderly people directly. Our study revealed under-activation in both younger and older patients with AD, in an area considered to be used in phonological storage, as well as the activation of an additional attentional area recruited by the younger patient group. Yetkin et al. (2006) also provide support for under-activation in patients with AD, in addition to the recruitment of extra brain regions. To summarize, patients with AD, when engaging in verbal working memory paradigms, appear to underactivate task relevant regions compared to normal elderly, as well as producing activation in additional areas. The activation found in additional areas might reflect compensatory processes.

NEUROIMAGING THE EFFECTS OF PRECLINICAL AD

Similar to that seen in patients with AD, non-demented carriers of the ApoE ε4 allele (with memory impairments), who are thought to be a population at risk of developing AD, have reduced cerebral metabolism in temporoparietal areas when compared to non-carriers (Small et al., 2000; Small et al., 1995). Reiman et al. (1996) also reported reduced metabolism in temporoparietal, prefrontal and posterior cingulate regions in cognitively normal ApoE ε4 homozygotes. The study by Reiman et al. (1996) may be particularly informative as it shows that people at risk of dementia are exhibiting altered patterns of metabolism which are preceding any cognitive impairment.

Small et al. (2000) assessed non-demented individuals that were either carriers or non-carriers of the ApoE ε4 allele, using PET. Most of these people were aware of a gradual onset of memory problems (e.g. difficulty in remembering names). Region of interest analysis showed that the carriers had significantly lower metabolism in the inferior parietal region, bilaterally. Small and colleagues also followed up 10 carriers and 10 non-carriers longitudinally and rescanned them using PET. Memory testing revealed no significant differences between the carriers and non-carriers at baseline or at follow-up. The region of interest analysis showed that the ApoE ε4 carriers had significantly reduced glucose metabolism in the posterior cingulate. A further analysis using Statistical Parametric Mapping revealed significant metabolic reductions in the inferior parietal and lateral temporal cortices in the carriers. The decrease of greatest magnitude was found in the right temporal cortex (5%), and all the carriers had a decrement in this area. The non-carriers had no significant metabolic decline in this area, but they did have significant decline primarily in the frontal cortex, which is consistent with normal ageing (Small et al., 2000). Significant correlations were also found between glucose metabolism (at baseline) and memory assessment scores (baseline minus follow up) for carriers, but not for non-carriers. The patterns of baseline metabolism appeared to predict future cognitive and metabolic decline.

Bookheimer et al. (2000) carried out an fMRI study which compared two groups (matched for age and education), one of which contained carriers of the ApoE-ε4 allele, the other of which did not (ApoE-ε3). The task required participants to memorise and recall pairs of words. The group at risk of developing AD exhibited greater levels of activation in the left hippocampus, the left parietal and the left prefrontal regions. In a similar study by Wishart et al. (2006) that investigated carriers and non-carriers of the ApoE ε4 allele using an fMRI WM task, carriers had greater activity in frontal and parietal regions compared to non-carriers. No areas were activated to a significantly higher level in the non-carriers compared to the carriers.

A study by Saykin et al. (2004) investigated the response that individuals with MCI had to the drug therapy donepezil. The researchers used an n-back task in conjunction with fMRI. The control group of elderly participants activated the frontal and parietal cortex bilaterally, in addition to other regions. The individuals with MCI had under-activation in frontoparietal areas before treatment. After treatment with donepezil, increased frontal activation was observed. The drug treatment seemed to boost activation in areas which were deficient at baseline.

On a single WM task individuals with MCI can also be seen to overactivate certain brain regions and underactivate others. In the study by Yetkin et al. (2006) which was described above, individuals with MCI were tested alongside the patients with AD and healthy controls. On the visual working memory paradigm, the individuals with MCI had increased activation compared to controls, in similar areas to the patients with AD, e.g. frontal and temporal regions. The MCI also had areas of significant under-activation compared to controls, e.g. in medial temporal and midline cortical regions.

The studies on individuals at risk of AD show that recruitment of extra areas and a greater extent of activation can occur on working memory tasks, as well as under-activation in task relevant areas. The differences in activation may depend on the number of years left before conversion to AD, the variations in WM tasks used (the difficulty and the brain areas involved) and the groups who are studied who are considered to be at risk (i.e. MCI or ApoE ε4 carriers). Further research is needed to identify which tasks induce the most reliable differences in brain activation.

Converters and non-converters should specifically be focused upon in future research as, although the study of groups at risk of AD can be informative, having e.g. an ApoE ε4 allele does not guarantee AD (only approximately 50% of carriers who are homozygous for the ε4 allele develop AD by the age of 90; Henderson et al., 1995). The people that do not convert to AD may be, therefore, diluting the significance of the findings of those who do convert. Furthermore, there are ApoE ε4 non-carriers who develop AD (only around 60% of patients with AD carry an ε4 allele; Mayeux et al., 1998). The ApoE non-carriers who develop AD may, therefore, be contaminating the group who is supposedly not at risk. Longitudinal studies may, therefore, be very beneficial in determining both cognitive and neuroimaging markers of AD.

Differences in brain activation patterns appear to be present in at risk groups before they convert to AD. In theory, it should be possible to use brain imaging techniques to identify individuals who will convert to AD from those who will not. As proof of concept for this hypothesis, in our laboratory a small number of participants with MCI were investigated on the n-back working memory fMRI paradigm. The MCI group in the present study included 4/6 converters (two out of six did not convert to AD by the time of this writing, but of course may still convert). If markers of preclinical AD could be identified before any behavioural signs were detectable, this would be an opportunity for very early treatment, at the time when patients might benefit most.

The MCI group who converted to AD and the group who remained stable both activated similar areas (figure 3).

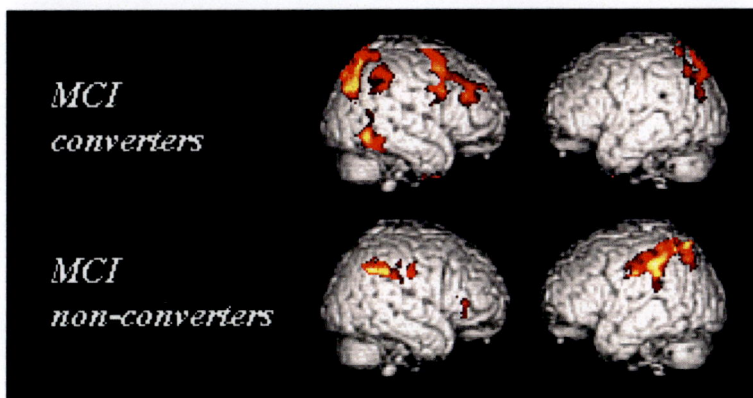

Figure 3. Areas activated on the WM task by groups with MCI. Retrospective analysis of converters and non-converters (p<0.01).

The pattern of activation appeared more widespread in the converter group in the frontal and right parietal regions. Similar to the group of younger AD patients, who, on average, had slightly lower scores than the older AD patients or elderly controls (although these differences were not significant), the more widespread activation in the right parietal lobule of the MCI converter group may reflect the activity of compensatory mechanisms for early disease related changes (e.g. left parietal atrophy and hypometabolism/perfusion).

The non-converters exhibited a much larger area of activation in the left parietal region than seen in the converters. This area, associated with phonological storage, was not activated by either the younger or older AD groups (but was an area activated by the young and elderly control groups). The converting group may have had a smaller cluster of activation in this area because of the increasing neuropathological burden that is likely to have been occurring in these individuals. Caution must be taken when interpreting these results, however, as the groups were small (4 MCI converters and 2 MCI non-converters). The study of larger groups of people with MCI should be very informative if followed up longitudinally with this method. Using fMRI derived differences such as those seen above as a diagnostic aid may present an earlier (and accurate) method of diagnosis that could precede traditional clinical methods and potentially identify people likely to benefit from early intervention. Although a step in the right direction, this type of WM paradigm, however, does not seem to provide results that can give a clear-cut distinctive pattern between MCI converters and non converters.

The above studies show that people at risk of developing AD can have different patterns of brain activation compared to controls. If appropriate cognitive paradigms are applied during brain imaging, it might be possible to identify patterns of activation that are unique to preclinical AD. If this is the case, the combination of brain imaging during cognitive testing may be a useful diagnostic tool. Imaging the brain activation patterns of patients with AD can also investigate if drug treatments are targeting the appropriate areas.

CONCLUSION

The WM problems found in AD to some extent overlap with those in normal physiological ageing. In normal ageing, a reduced capacity often occurs that is likely due to disruption in the central executive system. Similar deficits exist in AD, which causes problems when attempting to make an early diagnosis. Fortunately, the impairments tend to be more severe in AD and if the correct tests are used, the effects of normal ageing can be minimized and those of AD maximised. Patients with AD often have a lower WM capacity than age-matched controls and the central executive system is impaired to a greater degree. The patients may have deficits on more types of central executive control than are found in normal ageing. For example, patients with AD are impaired when dividing attention between tasks. Patients also appear to have a faster rate of forgetting and are influenced more by irrelevant stimuli than age-matched controls. The evidence, therefore, points towards the central executive system as a potential target for tests that aim to diagnose AD in the early stages.

There is some indication that the problems underlying the WM deficits found in normal ageing appear to be different to those found in AD. In normal ageing reduced white matter in the frontal lobes, a compromised dopaminergic system and/or metabolism reductions may contribute to the impairment. In AD, neuropathological and functional changes often occur for many years before the clinical signs of AD emerge. These changes take the form of grey matter atrophy in the frontal lobes, reduced temporoparietal perfusion/metabolism, cholinergic depletion and neurofibrillary plaque and tangle formations. These wide-ranging changes in the brains of patients with AD may contribute to the WM and attentional deficits. Brain imaging can advance our knowledge of the problems that occur in AD and help to identify useful cognitive tests to predict decline.

On WM brain imaging paradigms, similar brain areas are often activated in younger and older adults. The effects of normal ageing tend to be under-activation in certain areas. In our laboratory, using a 1-back task, the elderly group did not have any significant activation in the right parietal region, but this area was activated in the young group. This is an example of under-activation in older adults. Older individuals also often recruit bilateral frontal regions compared to younger people, although this was not seen in our study. These increases in bilateral activation are often attributed to compensatory mechanisms. The elderly group in our study did recruit an additional area that is generally used in visual discrimination however, and this was not activated significantly in the young group. Differences in patterns of activation between young and elderly adults may reflect compensation, different strategy usage or changes in neural architecture.

Patients with AD tend to underactivate certain brain regions on WM tasks. For example, in our study, neither the young AD group nor the old had activation in the left parietal region, but significant activation was found for both the young and elderly controls. Other differences that occur in patients with AD include the activation of additional areas and greater extents of activation.

A reasonable assumption may be that in younger elderly people (or middle-aged adults) the physiological effects on working memory should not be as prominent as in older elderly. We could, therefore, be more confident that any deficits observed would be signs of pathological ageing rather than effects of physiological ageing. To extend this point further, the identification of pathological ageing using psychometric testing and/or brain imaging might be more reliable for early onset AD rather than for late onset AD. This may be true of cognitive testing, however; in brain imaging one must be more careful, as patients that are younger may have more cognitive reserve than those that are older. Greater cognitive reserve could potentially lead to compensatory mechanisms that result in altered patterns of activation. Further research using control groups of appropriate ages will help to identify which cognitive and brain imaging alterations should occur reliably in AD.

Individuals at risk of AD (i.e. those who either have MCI or carry an ApoE ε4 allele) often have impairments similar to patients with AD. The at risk populations show impairments in central executive function when compared to populations considered not to be at risk and patients with AD tend to have a more compromised attentional system. Evidence also exists which suggests that central executive and attentional impairment can predict conversion to AD.

With regards to brain imaging, several studies have reported differences in the patterns of activation found in groups at risk of AD when compared to populations not known to be at risk. Some have shown under-activation in these populations, but others have demonstrated increased activation. The MCI individuals from our study who later converted to AD had a very limited cluster of activation in the left parietal area, whereas the non-converters had a large cluster. Both groups of patients with AD (young and old) lacked activation in this area, whereas the young and elderly control groups both activated the area substantially. The small amount of activation in the converting group may reflect dysfunction in the region due to an increasing neuropathological and functional burden. The converters in our study also had a large cluster of activation in the right parietal region (not seen in our normal elderly control group). Increased activation may occur due to compensation and extra effort that is employed to offset the effects of disease and cope with a struggling attention and WM system. The interaction between disease staging, potential for compensation and the type of task used may create the differential patterns of activation seen across studies.

Further research will identify which tasks induce patterns of activation that are most reliable in at risk populations. The challenge is to create paradigms that target areas associated with early and especially specific disease-related changes. Using a method of longitudinal assessment on at risk populations and even on healthy elderly controls, although more cumbersome than a cross-sectional approach, could have major breakthroughs in identifying those people on course for developing AD and would enable drug therapy intervention at the earliest stages. Paradigms that do not share impairments across normal and pathological ageing would obviously be the most useful in facilitating diagnosis and a range of tests assessing various abilities may be the best way to predict disease. Due to the reliance of WM and attention on the cholinergic system and the therapies that aim to enhance this system, paradigms of this nature may also be useful in identifying which individuals will respond to the drugs and to monitor drug efficacy.

It is possible, however, that, given the difficulties of finding appropriate ways to tackle central executive failure, the diagnostic potential of a wider range of cognitive tasks should be explored, focusing on abilities which are largely unaffected by the physiological processes of ageing and for which robust evidence of a strong association with the presence of the disease exist. Some progress in this respect has been made and there are a number of studies already pointing in this direction (Adlam, Bozeat, Arnold, Watson, and Hodges, 2006; Forbes-McKay, Ellis, Shanks, and Venneri, 2005; C. D. Smith et al., 2002; Venneri, Forbes-Mckay, and Shanks, 2005; Venneri et al., 2008). Preclinical work on populations at risk and evidence from functional neuroimaging studies is still limited, however, and substantial research investments are needed to obtain reliable findings which might translate into useful clinical diagnostic aids in the near future.

ACKNOWLEDGMENTS

The authors thank Michael F Shanks for his helpful comments and contribution in the original studies included in this chapter. AV received funding from MIUR at the time of this writing.

REFERENCES

Adlam, A. L., Bozeat, S., Arnold, R., Watson, P., and Hodges, J. R. (2006). Semantic knowledge in mild cognitive impairment and mild Alzheimer's disease. *Cortex, 42*, 675-684.

Almkvist, O. (2000). Functional brain imaging as a looking-glass into the degraded brain: reviewing evidence from Alzheimer disease in relation to normal aging. *Acta Psychologica (Amst), 105*, 255-277.

Almor, A., Kempler, D., MacDonald, M. C., Andersen, E. S., and Tyler, L. K. (1999). Why do Alzheimer patients have difficulty with pronouns? Working memory, semantics, and reference in comprehension and production in Alzheimer's disease. *Brain and Language, 67*, 202-227.

Awh, E., Jonides, J., Smith, E. E., Schumacher, E. H., Koeppe, R. A., and Katz, S. (1996). Dissociation of storage and rehearsal in verbal working memory. *Psychological Science, 7*, 25-31.

Babcock, R. L., and Salthouse, T. A. (1990). Effects of increased processing demands on age differences in working memory. *Psychology of Aging, 5*, 421-428.

Baddeley, A. D. (1986). *Working Memory*: Oxford: Oxford Scientific Publications.

Baddeley, A. D. (1996). Exploring the central executive. *Quarterly Journal of Experimental Psychology, 49A*, 5-28.

Baddeley, A. D. (1998). Working memory. *C R Acad Sci III, 321*, 167-173.

Baddeley, A. D. (2000). The episodic buffer: a new component of working memory? *Trends in Cognitive Science, 4*, 417-423.

Baddeley, A. D., Bressi, S., Della Sala, S., Logie, R., and Spinnler, H. (1991). The decline of working memory in Alzheimer's disease. A longitudinal study. *Brain, 114*, 2521-2542.

Baddeley, A. D., and Hitch, G. J. (1974). *Working Memory*: Academic Press, New York.

Baddeley, A. D., Logie, R., Bressi, S., Della Sala, S., and Spinnler, H. (1986). Dementia and working memory. *Quarterly Journal of Experimental Psychology A, 38*, 603-618.

Bartzokis, G., Cummings, J. L., Sultzer, D., Henderson, V. W., Nuechterlein, K. H., and Mintz, J. (2003). White matter structural integrity in healthy aging adults and patients with Alzheimer disease: a magnetic resonance imaging study. *Archives of Neurology, 60*, 393-398.

Becker, J. T., Mintun, M. A., Aleva, K., Wiseman, M. B., Nichols, T., and Dekosky, S. T. (1996). Alterations in functional neuroanatomical connectivity in Alzheimer's disease. Positron emission tomography of auditory verbal short-term memory. *Annals of the New York Academy of Science, 777*, 239-242.

Belleville, S., Chertkow, H., and Gauthier, S. (2007). Working memory and control of attention in persons with Alzheimer's disease and mild cognitive impairment. *Neuropsychology, 21*, 458-469.

Belleville, S., Peretz, I., and Malenfant, D. (1996). Examination of the working memory components in normal aging and in dementia of the Alzheimer type. *Neuropsychologia, 34*, 195-207.

Bookheimer, S. Y., Strojwas, M. H., Cohen, M. S., Saunders, A. M., Pericak-Vance, M. A., Mazziotta, J. C., et al. (2000). Patterns of brain activation in people at risk for Alzheimer's disease. *New England Journal of Medicine, 343*, 450-456.

Braak, H., and Braak, E. (1991). Neuropathological stageing of Alzheimer-related changes. *Acta Neuropathologica, 82*, 239-259.

Braver, T. S., and Barch, D. M. (2002). A theory of cognitive control, aging cognition, and neuromodulation. *Neuroscience Biobehavioural Review, 26*, 809-817.

Braver, T. S., and Cohen, J. D. (2000). On the control of control: the role of dopamine in regulating prefrontal function and working memory. In S. Monsell and J. Driver (Eds.), *Attention and Performance XVIII* (pp. 713-738): Cambridge, MA: MIT Press.

Braver, T. S., Cohen, J. D., Nystrom, L. E., Jonides, J., Smith, E. E., and Noll, D. C. (1997). A parametric study of prefrontal cortex involvement in human working memory. *Neuroimage, 5*, 49-62.

Cabeza, R. (2002). Hemispheric asymmetry reduction in older adults: the HAROLD model. *Psychology of Aging, 17*, 85-100.

Carlesimo, G. A., Mauri, M., Graceffa, A. M. S., Fadda, L., Loasses, A., Lorusso, S., et al. (1998). Memory performances in young, elderly, and very old healthy individuals versus patients with Alzheimer's disease: Evidence for discontinuity between normal and pathological aging. *Journal of Clinical and Experimental Neuropsychology, 20*, 14-29.

Carlomagno, S., Iavarone, A., Nolfe, G., Bourene, G., Martin, C., and Deloche, G. (1999). Dyscalculia in the early stages of Alzheimer's disease. *Acta Neurologica Scandinavica, 99*, 166-174.

Caselli, R. J., Graff-Radford, N. R., Reiman, E. M., Weaver, A., Osborne, D., Lucas, J., et al. (1999). Preclinical memory decline in cognitively normal apolipoprotein E-epsilon 4 homozygotes. *Neurology, 53*, 201-207.

Chase, T. N., Foster, N. L., Fedio, P., Brooks, R., Mansi, L., and Di Chiro, G. (1984). Regional cortical dysfunction in Alzheimer's disease as determined by positron emission tomography. *Annals. of Neurology, 15 Suppl*, S170-174.

Cherry, B. J., Buckwalter, J. G., and Henderson, V. W. (1996). Memory span procedures in Alzheimer's Disease. *Neuropsychology, 10*, 286-293.

Collette, F., Van der Linden, M., Bechet, S., and Salmon, E. (1999). Phonological loop and central executive functioning in Alzheimer's disease. *Neuropsychologia, 37*, 905-918.

Dal Forno, G., Rasmusson, D. X., Brandt, J., Carson, K. A., Brookmeyer, R., Troncoso, J., et al. (1996). Apolipoprotein E genotype and rate of decline in probable Alzheimer's disease. *Archives of Neurology, 53*, 345-350.

Economou, A., Papageorgiou, S. G., Karageorgiou, C., and Vassilopoulos, D. (2007). Nonepisodic memory deficits in amnestic MCI. *Cognitive and Behavioral Neurology, 20*, 99-106.

Estevez-Gonzalez, A., Garcia-Sanchez, C., Boltes, A., Otermin, P., Baiget, M., Escartin, A., et al. (2004). Preclinical memory profile in Alzheimer patients with and without allele APOE-epsilon4. *European Neurology, 51*, 199-205.

Fisk, J. E., and Sharp, C. A. (2004). Age-related impairment in executive functioning: updating, inhibition, shifting, and access. *Journal of Clinical and Experimental Neuropsychology, 26*, 874-890.

Foos, P. W. (1989). Adult age differences in working memory. *Psychology of Aging, 4*, 269-275.

Forbes-McKay, K. E., Ellis, A. W., Shanks, M. F., and Venneri, A. (2005). The age of acquisition of words produced in a semantic fluency task can reliably differentiate normal from pathological age related cognitive decline. *Neuropsychologia, 43*, 1625-1632.

Fox, N. C., Crum, W. R., Scahill, R. I., Stevens, J. M., Janssen, J. C., and Rossor, M. N. (2001). Imaging of onset and progression of Alzheimer's disease with voxel- compression mapping of serial magnetic resonance images. *Lancet, 358*, 201-205.

Frisoni, G. B., Testa, C., Sabattoli, F., Beltramello, A., Soininen, H., and Laakso, M. P. (2005). Structural correlates of early and late onset Alzheimer's disease: voxel based morphometric study. *Journal of Neurology, Neurosurgery and Psychiatry, 76*, 112-114.

Gazzaley, A., and D'Esposito, M. (2007). Top-down modulation and normal aging. *Annals of the New York Academy of Science, 1097*, 67-83.

Germano, C., and Kinsella, G. J. (2005). Working memory and learning in early Alzheimer's disease. *Neuropsychological Review, 15*, 1-10.

Geula, C., and Mesulam, M. M. (1994). Cholinergic systems and related neuropathological predilection patterns in Alzheimer's disease. In R. D. Terry, R. Katzman and K. L. Bick (Eds.), *Alzheimer's disease* (pp. 263-294). New York: Raven Press.

Gomez-Isla, T., West, H. L., Rebeck, G. W., Harr, S. D., Growdon, J. H., Locascio, J. J., et al. (1996). Clinical and pathological correlates of apolipoprotein E epsilon 4 in Alzheimer's disease. *Annals of Neurology, 39*, 62-70.

Gregoire, J., and Van der Linden, M. (1997). Effects of age on forward and backward digit spans. *Aging, Neuropsychology, and Cognition, 4*, 140-149.

Growdon, J. H., Locascio, J. J., Corkin, S., Gomez-Isla, T., and Hyman, B. T. (1996). Apolipoprotein E genotype does not influence rates of cognitive decline in Alzheimer's disease. *Neurology, 47*, 444-448.

Hasher, L., and Zacks, R. T. (1988). Working memory, comprehension and aging: a review and a new view. In G. H. Bower (Ed.), *The Psychology of Learning and Motivation* (pp. 193-225). New York: Academic Press.

Hashikawa, K., Matsumoto, M., Moriwaki, H., Oku, N., Okazaki, Y., Seike, Y., et al. (1995). Three-dimensional display of surface cortical perfusion by SPECT: application in assessing Alzheimer's disease. *Journal of Nuclear Medicine, 36*, 690-696.

Henderson, A. S., Easteal, S., Jorm, A. F., Mackinnon, A. J., Korten, A. E., Christensen, H., et al. (1995). Apolipoprotein E allele epsilon 4, dementia, and cognitive decline in a population sample. *Lancet, 346*, 1387-1390.

Hester, R. L., Kinsella, G. J., and Ong, B. (2004). Effect of age on forward and backward span tasks. *Journal of the International Neuropsychological Society, 10*, 475-481.

Jonides, J., Marshuetz, C., Smith, E. E., Reuter-Lorenz, P. A., Koeppe, R. A., and Hartley, A. (2000). Age differences in behavior and PET activation reveal differences in interference resolution in verbal working memory. *Journal of Cognitive Neuroscience, 12*, 188-196.

Jonides, J., Schumacher, E. H., Smith, E. E., Lauber, E., Awh, E., Minoshima, S., et al. (1997). Verbal-working-memory load affects regional brain activation as measured by PET. *Journal of Cognitive Neuroscience, 9*, 462-475.

Kopelman, M. D. (1985). Rates of forgetting in Alzheimer-type dementia and Korsakoff's syndrome. *Neuropsychologia, 23*, 623-638.

Lemaire, P., Arnaud, L., and Lecacheur, M. (2004). Adults' age-related differences in adaptivity of strategy choices: evidence from computational estimation. *Psychological Aging, 19*, 467-481.

Logie, R. (1995). *Visuo-spatial Working Memory*: Lawrence Erlbaum Associates.

MacPherson, S. E., Della Sala, S., Logie, R. H., and Wilcock, G. K. (2007). Specific ad impairment in concurrent performance of two memory tasks. *Cortex, 43*, 858-865.

Mayeux, R., Saunders, A. M., Shea, S., Mirra, S., Evans, D., Roses, A. D., et al. (1998). Utility of the apolipoprotein E genotype in the diagnosis of Alzheimer's disease. Alzheimer's Disease Centers Consortium on Apolipoprotein E and Alzheimer's Disease. *New England Journal of Medicine, 338*, 506-511.

McDowd, J. M., and Craik, F. I. (1988). Effects of aging and task difficulty on divided attention performance. *Journal of Experimental Psychology: Human Perception and Performance, 14*, 267-280.

Mesulam, M. M. (2000). *Principles of Behavioural and Congitive Neurology* (2nd ed.): Oxford University Press.

Morris, R. G. (1984). Dementia and the Functioning of the Articulatory Loop System. *Cognitive Neuropsychology, 1*, 143-157.

Morris, R. G. (1986). Short-term forgetting in senile dementia of the Alzheimer's type. *Cognitive Neuropsychology, 3*, 77-97.

Moss, M. B., and Albert, M. S. (1988). *Geriatric Neuropsychology*: Guilford, New York.

Moss, M. B., Albert, M. S., Butters, N., and Payne, M. (1986). Differential patterns of memory loss among patients with Alzheimer's disease, Huntington's disease, and alcoholic Korsakoff's syndrome. *Archives of Neurology, 43*, 239-246.

Naveh-Benjamin, M., Cowan, N., Kilb, A., and Chen, Z. (2007). Age-related differences in immediate serial recall: dissociating chunk formation and capacity. *Memory and Cognition, 35*, 724-737.

Parasuraman, R., Greenwood, P. M., Haxby, J. V., and Grady, C. L. (1992). Visuospatial attention in dementia of the Alzheimer type. *Brain, 115*, 711-733.

Parasuraman, R., Greenwood, P. M., and Sunderland, T. (2002). The apolipoprotein E gene, attention, and brain function. *Neuropsychology, 16*, 254-274.

Parasuraman, R., and Haxby, J. V. (1993). Attention and brain function in Alzheimer's disease: A review. *Neuropsychology, 7*, 242-272.

Petersen, R. C., Smith, G. E., Waring, S. C., Ivnik, R. J., Tangalos, E. G., and Kokmen, E. (1999). Mild cognitive impairment: clinical characterization and outcome. *Archives of Neurology, 56*, 303-308.

Petit-Taboue, M. C., Landeau, B., Desson, J. F., Desgranges, B., and Baron, J. C. (1998). Effects of healthy aging on the regional cerebral metabolic rate of glucose assessed with statistical parametric mapping. *Neuroimage, 7*, 176-184.

Plude, D. J., and Hoyer, W. J. (1986). Age and the selectivity of visual information processing. *Psychology of Aging, 1*, 4-10.

Polk, T. A., and Farah, M. J. (1998). The neural development and organization of letter recognition: evidence from functional neuroimaging, computational modeling, and behavioral studies. *Proceedings of the National Academy of Science U S A, 95*, 847-852.

Polk, T. A., Stallcup, M., Aguirre, G. K., Alsop, D. C., D'Esposito, M., Detre, J. A., et al. (2002). Neural specialization for letter recognition. *Journal of Cognitive Neuroscience, 14*, 145-159.

Puckett, J. M., and Lawson, W. M. (1989). Absence of adult age differences in forgetting in the Brown-Peterson Task. *Acta Psychologica (Amst), 72*, 159-175.

Rapp, M. A., and Reischies, F. M. (2005). Attention and executive control predict Alzheimer disease in late life - Results from the Berlin Aging Study (BASE). *American Journal of Geriatric Psychiatry, 13*, 134-141.

Reiman, E. M., Caselli, R. J., Yun, L. S., Chen, K., Bandy, D., Minoshima, S., et al. (1996). Preclinical evidence of Alzheimer's disease in persons homozygous for the epsilon 4 allele for apolipoprotein E. *New England Journal of Medicine, 334*, 752-758.

Reuter-Lorenz, P. A. (2002). New visions of the aging mind and brain. *Trends in Cognitive Science, 6*, 394.

Reuter-Lorenz, P. A., Jonides, J., Smith, E. E., Hartley, A., Miller, A., Marshuetz, C., et al. (2000). Age differences in the frontal lateralization of verbal and spatial working memory revealed by PET. *Journal of Cognitive Neuroscience, 12*, 174-187.

Ridderinkhof, K. R., Span, M. M., and van der Molen, M. W. (2002). Perseverative behavior and adaptive control in older adults: performance monitoring, rule induction, and set shifting. *Brain and Cognition, 49*, 382-401.

Rombouts, S. A., Barkhof, F., Van Meel, C. S., and Scheltens, P. (2002). Alterations in brain activation during cholinergic enhancement with rivastigmine in Alzheimer's disease. *Journal of Neurology, Neurosurgery and Psychiatry, 73*, 665-671.

Salat, D. H., Kaye, J. A., and Janowsky, J. S. (1999). Prefrontal gray and white matter volumes in healthy aging and Alzheimer disease. *Archives of Neurology, 56*, 338-344.

Salat, D. H., Kaye, J. A., and Janowsky, J. S. (2001). Selective preservation and degeneration within the prefrontal cortex in aging and Alzheimer disease. *Archives of Neurology, 58*, 1403-1408.

Salthouse, T. A. (1991). Mediation of adult age differences in cognition by reductions in working memory and speed of processing. *Psychological Science, 2*, 179-183.

Salthouse, T. A. (1996). General and specific speed mediation of adult age differences in memory. *Journals of Gerontology Series B-Psychological Sciences and Social Sciences, 51*, P30-P42.

Saykin, A. J., Wishart, H. A., Rabin, L. A., Flashman, L. A., McHugh, T. L., Mamourian, A. C., et al. (2004). Cholinergic enhancement of frontal lobe activity in mild cognitive impairment. *Brain, 127*, 1574-1583.

Schumacher, E. H., Lauber, E., Awh, E., Jonides, J., Smith, E. E., and Koeppe, R. A. (1996). PET evidence for an amodal verbal working memory system. *Neuroimage, 3*, 79-88.

Small, G. W., Ercoli, L. M., Silverman, D. H., Huang, S. C., Komo, S., Bookheimer, S. Y., et al. (2000). Cerebral metabolic and cognitive decline in persons at genetic risk for Alzheimer's disease. *Proceedings of the National Academy of Science U S A, 97*, 6037-6042.

Small, G. W., Mazziotta, J. C., Collins, M. T., Baxter, L. R., Phelps, M. E., Mandelkern, M. A., et al. (1995). Apolipoprotein E type 4 allele and cerebral glucose metabolism in relatives at risk for familial Alzheimer disease. *Jama, 273*, 942-947.

Smith, C. D., Andersen, A. H., Kryscio, R. J., Schmitt, F. A., Kindy, M. S., Blonder, L. X., et al. (2002). Women at risk for AD show increased parietal activation during a fluency task. *Neurology, 58*, 1197-1202.

Smith, G. S., de Leon, M. J., George, A. E., Kluger, A., Volkow, N. D., McRae, T., et al. (1992). Topography of cross-sectional and longitudinal glucose metabolic deficits in Alzheimer's disease. Pathophysiologic implications. *Archives of Neurology, 49*, 1142-1150.

Stuart-Hamilton, I. A. (2000). *The Psychology of Ageing: An Introduction.* (3rd ed.): Jessica Kingsley Publishers: London and Philadelphia.

Stuart-Hamilton, I. A., Rabbitt, P. M., and Huddy, A. (1988). The role of selective attention in the visuo-spatial memory of patients suffering from dementia of the Alzheimer type. *Compr Gerontology [B], 2*, 129-134.

Vecchi, T., Saveriano, V., and Paciaroni, L. (1998). Storage and processing working memory functions in Alzheimer-type dementia. *Behavioural Neurology, 11*, 227-231.

Veltman, D. J., Rombouts, S. A., and Dolan, R. J. (2003). Maintenance versus manipulation in verbal working memory revisited: an fMRI study. *Neuroimage, 18*, 247-256.

Venneri, A., Forbes-Mckay, K. E., and Shanks, M. F. (2005). Impoverishment of spontaneous language and the prediction of Alzheimer's disease. *Brain, 128*, E27.

Venneri, A., McGeown, W. J., Hietanen, H. M., Guerrini, C., Ellis, A. W., and Shanks, M. F. (2008). The anatomical bases of semantic retrieval deficits in early Alzheimer's disease. *Neuropsychologia, 46*, 497-510.

Venneri, A., Shanks, M. F., Staff, R. T., Pestell, S. J., Forbes, K. E., Gemmell, H. G., et al. (2002). Cerebral blood flow and cognitive responses to rivastigmine treatment in Alzheimer's disease. *Neuroreport, 13*, 83-87.

Verhaeghen, P., and Basak, C. (2005). Ageing and switching of the focus of attention in working memory: results from a modified N-back task. *Quarterly Journal of Experimental Psychology A, 58*, 134-154.

Verhaeghen, P., Marcoen, A., and Goossens, L. (1993). Facts and fiction about memory aging: a quantitative integration of research findings. *Journal of Gerontology, 48*, P157-171.

Wechsler, D. (1997). *Wechsler Memory Scale* (3rd ed.). San Antonio, TX: The Psychological Corporation.

Wishart, H. A., Saykin, A. J., Rabin, L. A., Santulli, R. B., Flashman, L. A., Guerin, S. J., et al. (2006). Increased brain activation during working memory in cognitively intact adults with the APOE epsilon4 allele. *Americal Journal of Psychiatry, 163,* 1603-1610.

Yetkin, F. Z., Rosenberg, R. N., Weiner, M. F., Purdy, P. D., and Cullum, C. M. (2006). FMRI of working memory in patients with mild cognitive impairment and probable Alzheimer's disease. *European Radiology, 16,* 193-206.

In: Alzheimer's Disease in the Middle-Aged
Editor: Hyun Sil Jeong, pp. 97-116

ISBN: 978-1-60456-480-8
© 2008 Nova Science Publishers, Inc.

Chapter 3

COGNITIVE REHABILITATION IN MIDDLE-AGED ALZHEIMER PATIENTS

Elisabetta Farina and Fabiana Villanelli

Neurorehabilitation Unit, IRCCS Don Gnocchi Foundation,
University of Milan, Milan, Italy

INTRODUCTION

GENERAL PRINCIPLES OF COGNITIVE REHABILITATION TREATMENT OF MIDDLE-AGED AD PATIENTS

Literature data support the notion that Alzheimer Disease (AD) patients show some sort of cognitive reserve capacity that can be exploited in cognitive training. In fact, recently some randomized controlled trial have demonstrated the efficacy of cognitive stimulation treatments in order to improve cognitive status and quality of life in people affected by dementia (Spector, 2003; Olazaran, 2004). On the other hand, in AD clinical heterogeneity is the rule, not the exception, and the disease is invariably progressive. For these reasons, cognitive rehabilitation interventions must be accurately tailored to the clinical characteristics of the patients. It must also be considered that AD affects family as well as the patient, and these interventions must take into account the needs of both patients and caregivers. Interventions must try to reduce disability, preserving residual cognitive, affective and physic abilities as long as possible. A multidimensional evaluation, taking into account residual cognitive and functional abilities, the possible presence of psychobehavioural disturbances, of associated general illnesses, and of the familiar and social support is necessary to establish reasonable goals for the cognitive rehabilitation program. This evaluation should include:

1) A complete battery of neuropsychological tests, covering all main cognitive functions (short and long term memory) better if tests of "ecological" memory are included, such as the Rivermead Behavioral Test, (Wilson et al., 1990), semantic memory, language comprehension and production, visuospatial and visuoperceptive functions, constructive and ideomotor praxia;

2) Scales to evaluate psychobehavioural disturbances, e.g. the Neuropsychiatric Inventory (Cummings et al, 1994) or the Revised Memory and Behaviour Checklist (Teri et al., 1992), and depression (e.g., the Geriatric Depression Scale) (Yesavage et al. 1982-83) or the Cornell Depression Scale for Dementia (Alexopoulos et al, 1988);

3) Tools to evaluate functional disability. Traditional "generic" functional scales, such as ADL and IADL (Lawton et al, 1969) are insensitive to the large variety of impairment shown by middle-aged AD patients in everyday life, and they do not reflect adequately the kind and the amount of help that is needed for cognitively impaired persons to plan and perform an action, a variable that can be modified by treatment. Therefore we recommend the use of more sensitive tools, such as the Alzheimer's Disease Activities of Daily Living International Scale (ADL-IS), that covers a large sample of activities of daily living, and shows high correlations with measures of cognitive functions and stage of dementia (Reisberg et al., 2001). A good option may be the use of performance measures of functional abilities: these are tools in which an individual is asked to perform or simulate an activity and is evaluated in a formal manner on that performance with standardized criteria. They have been used in medical rehabilitation for diagnosis and to demonstrate therapeutic progress, and have shown to predict survival, hospitalization, use of assistance, long-term-care and nursing home placement (Kuriansky and Gurland, 1976; Jette and Branch, 1985, Williams, 1987; Guralnik et al., 1989; Reuben et al., 1992). Other claimed advantages are good patient's acceptability, and good interrater reliability (Guralnik, et al., 1989; Reuben and Siu 1990; Mahurin et al., 1991). An example of performance measure is the Direct Assessment of Functional Status (DAFS, Lowenstein et al., 1989): the DAFS features mainly IADL skills (communication abilities, transportation, financial skills, shopping skills), along with two BADL skills (eating and dressing/grooming skills), and time orientation. Performance is rated as correct or incorrect. Our group has recently standardized another performance measure, The Functional Living Skills Assessment (FLSA) focused on mild ambulatory AD patients, which explores 8 areas of interest (Resources, Consumer Skills, Public Transportation, Time Management, Leisure, Telephone Skills, Self-Care and Health) and assesses a large range of functions, allows us to follow the patient evolution in an analytical manner (but it also provides a total score, that it easy to calculate and to follow serially) (Farina et., 1999; Farina et al., submitted). In two studies about cognitive rehabilitation in dementia, we demonstrated that the FLSA was the most sensitive instrument to detect functional changes in AD patients after performing a cognitive training of a 5-week duration (Farina et al., 2002; Farina et al., 2006 a)

4) Specific scales to evaluate comorbidities (even if they are less often present in middle-aged AD patients than in older ones) e.g. the CIRS (Parmalee PA et al 1995).

5) Tools to assess the impact of providing care to AD patients on family members' life, such as the Caregiver Burden Inventory (CBI, Novak et al., 1980), and to detect depressive symptoms in caregivers (e.g. Beck Depression Scale, Beck et al., 1961).

New diagnostic criteria for dementia consider not tenable the distinction between presenile and senile dementia (Reisberg, 2006), and even if some studies about the epidemiology of AD have claimed the younger AD patients have a disease evolution more rapid than the oldest, these data have been denied by other studies (with the exception of genetic dominant forms- Reisberg et al, 1989-). On the other hand, the clinical impression and the problems shown by middle aged AD patients in clinical practice are really different from older patients: a temporary stabilization of the cognitive status after starting a treatment with cholinesterase inhibitors is rarer than in older patients, the evolution of the disease is usually rather quick, and atypical forms of AD (e.g. with early and or relatively selective involvement of language or visuoperceptive functions) are frequently seen. This raises the possibility that the patient might be affected by other dementias (above all dementias of the frontotemporal spectrum). Middle-aged AD patients are also different as far as cognitive rehabilitation or stimulation is concerned.

In our practical experience of several years, we rarely saw clear improvement at neuropsychological tests or in functional tasks of middle-aged AD patients treated with cognitive rehabilitation or stimulation. On the contrary, this was the case for a good percentage of older patients recruited in our studies (Farina et al., 2006 a e b). Mostly middle-aged patients seem to follow a steady slope of deterioration, with almost every technique used (training of functions relatively conserved in the first phase of the disease, both with paper-and pencil and with computerized tasks; use of external aids or devices; training of the procedural memory in the activities of daily living; training with techniques based on implicit memory, such as errorless learning, spaced retrieval and forward or backward cueing. For most patients, cognitive-oriented techniques must be abandoned relatively quickly for more "generic" and simpler methods, such as occupational and recreational activities, which can give some results, more as far as behavioral problems are concerned rather than from the cognitive or functional point of view. To this aim, the choice of occupational/recreational activities must be accurately tailored on the past occupations and on the preference of the patient. It is necessary to question the patient, the spouse and/or other relatives about that, grading the degree of satisfaction that the patient seemed to find in a certain activity, and how frequently and from how long the patient practiced the activity. It is also necessary to test whether the patient is still able to perform the chosen activity without aid, or with minor aid. These are patients that are cruelly struck by the disease while still working and living a life with plenty of things to do and with social contacts. They rapidly loose their social and financial status, must retire from work and driving (not always voluntarily) and are often obliged to live a retired life at home (families of middle-aged dementia patients are usually shamed to show the patients to previous neighbors and friends). Therefore, they are easily frustrated if they realize that are no longer able to perform occupational activities, which would have been very easy for them before the disease started.

It has been underlined that collaboration with the patient's family is an important part of the rehabilitation program: younger AD patients are different from the older ones also from this point of view, e.g. for the possible presence in the family of children in their teens (and even in their childhood), or in any case too young in order to understand the disease and accept it. Psychological intervention extended to all the family (patient, spouse, children, and others) can be particularly important in middle-aged patients. Performing sessions in the clinical setting does not exhaust the whole rehabilitation program: on the contrary, it is the point of departure for activities that, once planned during the sessions at the hospital, must be implemented and continued at home with the aid of the family. To this aim, familiar persons must be instructed relative to the specific techniques used in this kind of patient (e.g. errorless learning and forward cueing) and psychologically supported in order to face and manage possible difficulties that can take place during the home sessions: e.g. the excessive confidence between the patient and his/her caregiver may reduce the patient's compliance and cause irritability: in this case the time of each home session must be reduced: sessions for collaborating patients may be 30-45 minutes long, while in the case of reduced compliance they must be 20 minutes maximum. The family collaboration with the rehabilitation program is essential from other points of view: the family must motivate the patient to take part in the hospital sessions and must assure a regular frequency; relatives must favor the birth of a therapeutic alliance between the patient, his/her family and therapists; they must stimulate the patient to generalize learning obtained in rehabilitation sessions to daily life.

Group intervention of cognitive stimulation can be particularly indicated in AD patients because it allow socialization, which has a positive effect on mood; however, AD is not common in middle age, and it is difficult to form groups. Therefore, in most cases patients receive rehabilitation in individualized sessions, or in groups formed by a very few patients (2-3), at least in our center.

DIFFERENT TECHNIQUES IN COGNITIVE REHABILITATION

In the following paragraph, we will give some details about the different techniques that can be used with patients affected by dementia.

In the first stage of AD, "specific" techniques, favoring relearning (or new learning) of a limited amount of information (e.g. the association face-name) can be proposed, such as spaced retrieval, the method of vanishing cues and errorless learning. These methods have been originally proposed as focusing on implicit memory, a type of memory preserved in early AD.

With the *spaced retrieval* technique, the patient is asked to retain an object that is presented at very short (few seconds) but increasingly longer intervals (5, 10, 20, 40, 60, 90, 120'' etc.). Intervals are filled with interfering tasks (such as a conversation). When the patient is unable to recall an item (for example after a 120 s interval), he/she receives a feedback and the retention interval is shortened to the previous step when the patient managed to recall a piece of information (90 s in this case). Spaced retrieval has shown its effectiveness in allowing AD patients to retain face-name associations (Camp and Foss, 1997), to localize objects (Bird and Kinsella, 1996) and to carry out prospective memory-related tasks (Mc Kitrick et al., 1992; Kixmiller 2002). Clare et al. (1999, 2000, 2002) administered spaced retrieval, in association with errorless learning and vanishing cues, to some AD patients who had to retain ecologically relevant face-name associations or personal information (see later on). Another implicit memory-oriented learning approach is the method of *vanishing cues* (previously successfully administered to amnesics): the patient is required to retrieve a verbal piece of information and he receives all the letters (cues) he needs to meet this goal. There are two different procedures: patient is asked to spontaneously retrieve a verbal piece of information (for example the name of a person). If he/she does not recall it, he/she is provided with an increasing number of letters to get the right word until the patient manages to retrieve it ("forward cueing"). At the second step, the patient is provided with a number of letters equal to the letters he previously needed to retrieve the item, but one less, and so on. The alternative procedure ("backward chaining"), initially provides the patient with all the letters composing a to be recalled item. The letters are then progressively decreased according to the patient's ability to retain the piece of information. The method of vanishing cues has shown to be effective in teaching AD patients face-name associations (Van der Linden and Juillerat, 1998), addresses and telephone numbers (De Vreese, 1999). Bird at al. (1995) managed to reduce behavioral disturbances in some demented patients by combining spaced retrieval with the method of vanishing cues. The studies of Clare et al. (1999, 2000, 2002) have been already mentioned.

Errorless learning has been derived by studies on amnesic subjects and focus on minimizing the number of errors during the learning process. This technique appears to be more beneficial in improving the ability of patients with explicit memory impairment to acquire new pieces of information than the errorful learning method. According to Wilson and Evans (1996), errorless learning improves learning by relying on implicit memory, which is very likely to be affected by errors, as it is perseverative and poorly flexible. Clare et al. (1999) successfully administered the errorless learning technique to a mild AD patient who had to learn 11 face-name associations concerning her club companions. However in this study, the errorless learning technique was combined with a language processing strategy, and with the vanishing cues spaced retrieval methods. The same authors (Clare et al., 2000) have then presented, together with the previous study, the results they obtained by administering the same combination of procedures to other 2 subjects. In this case, the patients were successfully trained to learn face-name associations or personal information. Another patient was trained to learn face-name associations of well-known people by using the errorless learning principle in association with one of the other techniques at a time. In the same article, the authors also administered the errorless learning technique to teach the use of external aids (calendar, diary, black board) to two AD patients in order to reduce the number of their repetitive questions (see later on).

However, in spite of these promising premises, more recent studies have questioned the usefulness of errorless learning in patients with dementia (Dunn and Clare, 2007; Haslam et al., 2006; Metzler-Baddeley and Snowden, 2005). From these studies, it seems that advantages of the errorless learning technique are limited (e.g., it can be useful to learn general information rather than specific ones), and that only some patients can benefit from it. Moreover, if the patient has still a residual of explicit memory, he/she will learn more throughout this residual than by using implicit memory.

It must also be recognized that most studies focusing on spaced retrieval, vanishing cues and errorless learning are small and there is poor evidence of a generalization in daily living tasks. More, it can be difficult to determine what kind of information may be useful to (re)learn for AD patients in everyday life, and the errorless learning technique can be difficult to use with some patients to their impulsiveness.

Another possibility with AD patients in the first stage is the use of external aids and supports, such as alarm clocks, place cards, diaries, boards, colored posters, and electronic aids. However, available data on this subject are limited, and further investigation is necessary.

Bourgeois et al. (1997) obtained a reduction of repetitive questions in a group of mild to moderate AD patients thanks to the use of a "memory book" they produced with the caregiver's help and containing family pictures, a checklist of daily living activities and drawings of to be done activities with time schedule. Also Clare et al. (2000) obtained a reduction of repetitive questions by using external aids (calendar, diary, board) with two mildly affected AD patients and administering errorless learning. However, only one patient did not loose the improvement at the follow up. Zanetti et al. (2000) trained 5 mild to moderate AD patients to learn 7 ecologic prospective memory-related tasks by the means of an electronic diary. The results produced by the use of the electronic diary were then compared with two control conditions (free retrieval following "spontaneous" learning and retrieval supported by a written list of cues). Patients performed significantly better in the first case than in the control conditions.

The most important prerequisite of studies on external aids is that thanks to the use of environmental supports, the to be done activity becomes less episodic and semantic memory dependent (the two compromised memories) and more procedural memory dependent. For example, by combining the use of big boards showing the name of given objects or places with oral instructions and practical demonstrations, it is possible to improve patients' performances in instrumental activities of daily living such as preparing breakfast, a coffee and so on.

Patients must be motivated to use external aids in their activities of daily living until they become part of their daily routine and increase their independence. For this reason, this intervention must be individually tailored and the method that encourages the patient to use aids must be carefully studied and administered (for example by dividing the learning process into different steps, by detecting the most effective way to elicit the appropriate reaction, by using errorless learning).

Very recently, preliminary data indicate that patients with Alzheimer disease can benefit also from the stimulation of "residual" neuropsychological functions carried out through *computerized programs* (Cipriani et al., 2005). In a pilot study, Tàrraga and coworkers (2006) compared an experimental group of AD patients, treated with a multimedia internet-based system (Smartbrain) and an integrated psychostimulation program, and two control groups, the first treated only with the psychostimulation program, and the second one not submitted to cognitive stimulation. Both groups received acetylcholinesterase inhibitors. After 12 weeks of treatment, the experimental group improved in two measures of cognitive global function (MMSE and ADAS-Cog), and this improvement was maintained at the follow-up. Another recent study, including patients with AD and with MCI (Talassi et al., 2007) compared a rehabilitation program including a computerized training along with a more generic and global approach, and a program including only the last one.

Both MCI and AD patients improved with the program including also the computerized approach from the cognitive and psychiatric point of view. AD patients treated only with the global approach showed minor cognitive improvement.

In the mild to moderate phase of dementia, more "global" and less specific interventions must be proposed.

Reality Orientation Therapy is the most known cognitive stimulation technique in AD, developed in the 50's and then improved during the following ten years (Taulbee and Folsom, 1966).

It is a technique that, through a focused and continuous stimulation, helps the patient to reorient himself/herself towards the environment: this leads the patient to a better comprehension of what surrounds him improving his/her sense of control and self-esteem. The theoretical foundations of the ROT are multiple. However, all the authors seem to agree in founding the rehabilitation process on the stimulation of the parts still partially integral of the individual mental state, with the aim to develop some form of independence (Brook, 1975; Florenzano, 1988).

There are two forms of ROT: formal ROT and informal ROT. Informal ROT approach is double: it involves a reorganization of the environment by the means of aids, such as calendars, clocks, signs (indicating toilets, kitchen etc.) and a repetitive reality reorientation through direct stimulation. The staff throughout the day carries out these activities in order to let patients recall basic information such as present day, month, year, age, location etc. Formal ROT is a structured group therapy. Formal ROT group sessions (composed by a maximum of five people at the same involutional stage) take place in a room built as a common house, and equipped with a big clock, a calendar and a black board; they usually last one-hour maximum. The first part of the session is devoted to acclimatization following the daily space-time orientation criteria (present day, month, year and location), while during the second part some exercises are proposed (dealing with space, time and personal orientation).

According to literature, ROT has been found to improve verbal orientation and memory for personal facts; other studies have reported slight improvements also in other cognitive measures, behavior and social interaction. However, it is uncertain whether ROT produces a positive impact on daily living activities and what is the persistence of its effects.

In last the 20 years, various researches have analyzed ROT efficacy in AD. The metanalysis carried out from the Cochrane Collaboration (Spector et al., 2000) has concluded that there is a sure evidence of effectiveness both for cognitive and behavioral aspects (even if the positive effect seems of short duration); the author thinks therefore that the ROT would have to be considered like part of the treatment of people with dementia. A recent controlled randomized multicentric study (Spector et al., 2003) in which patients received a treatment inspired mainly to the ROT and to the cognitive stimulation has confirmed the possible benefits for the patients affected by dementia, who in this study improved regarding to controls in several parameters (MMSE, ADAS-Cog, Quality of life-Alzheimer' s Disease scales). Authors have calculated that the amplitude of the improvement was substantially comparable to those obtainable with inhibitors of cholinesterase in clinic trials. Unfortunately, the effect does not last a long time. However, there is some evidence that a program supported in the time can maintain the advantages acquired (Orrell et al., 2005). A retrospective study has concluded that the application of repeated cycles of ROT during initial and intermediate stages of disease could delay the cognitive decline and institutionalization (Metitieri et al., 2001).

ROT appears effective also when administered by a caregiver trained to offer the program at home (Onder et al., 2005).

Reality orientation enhances the effects of donepezil on cognition in Alzheimer's disease. ROT approach is often combined with two emotion-oriented techniques (Ishizahi et al., 2002; Onor et al., 2007): Reminiscence Therapy and Remotivation Therapy. They are, in fact, called 3R therapies.

The *Reminiscence* technique aims to bring into consciousness past experiences and unresolved conflicts, thus helping elderly people to put their experiences into perspective and preparing for death (Head at al., 1990; Burside and Haight; 1994). The idea is that, since remote memory is usually the last to deteriorate, RT could be an effective means of communication for demented patients. This therapy usually involves group meetings, in which participants are encouraged to talk about past events (e.g., aspects from their childhood, love relationships and marriage, education and work life, anniversaries and celebrations of historic events); they are often assisted with aids such as music or objects associated with those events in order to stimulate memory and mood. According to the Cochrane Review, the randomized (or almost randomized) trials that have been carried out on this subject (Baines et al., 1987; Goldwasser et al., 1987; Orten et al., 1989) are not sufficient to reach any conclusions on the efficacy of the Reminiscence Therapy, although the best trial (Baines et al., 1987) reports a slight but statistically insignificant improvement in behavior.

(Spector et al., 1999). A more general literature review on emotion-oriented approaches in the care for persons suffering from dementia concluded that mainly positive results (including increased social interaction and decrease of behavior problems) are achieved with these kinds of approaches. Unfortunately many studies have methodological limitations and are done independently, which makes comparison difficult (Finnema et al., 2000).

The *Remotivation Therapy* was initially developed to treat schizophrenic patients but was then administered also to institutionalized elderly patients with psychogeriatric problems (Abrahams et al., 1979; Levy, 1987). The therapist aims to mobilize patient's interest in his environment by stimulating him every day, individually or in a group session, and leading him to focus his attention on simple subjects and/or events (history, holidays, food, money etc.). Unlike what happens in psychotherapy sessions, subjects concerning emotional problems such as the relationship with the family, diseases, institutionalization, religion and so on, are avoided as much as possible. The Remotivation therapy involves a highly structured method in its group sessions. However, the studies about the effectiveness of this technique in patients with dementia are scanty. Janseen and Giberson (1988) outlined that after a Remotivation therapy training, patients affected by various degrees of dementia showed a greater interest in group activities and an increased verbal and emotional communication level.

With the progression of dementia, treatments with *recreational activities*, such as games and art therapies (e.g., music, dance, art), that are frequently offered to people with dementia in nursing homes or day-care centers, can be useful to ameliorate mood and avoid social isolation of people with dementia. As discussed above, this kind of treatments can be particularly useful in the practical management of middle-aged AD patients. The primary purposes of recreational activities, according to the American Therapeutic Recreation Association (ATRA) guidelines, are to restore, remediate or rehabilitate in order to improve functioning and independence as well as reduce (or eliminate) the effect of illness or disability. Activity is a basic human need expressed in leisure and work pursuits; unfortunately, dementia leads to boredom and isolation due to a low rate of activity participation, and this results in agitated or passive behaviors, and in functional loss. Recreational Services are thought to provide recreation resources and opportunities in order to improve patients' health and well being (Fitzsimmons, 2003). Chosen interventions of recreational activities for AD patients must match the functional skills of the persons with dementia and their personality style of interest to provide stimulation and enrichment to the patient and thus mobilize the patient's available cognitive resources. However, only a few controlled studies have been performed to demonstrate efficacy of recreational activities in AD: there is some evidence that these interventions decrease behavioral problems, improve mood and increase socialization (Karlsson et al., 1988; Gerber et al., 1991; Rovner et al., 1996). Recently, it has been suggested that even some extremely easy activities, such as Bingo, can significantly improve cognitive performances in AD patients (unlike motor activity) (Sobel, 2001) Additional support for this recreational approach in AD treatment comes from the works of Teri and Logsdon (Teri et al., 1992; Teri, 1994), who have developed a protocol that includes behavior psychotherapy and a number of interventions aimed at increasing the number of pleasant activities. This protocol has shown to improve the mood of patients and caregivers alike.

Recreational activities can be combined with occupational interventions: some data suggest a positive effect on functional abilities of demented patients by programs based on procedural learning (Zanetti et al., 1997, 2001): a significant reduction of time spent to perform selected activities of daily living was noted. On the other hand, educating caregivers about the impact of the environment on dementia-related behaviors, and about the relationship between excess stimulation and behavioral disturbances, has been shown to slow functional decline and to reduce behavior problems in a randomized, controlled trial (Gitlin et al., 2001). In another study, a brief structured intervention at home by an occupational therapist (suggesting adaptation of the environment, and strategies for control of reactive behaviors and improvement of residual functional abilities), and by a psychologist (giving psychological support to caregivers, and giving advice on family relationships, psychological consequences of caring and verbal and non-verbal communication) led to a significant reduction of the frequency of problem behavior and, to a lesser extent, of time spent for caring (Nobili et al., 2004). Adherence to occupational therapy recommendations can improve quality of life of AD patients living in the community and diminish caregiver burden (Dooley and Hinojosa J, 2004).

Our group has recently demonstrated cognitive and functional gains in demented patients treated with training of activities of daily living (based on stimulation of procedural memory) or recreational-occupational activities (plus support psychotherapy for patients and caregivers Farina et al., 2002, 2006 a). Patients treated with recreational-occupational activities also showed a significant improvement in behavior. A limitation of our studies was that in both cases we compared mentioned techniques to other non-pharmacological treatments; therefore, we had no control (not-treated) group. Therefore, we performed an additional aimed to overcome this limitation, by comparing a control group (AD subjects receiving only standard medical care) with AD patients taking part to a stimulation program based on recreational and occupational activities, associated to a brief cycle of support psychotherapy for patients and caregivers. When comparing baseline with post-training condition, patients displayed a substantial reduction in disruptive behavior, and a tendency to a general reduction of behavioral symptoms compared to controls. This reduction was mirrored by a significant reduction of caregiver reaction to behavioral disturbances (Farina et al., 2006 b).

Patients in the moderate to severe phase of dementia can benefit of *music therapy*, even if this kind of treatment has been proposed also in the early phases of the disease. Music therapy is a potential non-pharmacological treatment for the behavioral and psychological symptoms of dementia. It is, in fact, a safe and effective method for treating agitation and anxiety in moderately severe and severe AD. This is in line with the result of some studies on music therapy in dementia (Sherratt et al., 2004; Svansdottir HB et al 2006), even if a recent Cochrane report concluded that more and better quality research is required to investigate the effectiveness of music therapy in reducing problems in behavioral, social, emotional and cognitive domains in patients with dementia (Vink et al., 2004). But the effect of music therapy could not be limited to reduction of agitation and anxiety: a randomized placebo-controlled trial with blinded observer rater aimed to explore whether music, live or pre-recorded, is effective in the treatment of apathy in subjects with moderate to severe dementia, concluded that live interactive music has immediate and positive engagement effects in dementia subjects with apathy, regardless of the severity of their dementia, while pre-recorded music is non-harmful but less clearly beneficial (Holmes et al., 2006).

Other studies have claimed that music could enhance cognitive performances of AD patients (Van de Winkel et al., 2004). In a recent study considerable improvement was found as far as autobiographical memory is concerned in the music condition, associated with a significant reduction in state anxiety, suggesting anxiety reduction as a potential mechanism underlying the enhancing effect of music on autobiographical memory recall (Irish et al., 2006).

For patients with severe dementia, *Validation Therapy* (VT), which was developed by Naomi Feil (1993, 1996) between 1963 and 1980 to offer an alternative to ROT and particularly for older demented patients living in care retirement communities, is frequently proposed as non-pharmacological treatment. Feil describes VT as a method to encourage the intellectual development in elderly people with mild or severe orientation disorders, that is aimed at restoring patients' self-esteem, reducing stress, anxiety and isolation from the external world, decreasing the need of safety measures, promoting contacts with other people, facilitating their independence and helping them to carry out unsolved vital tasks. According to the author, when more recent memory fails, elderly people try to restore balance to their life by retrieving earlier memories. Painful feelings that are expressed and "validated" by a trusted listener will diminish, while painful feelings that are ignored will gain strength, leading the elderly individual to social isolation and vegetative state. Feil classifies individuals with cognitive impairment as having one of four stages of a continuum of dementia: Malorientation, Time Confusion, Repetitive Motion and Vegetation. Each stage is identified by sets of both cognitive and behavioral characteristics: through the empathic listening, eye and physical contact, the therapist tries to understand the patient's point of view to establish an emotional contact with him or her; the goal is not to reach awareness of reality but to understand the meaning of the patient's behavior. The therapist of Validation accepts that a confused old man retires into his shell as a consequence of aging, and accepts his going back to the past as a survival mean, and a healthy process that lessens the age-related burden. In this way, the therapist "validates" the elderly individual's feelings and uses the empathy to be on the same wavelength with his interior reality. VT can be administered to the single patient, but whenever possible, it involves group meetings.

Various observational studies have indicated that there are positive effects in using VT with regard to the interactions that patients are able to make during validation groups (Bleathman and Morton, 1988; Babins et al., 1988). However, although the Cochrane Collaboration review has identified 18 studies on the efficacy of this technique, only two of them were randomized controlled trials (Robb et al., 1986; Toseland et al., 1997); these studies indicate that there is no statistically significant benefit but only a positive trend of Validation Therapy concerning some outcomes; in addition, the potential advantage of this therapy could depend only on a greater attention to the patient (Neal and Briggs, 1999).

Multisensory environments such as *Snoezelen®* rooms are becoming increasingly popular in health care facilities for individuals with moderate-severe dementia. Snoezelen® provides sensory stimuli to stimulate the primary senses of sight, hearing, touch, taste and smell, through the use of lighting effects, tactile surfaces, meditative music and the odor of relaxing essential oils (Pinkney 1997). The clinical application of snoezelen has been extended from the field of learning disability to dementia care over the past decade. The rationale for its use lies in providing a sensory environment that places fewer demands on intellectual abilities but capitalizes on the residual sensorimotor abilities of people with dementia (e.g. Hope 1998). Some encouraging results have been documented in the area of promoting adaptive behaviors (e.g. Baker et al 2001, Long 1992, Spaull 1998), reducing agitation (Baillon et al., 2004), or apathy (Verkaik et al., 2005). However, the clinical application of Snoezelen® often varies in form, nature, principles and procedures. Such variations not only make examination of the therapeutic values of Snoezelen® difficult, but also make difficult the clinical development of Snoezelen® in dementia care. A Cochrane review of evidence for the efficacy of Snoezelen® in the care of people with dementia concluded that data were too limited to reach a firm conclusion (Chung et al., 2002) Acrossover randomised controlled study aimed to evaluate the effect of Snoezelen® on the mood and behavior of patients with dementia, in comparison to Reminiscence Therapy concluded that both interventions had a positive effect (Baillon et al., 2004)

Gentle Care® is a prosthetic life care system developed by Moyra Jones (1996). The aim of this system is to help families and professional carers in understanding the diseases that cause dementia, thus allowing caregivers to develop a "prosthesis of care" based on the premise of carefully defining the deficit the person is experiencing: this "prosthesis of care" will seek to arrange an environmental fit between the person with dementing illness and the physical space, the programs, and the significant people with whom the person must interact. The Gentle Care® system accommodates and supports existing levels of function and development, rather than challenging the person with dementia to adapt and perform in ways no longer possible. Carers are assisted to evaluate the functional deficits and strengths of the client, they are provided with problem solving strategies, and they are taught to integrate daily activities with programs that exploit the patient's residual abilities (Vitali, 2004). The physical space must assure security, mobility, easiness of access, privacy, comfort, and socialization; it must suggest to the patient its own function, and it must be flexible to adapt to patient and carer changes. Meaningful activities, that aim to satisfy fundamental psychological needs, are integrated to build a daily routine, specific for each patient (according to his/her moral and cultural background, attitude, capability).

Finally, it deserves a mention the positive effects that *physical activity* and exercise can have in patients with dementia. In the last years, many data have accumulated on this point. Exercise training combined with teaching caregivers behavioral management techniques improved physical health and depression in patients with Alzheimer disease in a randomized controlled trial (Teri et al., 2003). A recent work, comparing supervised walking, comprehensive exercise (walking plus strength training, balance, and flexibility exercises), and social conversation (casual rather than therapeutic themes) found that participants receiving comprehensive exercise exhibited higher positive and lower negative affect and mood. (Williams and Tappen, 2007). In another study, a simple exercise program, 1 hour twice a week, led to significantly slower decline in ADL score in patients with AD living in a nursing home than routine medical care (Rolland et al., 2007).

A recent review suggests that literature supports the claim that physical activity enhances cognitive and brain function, and protects against the development of neurodegenerative diseases (Kramer and Erickosn, 2007)

Another article reports the effects of language-enriched physical fitness interventions provided by universitary undergraduate students to 24 mild- to moderate-stage Alzheimer's disease patients. Socialization experiences consisted of supervised volunteer work and cultural/recreational activities. Changes in global functioning and neuropsychological test performance were evaluated and compared to those of a similar group of untreated patients from the Consortium for the Establishment of a Registry for Alzheimer's Disease (CERAD). Cohorts completing 4 semesters or longer showed no significant between-year changes after their first year on the Clinical Dementia Rating, a measure of global functioning, and on 5 or 6 of the cognitive and language measures. Comparisons with the CERAD sample suggested a slower rate of decline for the AD treated group. The stabilization of global and cognitive performance was not apparent among participants who completed only 2 semesters. (Arkin 2007) Exercise sessions consisted of flexibility, balance, aerobic, and weight resistance activities. Highly significant fitness gains were achieved in the six-minute walk test, upper and lower body strength, and duration of aerobic exercise (Arkin, 2003).

This work is also notable for other reasons: it is an example of the most recent tendency in the literature about cognitive rehabilitation in AD, that is the combination of interventions of different nature (global/aspecific interventions are associated to selective/specific training): another example is a randomized study on AD and Mild Cognitive Impairment patients comparing a psychomotor intervention associating spatial-temporal reorientation, ADL training, socialization, and specific cognitive exercises (to train attention, language, visuospatial abilities, calculation, and frontal functions) with psychosocial intervention alone, and showing that the experimental group appears cognitively stable after six months, and less depressed after twelve months (Olazarán et al., 2004)

Arkin (2007) comments in this manner why she chose to perform a combined intervention (page 73): "Clinically, there is much to said for leaving the combined intervention intact. By offering a variety of activities, you are providing multiple and different opportunities for participants to be successful. Someone whose language skills are seriously compromised and resist improvement can still achieve pleasure and satisfaction from rocking babies at a day care center and/or make tangible and esteem-building gains in speed or duration of aerobic activity or increases in amounts of weight lifted. A frail individual who cannot do well on the physical activities may benefit from the cognitive activities and be able to read stories to preschoolers or newspapers to a blind person".

Another reason for which the Arkin's work is interesting is that she included in her study two middle-aged AD patients. A 59 years old patient completed 4 years of treatment, thus entering in a small (4 persons) group showing stabilization in language measures, and less marked decline than CERAD controls at MMSE. On the whole, however, it is very difficult to extract information about middle-aged patients in the existing literature about cognitive rehabilitation in AD: no work specifically mentions these patients.

CONCLUSION

A Clinical Experience

In our clinical experience, it is difficult to initiate middle-aged patients to "classical" group training, because of the age difference with most AD patients (they do not have the same social and cultural background as elderly patients). Therefore, these patients are often treated with individual rehabilitation sessions. We want to detail, however, an experience in which two patients, both of them age 58 at the beginning of training, were treated together twice a week for 40 sessions.

The objectives of the program and techniques used to attain these objectives were the following:

- Controlling the progression of the deficits:

    a) Temporal and spatial reorientation (use of external aid)
    b) Language: maintenance of the written and spoken language abilities (stimulation

of verbal initiative during conversation on subjects of interest for the patients)

c)   Attention and concentration (attentive matrices)
d)   Praxia: work with paper and pencil (copying or painting pictures, manual activities with different materials) or more ecological ones (connecting the buttons, putting on the shoes, connecting the shoe-strings, putting on the coat, opening and closing pens, opening and using common objects etc).
e)   Visuo-perceptive deficits (exploration of paintings and of the environment)

- Maintenance of the AVQ (stimulation of the procedural memory in the activity of daily living)
- Maintenance of autobiographic memory
- Improving mood and well-being

a)   Games (cards, domino, bingo, goose game)
b)   Pleasant home activities (care of the grandson or of the garden)

- Emotional management of the patients (anxiety, depression, anger)
- Psychological support of caregivers (planned conversations at the beginning and end of treatment, conversations upon caregiver's request or to educate the caregivers to stimulate the patients at home).

The activities for these patients had been chosen to respect the following criteria:

- Asserting the dignity of the patients
- Not emphasizing the difficulties of the patients but supporting their residual abilities
- Preferring pleasant activities
- Respecting individual personality (taste, preferences)
- Supporting spontaneous participation
- Aiding the patient to establish social roles (inside the family or the entourage of friends, and inside the group of cognitive stimulation)
- Favoring self-esteem

The clinical sessions were structured in the following way: greetings of the therapist to welcome the patients and their relatives (the wife for a patient and the daughter for the other). The greetings were very affectionate: the aim was to let the patient and their families know themselves, and to favour the relationship between the therapist and the patient and between the therapist and the relatives. The objective was, also, a global care of the patients in order to create positive feelings and motivate the patient to come to the hospital for the session of cognitive rehabilitation spontaneously. After the first greetings the therapist moved with the patients to a wide, luminous receiving room in order to begin the work.

The patients sat down one beside the other and the therapist took a place near them and not in the classic position from behind a writing desk, in order not to break the relaxing and pleasant atmosphere that had been created. The patients in the first stages of the disease are often aware of their cognitive deficits, they feel themselves defident towards the other people and therefore are victims of anxiety and depression much more than the older ones. That's why we underline the importance of maintaining a good and positive mood as the base of the therapy.

After a short talk to find out how they felt that day and how the last week went on, the therapist began a first session of temporal and spatial reorientation taking advantage of personal calendars that the patients took home and were used to consult daily with their relatives. This aspect must be emphasised because it evidences how much is important for the patient to continue the cognitive stimulation at home in order to create that positive routine that contributes to maintaining and increasing residual cognitive and functional abilities.

During the session the therapist stimulated one specific cognitive function or purposed recreational occupations (see above).

After 45 minutes, the dismissal was similar to the beginning of the training session: the therapist returned with the patients to the relatives who were in the waiting room. The therapist, with the aid of the patients, reviewed with the caregiver the activities carried out during the session and then said good-bye to all, reminding them of the next meeting date which was also written by the patients on their personal agenda.

Apart from the general objectives already mentioned, the training had the specific aim to favor the acquaintance between the two families (the patients and their relatives go out together during the week end in order to spend a little time taking walks or drinking coffee and talking together) to give psychological and psychoeducational support to the caregiver and to the patients as they request.

Even if the Alzheimer disease showed a rapid course in these two patients it demonstrated positive results improving patients' mood and self-esteem and ameliorating the caregivers abilities to cope with the disease.

The experience surely has, also, shown that the small group (2 or 3 people) is a profitable formula for the treatment of middle-aged AD patients. Other experiences would be useful in order to improve the protocol of treatment for this type of patient but we are sure that it's important to take total care of the person concerning his/her cognitive, social, relational, psychological and emotional aspects.

REFERENCES

Abrahams JP, Wallach HF, Divens S. Behavioral improvement in long-term geriatric patients during an age-integrated psychosocial rehabilitation program. *J. Am. Geriatr. Soc.* 1979;27:218-221.

Alexopoulos GA, Abrams RC, Young RC and Shamoian CA: Cornell scale for depression in dementia. *Biol. Psych.* 1988, 23:271-284.

Arkin SM. Student-led exercise sessions yield significant fitness gains for Alzheimer's patients. *Am. J. Alzheimers Dis. Other Demen.*. 2003 May-Jun;18(3):159-70.

Arkin S. Language-Enriched Excercice Plus Socoialization slows Cognitive Decline in Alzheimer's Disease. *Am. J. Alzheimers Dis. Other Demen.*, 2007 Feb/Mar; volume 22 Number 1, 62-77 ,

Babins LH, Dillon JP, Merovitz S. The effects of Validation Therapy on disorientated elderly. Activities, *Adaption and Aging* 1988;12:73-86.

Baillon S, Van Diepen E, Prettyman R, Redman J, Rooke N, Campell R A. comparison of the effects of Snoezelen and reminiscence therapy on the agitated behaviour of patients with dementia. *Int. J. Geriatr. Psychiatry.* 2004 Nov;19(11):1047-52.

Baines S, Saxby P, Ehlert K. Reality orientation and reminiscence therapy: a controlled cross-over study of elderly confused people. *Br. J. Psychiatry* 1987; 151:222-231.

Baker R, Bell, S, Thomas, P, Assey, J and Wareing LA. A randomized controlled trial of the effects of multisensory stimulation for people with dementia. *British Journal of Clinical Psychology* 2001; 40, pp. 81–96.

Beck AT, Ward CH, Mendelson M, Mock JE and Erbaugh JK.: An inventory for measuring depression. *Arch. Gen. Psychiatry* 1961;561-571.

Bird M, Alexopoulus P, Adamowicz J. Success and failure in five case studies: Use of cued recall to ameliorate behavior problems in senile dementia. *Int. J. Geriatr. Psychiatry* 1995;10:305-311.

Bird M, Kinsella G. Long term cued recall of tasks in senile dementia. *Psychol. Aging* 1996;11:45-56.

Bleathman C, Morton, I. Validation therapy with the demented elderly. *J. Adv. Nurs.* 1988;13:511-514.

Brook P, Degun G, Mather M. Reality Orientation, a therapy for psychogeriatric patients: a controlled study. *Brit. J. Psychiatry* 1975;127: 42-45.

Burgeois MS, Burgio LD, Schultz R, Beach S, Palmer B. Modifying repetitive verbalization of community-dwelling patients with AD. *Gerontologist* 1997;37:30-39.

Burnside I, Haight B. Reminiscence and life review: therapeutic interventions for older people.1994; 19:55-61.

Camp CJ, Foss JW. Designing ecologically valid intervention for persons with dementia. In: Payne DG, Conrad FG (eds): Intersection in basic and apllied memory research. *New York: Springer*, 1997, pp 311-315.

Cipriani G, Bianchetti A, Trabucchi M Outcomes of a computer-based cognitive rehabilitation program on Alzheimer's disease patients compared with those on patients affected by mild cognitive impairment. . 2006 Nov-Dec;43(3):327-35.

Chung JC, Lai CK, Chung PM, French HP. Snoezelen for dementia *Cochrane Database Syst. Rev.* 2002;(4):CD003152.

Clare L, Wilson BA, Breen K, Hodges JR.: Errorless learing of face-name association in early Alzheimer's disease. *Neurocase*1999; 5:37-46.

Clare L, Wilson BA, Carter G, Breen K, Gosses A, Hodges JR. Intervening with everyday memory problems in dementia of Alzheimer type: an errorless learning approach. *J. Clin. Exp. Neuropsychol.* 2000;22:132-146.

Clare L., Wilson B.A., Carter G., Roth I., Hodges J.R.. Relearning face-name associations in early Alzheimer's disease. *Neuropsychology* 2002 Oct;16(4):538-47.

Cummings JL, Mega M, Gray K, Rosenberg-Thompson S, Carusi DA, Gornbein J. The Neuropsychiatric Inventory: comprehensive assessment of psychopathology in dementia. Neurology 1994; 44:2308-2314.

De Vreese LP, Neri M. Ecological impact of combined cognitive training programs (CPT) and drug treatment (ChE-I) in Alzheimer's disease. *Int. Psychogeriat.* 1999 a; 11(suppl),S187.

De Vreese LP. Cognitive rehabilitation procedures in cognitively challenged elderly. Paper presented at the 3rd International Symposium on "Advances in geriatric psychiatry: instruments for diagnosis, prognosis and rehabilitation". Department of Psychiatry, University of Saõ Paolo, Brasil, 1999 b.

Dooley NR, Hinojosa J. Improving quality of life for persons with Alzheimer's disease and their family caregivers: brief occupational therapy intervention. *Am. J. Occupational Therapy.* 2004; 58:561-569.

Dunn J. e Clare L. Learning face-name association in early-stage dementia: Comparing the effects of errorless learning and effortful processing *Neuropsychol Rehabil.* 2007 Jul 7;:1-20

Farina, E, Fioravanti R, Chiavari L, Imbornone E, Pomati S., Pinardi G., Alberoni M.,. Mariani C. Functional Living Skills Assessment: A standardized instrument built to monitor activities of daily living in demented patients: preliminary data. *J. Neurol.* 1999;246 (suppl. 1): I/101.

Farina E, Fioravanti R, Chiavari L, Imbornone E, Alberoni M, Pomati S, Pinardi G, Pignatti R, Mariani C. Comparing two programs of cognitive training in Alzheimer's disease: a pilot study. *Acta Neurologica Scandinavica,* 2002;105(5):365, 371.

Farina E, Mantovani F, Fioravanti R Pignatti R, Chiavari L, Imbornone E, Olivotto F, Alberoni M, Mariani C, Nemni R. Evaluating two group programmes of cognitive training in mild to moderate AD: is there any difference between a "global" stimulation and a "cognitive-specific" one? Aging Ment Health. March 2006 a, 10(3): 1–8.

Farina E, Mantovani F, Fioravanti R, Rotella G, Villanelli F, Imbornone E, Olivotto F, Tincani M, Alberoni M, Petrone E, Nemni R, Postiglione A Efficacy of recreational and occupational activities associated to psychologic support in mild to moderate Alzheimer disease: a multicenter controlled study. *Alzheimer Dis. Assoc. Disord.* Oct-Dec 2006 b;20(4):275-82

Feil N. Il metodo Validation. Milano: Sperling and Kupfer, 1996.

Feil, N. The validation breakthrough: simple techniques for communicating with people with "Alzheimer's-type dementia". Baltimore: Health Promotion Press, 1993.

Finnema E, Dröes RM, Ribbe M, Van Tilburg W. The effects of emotion-oriented approaches in the care for persons suffering from dementia: a review of the literature. *Int. J. Geriatr. Psychiatry 2000 Feb;15(2):141-61.*

Fitzsimmons S. Dementia practice guidelines for recreation therapy. Alexandria, *VA: ATRA Publications*; 2003.

Florenzano F. *La Reality Orientation in Psicogeriatria.* Roma: Primerano, 1988.

Gerber GJ, Prince PN, Snider HG, Atchinson K, Dubois L, Kilgour JA. Group activity and cognitive improvement among patients with Alzheimer's disease. *Hosp. Community Psychiatry* 1991;42:843-845.

Gitlin LN, Corcoran M, Winter L, Boyce A, Hauck WW. A randomized, controlled trial of a home environmental intervention: effect on efficacy and upset in caregivers and on daily function of persons with dementia. *Gerontologist.* 2001; 41(1): 4-14.

Goldwasser AN, Auerbach SM, Harkins SW. Cognitive, affective and behavioural effects of Reminiscence Group Therapy on Demented elderly. *Int. J. Aging Hum. Dev.* 1987; 25:209-222.

Guralnik JM, Branch LG, Cummings SR, Curb JD. Physical performance measures in aging research. *J Gerontol* 1989;44:141-146.

Haslam C., Gilroy D., Black S., Beesley T. "How successful is errorless learning in supporting memory for high and low-level knowledge in dementia?" *Neuropsyc. Reha.* 2006, 16(5), 505-536.

Head DM, Portnoy S, Woods RT. The impact of reminiscence groups in two different settings. *In. J. Geriatr. Psychiatry* 1990; 5:292-302.

Holmes C, Knights A, Dean C, Hodkinson S, Hopkins V. Keep music live: music and the alleviation of apathy in dementia subjects. *Int. Psychogeriatr.* 2006 Dec;18(4):623-30.

Hope KW. "The effects of multisensory environments on older people with dementia". *Journal of Psychiatric and Mental Health Nursing* 1998;5:377-385

Irish M, Cunningham CJ, Walsh JB, Coakley D, Lawlor BA, Robertson IH, Coen RF. Investigating the enhancing effect of music on autobiographical memory in mild Alzheimer's disease. *Dement Geriatr. Cogn. Disord.* 2006;22(1):108-20.

Ishizaki J, Meguro K, Ohe K, Kimura E, Tsuchiya E, Ishii H, Sekita Y, Yamadori A.Therapeutic psychosocial intervention for elderly subjects with very mild Alzheimer disease in a community: the tajiri project. *Alzheimer Dis. Assoc. Disord.* 2002 Oct-Dec;16(4):261-9.

Janseen JA, Giberson DL. Remotivation therapy. *J. Gerontol. Nurs.* 1988;14:31-34.

Jette AM, Branch LG Impairment and disability in the aged. *J. Chronic Dis.* 1985;38:59-65.

Jones M. Gentle Care: *Changing the experience of Alzheimer's Disease in a positive way.* Moira Jones Resources, Barnaby BC, Canada, 1996.

Karlsson I, Brane G, Melin E, Nyth AI, Rybo E. Effects of environmental stimulation on biochemical and psychological variables in dementia. *Acta Psychiatr. Scand.* 1988; 77:207-213.

Kixmiller J.S. Evaluation of Prospective Memory Training for Individuals with Mild Alzheimer's Disease *Brain and Cognition.* 2002, Jul;49 (2):237-41.

Kramer AF, Erickson KI Capitalizing on cortical plasticity: influence of physical activity on cognition and brain function. *Trends Cogn. Sci.* 2007 Aug;11(8):342-8.

Koger SM, Brotons M. Music therapy for dementia symptoms (Cochrane Review). In: The Cochrane Library, Issue 4, 1999. Oxford: Update Software, 1999.

Koh K, Ray R, Lee J, Nair A, Ho T, Ang P. Dementia in elderly patients: can the 3R mental stimulation programme improve mental status? *Age Ageing* 1994; 23:195-199.

Kongable LG, Buckwalter KC, Stolley JM. The effects of pet therapy on the social behavior of instituzionalized Alzheimer's clients. *Arch. Psychiatric. Nurs.* 1989; 3:191-198.

Krebs-Roubicek EM. Group therapy with demented elderly. *Prog. Clin. Biol. Res.* 1989;317:1261-1272.

Kuriansky J, Gurland B The performance test of activities of daily living. *Int. J. Aging Hum. Dev.* 1976;7:343-352.

Lawton MP, Brody EM Assessment for older people: self-maintaining and instrumental activities of daily living. *Gerontologist* 1969;9:179-186.

Levy LL. Psychosocial intervention and dementia, Part 1: State of the art, future directions. *Occupational Therapy in Mental Health* 1987;7:69-107.

Long A.P. and Haig, L. "How do clients benefit from Snoezelen? An exploratory study". *British Journal of Occupational Therapy* 1992; 55, pp. 103–106.

Lowenstein DA, Amigo E, Duara R, Guterman A, Hurwitz D, Berkowitz N, Wilkie F, Weinberg G, Black B, Gittelman B, Eisdorfer C A new Scale for the assessment of functional status in Alzheimer's Disease and Related Disorders. *J. Gerontol.* 1989;44:114-121

Mahurin RK, De Bettignies BH, Pirozzolo FJ. Structured assessment of independent living skills: preliminary report of a performance measure of functional abilities in dementia. *J. Gerontol.* 1991;46:P-58-66.

McKitrick LA, Camp CJ, Black W. Prospective memory intervention in Alzheimer's disease. *J. Gerontology* 1992;47:337-343.

Metitieri T, Zanetti O, Geroldi C, Frisoni GB, De Leo D, Dello Buono M, Bianchetti A, Trabucchi M Reality orientation therapy to delay outcomes of progression in patients with dementia. A retrospective study. *Clin. Rehabil.* 2001 Oct;15(5):471-8.

Metzler-Baddeley C. e Snowden J.S. "Brief Report: Errorless versus Errorful Learning as a Memory Rehabilitation approach in Alzheimer's Disease" *J. Clin. Exp. Neuropsychol.* 2005; 27:1070-79.

Neal M, Briggs M. Validation therapy for dementia (Cochrane Review). In: The Cochrane Library, Issue 4, 1999. Oxford: Update Software, 1999.

Nobili A, Riva E, Tettamanti M, Lucca U, Liscio M, Petrucci B, Salvini Porro G. The effect of a structured intervention on caregivers of patients with dementia and problem behaviors. A randomized controlled pilot study. *Alzheimer Dis. Assoc. Disord.* 2004;18:75-82.

Novak, M., Guest, C. (1980). Application of a multidimensional caregiver burden inventory. *Gerontologist*, 29, 798-780.

Olazaràn J, Muñiz R, Reisberg B, Peña-Casanova J, del Ser T, Cruz- Jentoft AJ, Serrano P, Navarro E, Garcia de la Rocha ML, Frank A, Galiano M, Fernandez-Bullido Y, Serra JA, Gonzalez-Salvador MT, Sevilla C "Benefits of cognitive-motor intervention in MCI and mild to moderate Alzheimer disease". *Neurology.* 2004 Dec 28;63(12):2348-53

Onder G, Zanetti O, Giacobini E, Frisoni GB, Bartorelli L, Carbone G, Lambertucci P, Silveri MC, Bernabei R. Reality orientation therapy combined with cholinesterase inhibitors in Alzheimer's disease: randomised controlled trial. *Br. J. Psychiatry.* 2005 Nov;187:450-5.

Onor ML, Trevisiol M, Negro C, Signorini A, Saina M, Aguglia E. Impact of a multimodal rehabilitative intervention on demented patients and their caregivers. *Am. J. Alzheimers Dis. Other Demen.* 2007 Aug-Sep;22(4):261-72.

Orrell M, Spector A, Thorgrimsen L, Woods B A pilot study examining the effectiveness of maintenance Cognitive Stimulation Therapy (MCST) for people with dementia. *Int. J. Geriatr. Psychiatry* 2005 May;20(5):446-51

Orten JD, Allen M, Cook J. Reminiscence groups with confused nursing centre residents: An experimental study. *Soc. Work Health Care* 1989;14:73-86.

Parmalee PA, Thuras PD, Katz IR, Lawton MP: Validation of the Cumulative Illness Rating Scale in a geriatric residential population. *J Am Geriatr Soc* 1995;43:130-137)

Pinkney L. "A comparison of the Snoezelen environment and a music relaxation group on the mood and behaviour of patients with senile dementia". *British Journal of Occupational Therapy,* 1997; 60, 209–212.

Reisberg B, Ferris SH, Franssen E, Jenkins EC, Wisiniewski KE "Clinical features of a neuropathologically verified familial Alzheimer's cohort with onset in the fourth decade: comparison with senile onset Alzheimer's disease and etiopathogenic implications"Aging and Dementia Research Center, New York University Medical Center, New York 10016. *Prog. Clin. Biol. Res.*1989;317:43-54.

Reisberg B, Finkel S, Overall J, Schmidt-Gollas N, Kanowski S, Lehfeld H, Hulla F, Sclan SG, Wilms HU, Heininger K, Hindmarch I, Stemmler M, Poon L, Kluger A, Cooler C,

Bergener M, Hugonot-Diener L, Robert PH, Antipolis S, Erzigkeit H The Alzheimer's disease activities of daily living international scale (ADL-IS). *Int. Psychogeriatr.* 2001 Jun;13(2):163-81.

Reisberg B Diagnostic criteria in dementia: a comparison of current criteria, research challenges, and implications for DSM-V. *J. Geriatr. Psychiatry Neurol.* 2006 Sep;19(3):137-46. Review.

Reuben DB, Siu AL An objective measure of physical function of elderly outpatients The Physical Performance Test. *J. Am. Geriatr. Soc.* 1990;38:1105-1112.

Reuben DB, Siu AL, Kimpau S. The predictive validity of self-report and performance-based measures of function and health. *J. Gerontol.* 1992;47:M106-110.

Robb SS, Stegman CE, Wolanin MO. No research versus research with compromised results: a study of Validation Therapy. *Nurs. Res.* 1986;35:113-118.

Rolland Y, Pillard F, Klapouszczak A, Reynish E, Thomas D, Andrieu S, Rivière D, Vellas B "Exercise program for nursing home residents with Alzheimer's disease: a 1-year randomized, controlled trial". *J. Am. Geriatr. Soc.* 2007 Feb;55(2):158-65.

Rovner BW, Steel CD, Shmuely Y, Folstein MF. A randomized trial of dementia care in nursing homes. *J. Am. Geriatr. Soc.* 1996; 44:7-13.

Sherratt K, Thorton A, Hatton C. Music interventions for people with dementia: a review of the literature. *Aging Ment. Health* 2004 8(1):3-12.

Sobel, BP. Bingo vs. physical intervention in stimulating short-term cognition in Alzheimer's disease patients. *Am. J. Alzheimers Dis. Other Demen.* 2001 Mar-Apr;16(2):115-20.

Spaull, D., Leach, C. and Frampton, I. "An evaluation of the effects of sensory stimulation with people who have dementia". *Behavioural and Cognitive Psychotherapy*, 1998; 26, 77–86.

Spector A, Orrell M, Davies S, Woods B: Reality orientation for dementia (Cochrane Review). In: The Cochrane Library, Issue 4, 1999a. Oxford: Update Software, 1999.

Spector A, Orrell M, Davies S, Woods RT. Reminescence for dementia (Cochrane Review). In: The Cochrane Library, Issue 4, 1999b. Oxford: Update Software, 1999.

Spector A, Thorgrimsen L, Woods B, Royan L, Davies S, Butterworth M, Orrell M. Efficacy of an evidence-based cognitive stimulation therapy programme for people with dementia: randomised controlled trial. *Br. J. Psychiatry.* 2003 Sep;183:248-54.

Spector A, Orrel M, Davies S, Woods B. Reality orientation for dementia. Cochrane Database Syst Rev. 2000;(4):CD001119. Review. Update in: Cochrane Database Syst Rev. 2000; (3): CD001119

Svansdottir HB, Snaedal J Music therapy in moderate and severe dementia of Alzheimer's type. A case control study *Int. Psychogeriatr.* 2006 Dec;18(4):613-21.

Tarraga L, Boada M, Modinos G, Espinosa A, Diego S, Morera A, Guitart M, Balcells J, Lopez OL, Becker JT. A randomised pilot study to assess the efficacy of an interactive, multimedia tool of cognitive stimulation in Alzheimer's disease. *J. Neurol. Neurosurg. Psychiatry.* 2006 Oct;77(10):1116-21.

Talassi E, Guerreschi M, Feriani M, Fedi V, Bianchetti A, Trabucchi M. Effectiveness of a cognitive rehabilitation program in mild dementia (MD) and mild cognitive impairment (MCI): a case control study. *Arch. Gerontol. Geriatr.* 2007;44 Suppl 1:391-9.

Taulbee LR, Folsom JC. Reality orientation for geriatric patients. Hosp Commun Psychiatry 1966; 17,133-135.

Teri L, Gibbons LE, McCurry SM, Logsdon RG, Buchner DM, Barlow WE, Kukull WA, LaCroix AZ, McCormick W, Larson EB. Exercise plus behavioral management in patients with Alzheimer Disease. *JAMA* 2003;2015-2022.

Teri L, Truax P, Logsdon R, Uamoto J, Zarit S, Vitaliano PP. Assessement of behavioral problems in dementia: the Revised Memory and Behavior Problem Checklist. *Psychol. Aging* 1992;7:627-631.

Teri L. Behavioral treatment of depression in patients with dementia. Alzheimer *Dis. Assoc. Disord.* 1994;8(suppl. 3):66-74.

Toseland RW, Diehl M, Freeman K et al. The Impact of Validation Group Therapy on Nursing Home Residents with Dementia. *J. Appl. Gerontol.* 1997;16:31-50.

Van de Winckel A, Feys H, De Weerdt W, Dom R. Cognitive and behavioural effects of music-based exercises in patients with dementia. *Clin. Rehabil.* 2004 May;18(3):253-60

Van der Linden M, Juillerat AC. Prise en charge des déficits cognitifs chez les patients atteints de maladie d'Alzheimer. *Rev. Neurol.* 1998; 154:137-143.

Verkaik R., van Weert J.C., Francke A.L. "The effects of psychosocial methods on depressed, aggressive and apathetic behaviors of people with dementia: a systematic review". *Int. J. Geriatr. Psychiatry.* 2005 Apr;20(4):301-14. Review.

Vink AC, Birks JS, Bruinsma MS, Scholten RJ. Music therapy for people with dementia. *Cochrane Database Syst. Rew.* 2004;(3):CD003477.

Vitali S. La metodologia Gentle Care – Gentle Care model. G Gerontol 2004;52:412-417.

Williams ME Identifying the older person likely to require long-term care services. *J. Am. Geriatr. Soc.* 1987;35:761-766.

Williams C.L., Tappen R.M. "Effect of exercise on mood in nursing home residents with Alzheimer's disease". *Am. J. Alzheimers Dis. Other Demen.* 2007 Oct-Nov;22(5):389-97

Wilson B., Cockburn J., Baddeley A. *Test di memoria comportamentale Rivermead.* Organizzazioni Speciali, Firenze, 1990.

Wilson BA, Evans JJ. Error-free learning in rehabilitation of people with memory impairment. J. *Head Trauma Rehab.* 1996;11:54-64.

Yesavage JA, Brink TL, Rose TL, et al. Development and validation of a geriatric depression screening scale: a preliminary report. *J. Psychiatric Res.* 1982-83;17:37-49.

Zanetti O, Binetti G, Magni E, Rozzini L, Bianchetti A, Trabucchi M. Procedural memory stimulation in Alzheimer's disease: impact of a training programme. *Acta Neuro. Scand.* 1997a;95:152-157.

Zanetti O, Zanieri G, De Vreese LP, Frisoni G, Binetti G, Trabucchi M. Utilizing an electronic memory aid with Alzheimer's disease patients. A study of feasibility. Paper presented at the 6th International Stockolm/Springfield Symposium on advances in Alzheimer Therapy, Stockolm, Sweden, 2000.

Zanetti O, Zanieri G, Di Giovanni G, et al. Effectiveness of procedural memory stimulation in mild Alzheimer's disease: a controlled study. *Neurosychol. Rehabil.* 2001;11:263-272.

In: Alzheimer's Disease in the Middle-Aged
Editor: Hyun Sil Jeong, pp. 117-136

ISBN: 978-1-60456-480-8
© 2008 Nova Science Publishers, Inc.

Chapter 4

HELICOBACTER PYLORI INFECTION AND ALZHEIMER'S DISEASE: CORRELATION OF CEREBROSPINAL FLUID HELICOBACTER PYLORI IgG ANTIBODIES WITH DISEASE SEVERITY

Jannis Kountouras[*], Marina Boziki, Emmanuel Gavalas, Christos Zavos, Georgia Deretzi, Nikolaos Grigoriadis, Panagiotis Katsinelos and Dimitrios Tzilves
Department of Medicine, Second Medical Clinic,
Aristotle University of Thessaloniki, Ippokration Hospital,
Thessaloniki, Greece

ABSTRACT

Although degenerative diseases of the central nervous system, including Alzheimer's disease (AD), have an increasingly high impact in aged population, their association with *Helicobacter pylori* (*H. pylori*) infection has not as yet been thoroughly researched. This issue has only recently been addressed by two studies. A higher seropositivity for anti-*H. pylori*-specific IgG antibodies was reported in AD patients than in age-matched controls. Moreover, based on the histological analysis of gastric mucosa biopsy for the documentation of current *H. pylori* infection, a higher rate of infection was reported in AD patients compared to anemic controls. It is thus reasonable to further investigate the role of *H. pylori* in AD initiation, progression or susceptibility by documenting its qualitative and quantitative presence in the cerebrospinal fluid (CSF) of these patients. A prospective, non-randomized, comparative study was carried out to investigate the levels of anti-*H. pylori*-specific IgG antibodies in the CSF and serum of AD patients, compared with those of age-matched cognitively normal controls. CSF and serum samples were obtained from 27 patients with AD and 27 control participants. Anti-*H. pylori* IgG concentrations in the CSF and the serum were measured by means of an enzyme-linked

[*] Jannis Kountouras, MD, PhD; Professor of Medicine; Gastroenterologist; 8 Fanariou St, Byzantio; 551 33, Thessaloniki, Macedonia, Greece; Tel: +30-2310-892238, Fax: +30-2310-992794; E-mail: jannis@med.auth.gr

immunosorbent assay. The mean concentration of anti-*H. pylori*-specific IgG was significantly greater in: a) the CSF of AD patients (10.53±12.54 U/mL) than in controls (8.63±8.01 U/mL, *p*=0.047), and b) the serum of AD patients (30.44±33.94 U/mL) than in controls (16.24±5.77 U/mL, *p*=0.041). Anti-*H. pylori* IgG antibodies in the CSF correlated with the degree of severity of the disease. These findings further support a role for *H. pylori* infection in the pathobiology of AD.

Keywords: Alzheimer's Disease, *Helicobacter pylori*, cerebrospinal fluid, anti-*H. pylori*-specific IgG antibodies, autoantibodies, molecular mimicry.

INTRODUCTION

A. Alzheimer's Disease

Alzheimer's disease (AD) is the most common cause of dementia, accounting for 50-60% of all cases [1]. The dysregulation in the metabolism of amyloid precursor protein (APP) and consequent deposition of amyloid-β (Abeta) peptide has been envisaged as crucial for the development of neurodegeneration in AD [2,3]; key features include the deposition of the Abeta in the form of senile (or amyloid) plaques, the formation of neurofibrillary tangles, and the loss of neurons and synapses in specific brain regions [4]. Amyloid deposition begins 10-20 years before the appearance of clinical dementia. During this time, the brain is confronted with increasing amounts of toxic Abeta peptides and both the innate and the adaptive immune systems may play an important role in the disorder. Innate immunity in the brain is mainly represented by microglial cells [5-6], which phagocytose and degrade Abeta. As the catabolism of Abeta decreases, glial cells become overstimulated and damage or kill neurons by the release of inflammatory (neurotoxic) molecules such as tumor necrosis factor (TNF)-α, interleukin (IL)-1beta, IL-6, chemokines [IL-8, macrophage inflammatory protein-1α (MIP-1α), monocyte chemo-attractant protein-1], nitric oxide (NO) or reactive oxygen metabolites (ROMs) [7-10]. In this respect, glial activation and expression of cytokines may act in synergy with other genetic and acquired environmental risks to culminate in the development of this immune-mediated disease involved defective immune regulation and auroimmunity [11-14].

Specifically, microglia as well as astrocytes, macrophages and dendritic cells [(DCs), the most potent antigen-presenting cells (APCs)] are the immune effector cells in the central nervous system (CNS) concomitant with inflammatory brain disease and play a significant role in the host defense against invading agents including microorganisms [15,16]. Brain inflammation, characterized by reactive microglia and astrocytes, is noticed in close vicinity of amyloid plaques in AD and in transgenic mouse models of the disease [5,17]. Microglia contain several antigenic and functional markers similar to DCs and macrophages [18] and can function as main APCs within the CNS; microglia express immune-related antigens, constitutively HLA-DR in situ, the DC marker RFD1 upon activation [19,20] and, comparable to DCs [5], may also present antigen in the context of major histocompatibility complex (MHC) to CD4+ and CD8+ T lymphocytes (TLs). In this regard, MHC class II (HLA-DR) antigen -positive reactive microglia were observed throughout the cortex of post-mortem brains of patients with AD, particularly concentrated in the areas of senile plaque formation [21] and enriched microglial cultures alone were capable of stimulating TL responses or the CD4+ TL subset, a response which could be inhibited with an anti-MHC class II blocking antibody [22]. The interaction of activated CD4+T cells with microglia led to a pro-inflammatory T helper type 1 (Th1) response with a Th1-type cytokine expression profile involved in the pathogenesis of AD [11] via apoptosis representing an important contributor to induction, progression and pathology of neurodegeneration in AD [23-26]. Th1 response, by secreting substantial levels of pro-inflammatory Th1-type cytokine TNF-α [5,27] leads to TNF-α-related apoptotic neuronal cell death in neurodegenerative diseases including AD [26,28]; TNF death receptor pathway and caspases are activated in the early stages of neuronal degeneration in AD [29]. Moreover, the Fas-FasL pathways may contribute to mechanisms of neuronal loss and neuritic degeneration in AD [30]. Hyperexpression of Fas mRNA and surface Fas receptor on TLs may explain the occurrence of inflammatory cellular infiltrates in the CNS of AD patients [31] leading to apoptotic damage; the key apoptosis regulator FasL may participate in both neuronal and immune cell apoptosis in AD [32]. A CD8+ cell-mediated apoptotic mechanism (activated cytotoxic TLs) may also play a pathogenic role in AD [13]. Additional recent studies have identified novel pathways, including the Wnt pathway and the serine-threonine kinase Akt, as central modulators that oversee cellular apoptosis in AD and the formation of neurofibrillary tangles through their downstream substrates including Bad, and Bcl-xL, and glycogen synthase kinase-3beta [25]. Besides, Abeta directly induces neuronal apoptotic death (involving JNK activation, Bcl-w downregulation, and release of mitochondrial Smac), suggesting a role of Abeta neurotoxicity in AD neurodegeneration responsible in part for the cognitive decline found in AD patients [33,34]. Although there is evidence suggesting a role of autoreactive Abeta-specific TLs in the elimination of this peptide, this beneficial mechanism however seems to be impaired in the majority of patients with AD [35], thereby escalating the detrimental effect of TLs in AD [36]. Notably, apoptotic, rather than necrotic, microglia associated nerve cell death appears as likely to underlie a number of common neurological conditions including AD, Parkinson's disease, glaucoma (ocular AD) or multiple sclerosis [37-41]. The latter disease, for example, is also crucially dependent on activation of pro-inflammatory Th1Ls by APCs, resistance of TLs to Fas-mediated apoptosis is involved in its exacerbation, and auto-aggressive Th1 cells can be adoptively transferred to non-diseased recipient mice that subsequently develop disease [5,42]. Summarizing, the above mentioned data describe the current evidence for cellular immune defective and apoptotic mechanisms playing an important role in the neurodegenerative process in AD.

Regarding humoral immunity, recent evidence suggests that the possible presence of anti-neuronal antibodies and autoimmune mechanisms may be responsible for eliciting neuronal cell death in AD [43]. Therefore, apart from cellular immunity, abnormalities of humoral immunity appear to play a role in the pathogenesis of AD.

The early events underlying AD remain uncertain, although environmental factors may be involved. In this respect, the possibility that microorganisms can cause AD has recently been addressed [44,45]; infiltration of the brain by pathogens acts as a trigger or co-factor for AD, with *Herpes simplex* virus type 1 and *Chlamydophila* being most frequently implicated. [45,46]. These pathogens by eliciting inflammation, may cause the neurological damage that results in AD. In this regard, an infection-based animal model demonstrates that following intranasal inoculation of BALB/c mice with *C. pneumoniae*, amyloid plaques/deposits consistent with those observed in the AD brain develop, thereby implicating this infection in the etiology of AD [45].

B. *Helicobacter Pylori* Infection

H. pylori, a curved spiral gram-negative bacterium that colonizes the gastric mucosa of most humans worldwide (more than one half of the world's population is infected with this bacterium, mainly affecting older adults in the developed world), has been linked with a number of upper digestive diseases, particularly peptic ulcer disease that was viewed, like AD, as a classic degenerative condition, resulting from some toxic combination of *H. pylori* and/or stress, chemical irritants and bad genes [44,47,48]. Moreover, this bacterium has been associated with extradigestive disorders [49-52] such as functional vascular disorders caused by vascular dysregulation, atherosclerosis [53], hypertension, cardiovascular and/or cerebrovascular ischemia and stroke [54], all of which have been found to be risk factors for AD, mainly by impairing blood–brain barrier, a common denominator associated with various degrees of dementia, including AD [43,55-58]; these conditions contribute to the clinical manifestations and worsening of AD [59].

As in the case of AD, comparable cellular immune-mediated and apoptotic pathogenic features can also be introduced for *H. pylori* infection. Although *H. pylori* does not invade the gastric lamina propria, it induces an infiltrate of granulocytes and TLs playing a major role in the pathology of upper gastrointestinal diseases. Specific subsets of infiltrating TLs also play a central role in controlling the outcome of this pathogen via the cytokine response induced by the *H. pylori* infection [60,61]; while the type of host immune response against *H. pylori* is crucial for the outcome of the infection, this response does not enable the immune system to clear the infection and may instead be detrimental to tissue integrity [61,62]. This bacterium elicits complex immune responses, both innate and adaptive. The dense infiltration of the gastric mucosa with cells of the immune system suggests that a complex interplay between APCs and other immune cells may be important for the development of *H. pylori*-induced gastric pathologies [63]. The immune response is triggered by presentation of antigen peptides on the major histocompatibility assembly of the APCs with the assistance of costimulatory molecules such as B7-1 (CD80) and B7-2 (CD86) [64]. In view that DCs are professional APCs initiating T-cell responses and important mediators between the innate and cognate immune system [60,65], the initial immune response toward bacteria is characteristically dominated by DCs and other APCs; lamina propria macrophages also act as APC in the *H. pylori*-infected gastric mucosa [64]. Therefore, DC activation by *H. pylori* is essential for the development of an immune response [60], and stimulation/maturation of DCs are characteristically associated with the expression of bacterial epitopes on MHC on the surface together with costimulatory molecules [66]. *H. pylori* infection upregulates the expression of MHC class II antigens on gastric epithelium [67,68]; gastric epithelial cells may acquire APC properties in *H. pylori* infection by de novo expression of HLA-DR and costimulatory molecules [67]. Moreover, *H. pylori* induces DC activation, maturation as well as antigen presentation; its outer membrane proteins are capable of activating DCs, and DCs pulsed with *H. pylori* were shown to induce Th1 effector responses [60,65,66]. In this regard, *H. pylori* and its secreted products contribute to T-cell recruitment to the gastric mucosa and the responding TLs have an activated memory Th1 phenotype [61]. Therefore, *H. pylori*-

associated gastroduodenal pathologies can be regarded as a Th1-driven immunopathological response to a number of *H. pylori* antigens. Specifically (in *H. pylori*-related autoimmune gastritis), cytolytic TLs infiltrating the gastric mucosa cross-recognize different epitopes of *H. pylori* proteins and gastric H+/K+-ATPase autoantigen (a significant proportion of the CD4+ T cell clones proliferated in response to H+/K+-ATPase showing a Th1 profile) and this bacterium may lead to gastric autoimmunity via molecular mimicry [62,69]; activation of gastric H+/K+-ATPase-specific Th1 TLs is critical in the pathogenesis of gastric autoimmunity and atrophy in humans [69]. A predominant *H. pylori*-specific Th1 response is characterized by high TNF-α, interferon (IFN)-γ, IL-2 and IL-12 production [62,63] leading to gastric epithelial cell apoptotic damage. Several studies reported that the Fas/Fas ligand system is involved in *H. pylori*-induced apoptosis, and T cell-mediated cytotoxicity via Fas/Fas-L signaling may contribute to the induction of apoptosis in gastric epithelial cells in the context of *H. pylori* infection [62,63]. Inflammatory cytokines present during *H. pylori* infection, such as IFN-γ, enhance activation of the Fas signaling pathway in vitro [70]. In this regard, Fas and TNF-α-receptor type 1 (TNF-R1) expressed on gastric epithelial cells from *H. pylori*-infected patients are responsible for the accelerated cell apoptosis [71,72]; TNF-α induces apoptotic death of gastric parietal contributing to the atrophy and hypochlorhydria of the gastric mucosa noticed during chronic *H. pylori* infection [73]. Additional evidence indicates that *H. pylori* is capable of inducing apoptotic effects through the mitochondrial apoptotic pathway involved activation of the proapoptotic proteins Bax and Bak, activation of certain caspases or through inducible NO [74-79]; NO is a rapidly diffusing gas and a potent neurotoxin that may contribute to the apoptotic neuronal cell death in degenerative neuropathies, including AD [80] and glaucomatous optic neuropathy [81].

The above-mentioned data describe the evidence for the irregular cellular immune and apoptotic mechanisms playing an important role in the *H. pylori*-associated gastrointestinal pathologies and potentially affecting the neurodegenerative process in AD. In this respect, *H. pylori* infection induces cellular immune responses that, owing to the sharing of homologous epitopes (molecular mimicry), cross-react with components of nerves [52], thereby contributing to potential neural tissue damage in AD.

Comparable data to AD abnormalities of humoral immunity can also be considered for *H. pylori* infection. Indeed, gastric autoimmunity is well established in patients with *H. pylori* infection associated with induction of autoantibodies that cross-react with the gastric mucosa [82]. This type of autoreactivity is linked with the presence and degree of inflammation and atrophy of the glands [83]. Moreover, serum parietal cell autoantibodies correlate with anti-*H. pylori* antibody titers [84]. Therefore, the serological titer of anti-*H. pylori* seems to reflect the autoimmunity status that correlates with gastric mucosal atrophy, thereby indirectly offering evidence of the severity of histological inflammatory changes [85]. Interestingly, molecular mimicry of host structures by the saccharide portion of lipopolysaccharides of the gastrointestinal pathogens *Campylobacter jejuni* (*C. jejuni*) and *H. pylori* is thought to be connected with the development of autoimmune sequelae observed in neuropathies. *C. jejuni*, a principal cause of gastroenteritis, is the most common antecedent infection in Guillain-Barré syndrome, an inflammatory autoimmune neuropathy. Chemical analyses of the core oligosaccharides of neuropathy-associated *C. jejuni* strains have revealed structural homology with human gangliosides. Serum antibodies against gangliosides are found in one third of patients with Guillain-Barré syndrome, but are generally absent in enteritis cases. Collective data suggest that the antibodies are induced by antecedent infection with *C. jejuni*, and subsequently react with nerve tissue causing damage [86], possibly by apoptosis. In addition, several IgG antibodies against *H. pylori* proteins are found in the cerebrospinal fluid (CSF) in 57% of patients with Guillain-Barré syndrome. No cross reactivity against *C. jejuni* is observed and these antibodies may also be involved in the immune responses of patients with Guillain-Barré syndrome [87]. Similarly, 46% of patients with Guillain-Barré syndrome have specific IgG antibodies to VacA of *H. pylori* in the CSF, and the sequence homology found between VacA and human Na+/K+ ATPase A subunit suggests that antibodies to VacA involve ion channels in abaxonal Schwann cell plasmalemma resulting in demyelination in some patients within the CSF [88, 89]. In this regard, it is relevant to speculate that such anti-*H. pylori*–mediated apoptotic mechanisms might also lead to degeneration of ganglion cells, thereby contributing to AD neuropathy or other degenerative neuropathies such as achalasia [90] or glaucoma [41]. Support for this theory is provided by our recent observations indicating that the titer of anti-*H. pylori* IgG antibodies in the aqueous humor of patients with glaucoma may reflect the severity of glaucomatous damage [91]. Summarizing, the above-mentioned data describe the current evidence for abnormalities of humoral immunity playing a significant role in the *H. pylori*-associated gastric pathologies and potentially contributing to other degenerative neuropathies, including AD neuropathy.

C. Association of *H. Pylori* Infection with AD

Although degenerative diseases of the CNS, including AD, have an increasingly high impact in aged population, their association with *H. pylori* infection has not as yet been thoroughly researched. This issue has only recently been addressed by two studies [92,93]. A higher seropositivity for anti-*H. pylori* immunoglobulin (Ig) G antibodies was reported in 30 patients with AD than in age-matched controls [92]. However, this serological test has limitations because it does not discriminate between current and old infections [94]. Such a distinction is essential because current *H. pylori* infection, as mentioned, induces humoral and cellular immune responses that, owing to the sharing of homologous epitopes (molecular mimicry), cross-react with components of nerves [52], thereby affecting or perpetuating neural tissue damage. Moreover, eradication of *H. pylori* infection might delay AD progression, particularly at early disease stages.

Based on the histological analysis of gastric mucosa biopsy for the documentation of current *H. pylori* infection, we reported a higher rate of infection in AD patients compared to anemic controls [93]. It is thus reasonable to further investigate the role of *H. pylori* in AD initiation, progression or susceptibility by documenting its qualitative and quantitative presence in the CSF of these patients. We therefore investigated the presence of *H. pylori*-specific IgG antibodies in the CSF of patients with AD and compared their levels with those of age-matched controls to determine whether *H. pylori* plays a role in this disease.

MATERIALS AND METHODS

We prospectively investigated the presence of anti-*H. pylori*-specific IgG antibodies in CSF and serum samples obtained from 27 AD patients (group A). The control group consisted of 27 consecutive, age-matched, cognitively normal patients with prostate hyperplasia or long-bone fractures necessitating surgery after epidural anesthesia (Group B). All participants were enrolled consecutively between January 2005 and November 2006. Both groups were native Greek citizens living in Thessaloniki. They were of similar education and socioeconomic status, matched age and sex, and did not belong to high-risk professional groups such as nurses or physicians.

Patients fulfilled the NINCDS-ADRDA criteria for the diagnosis of AD [95]. All participants underwent a comprehensive neuropsychological examination including Mini-Mental State Examination (MMSE), Cambridge Cognitive Test (CAMCOG), Functional Rating Scale of the Severity of Dementia (FRSSD), Neuropsychological Inventory (NPI) and Geriatric Depression Scale (GDS). Inclusion of cognitively normal participants required MMSE score>24, CAMCOG score>85 and FRSSD score<5. Moreover, in addition to scores above cut-off in cognitive tests, subjective memory complaints should be absent for a participant in order to be regarded as cognitively normal.

Patients were excluded if they had taken H_2-receptor antagonists, proton pump inhibitors, antibiotics, bismuth compounds, or nonsteroidal anti-inflammatory drugs (excluding low doses of aspirin, i.e., 80 mg two to three times weekly) in the preceding 4 weeks. Patients were also excluded if they had undergone previous gastric surgery; were on anticoagulant therapy; were alcohol abusers; had allergy to penicillin and macrolides; had evidence of gastric cancer or other neoplasms; or had severe cardiac, pulmonary, kidney, or liver disease.

All patients and/or their relatives gave their informed consent and the study protocol was approved by the local ethics committee.

CSF samples 5 mL were obtained through lumbar puncture using a 24 gauge needle with special care to avoid blood contamination. The sample was transferred immediately and was stored in a freezer at $-70°C$ until assay for anti-*H. pylori* IgG antibody (within 20–25 days).

Anti-*H. pylori* IgG antibody levels in the serum were also determined in all AD patients and controls. For this purpose, blood samples were collected from the AD patients and on the day of surgery from controls; samples were centrifuged at 3,000 *g* for 10 min to obtain serum, then aliquoted and stored at $-70°C$ in the laboratory freezer until assay (within 20–25 days). This investigation included a total of 54 CSF and blood samples: 27 from AD patients and 27 from age-matched controls.

Anti-*H. Pylori* IgG Analysis

In the present study the concentrations of anti-*H. pylori* IgG in the CSF and the serum samples were measured with a commercial enzyme-linked immunosorbent assay (ELISA) kit (Enzywell DIESSE Diagnostica Senese, Siena, Italy). The *H. pylori* serological analysis status has already been described previously [51, 96]. The manufacturer's recommended cut-off value of 10 U/mL was used to define each patient's serological analysis as positive or negative.

The dilution of serum samples was 1:101 with sample buffer, whereas the dilution of CSF samples was 1:2 with sample buffer. In particular, 100 μL of the patient sample contained 50 μL of CSF diluted with the sample buffer (containing BSA and 0.09% (w/v) sodium azide). Intra-assay coefficient of variation (CV) was 4-8% and interassay CV was 10-12%.

The expected value in the CSF of the normal population is negative. However, in our laboratory, we have established our own normal range. The cut-off value to determine the *H. pylori*-positive cases in the CSF, according to the anti-*H. pylori*-specific IgG by measured ELISA was determined as follows: the mean of the corrected optical density (OD) values of the CSF samples (based on the negative ELISA assay in serum) was calculated and added to three times the standard deviation. Those CSF samples with an OD greater than the mean of negative CSF samples plus 3 standard deviations (SD) were considered to be positive, while those with an OD less than the mean of negative CSF samples plus 3 standard deviations were considered negative. According to this method, a cut-off value of 1.87 U/mL was established. Patients with a value less than 1.87 U/mL were considered as *H. pylori* negative [97].

Statistical Analysis

Clinical data and anti-*H. pylori* IgG titers in serum and CSF were expressed as mean ± SD. For comparisons of the age (years) of the patients versus controls, the nonparametric Mann–Whitney *U*-test was used, whereas for sex analysis, the two-tailed Fisher's exact test was applied. The latter test was also used to assess the difference in *H. pylori*-positive cases in serum and CSF between the groups. Anti-*H. pylori* IgG titers in serum and CSF were expressed as mean ± SD. Mann–Whitney *U*-test was applied to compare the anti-*H. pylori* IgG antibodies in CSF in groups A and B. Two independent samples' t-test was applied for the comparison of mean MMSE score between CSF anti-*H. pylori* IgG positive and negative cases. Significance was set at $p<0.05$.

RESULTS

Demographic, clinical data and levels of anti-*H. pylori* IgG antibodies in serum and in CSF are shown in table 1. There was no difference among the study groups in age and sex.

Table 1. Demographic, clinical data, and levels of anti-*Helicobacter pylori* (*Hp*) IgG antibodies in serum and in cerebrospinal fluid (CSF) (group A: Alzheimer's Disease patients; group B: cognitively normal controls; SD: standard deviation)

Characteristic	Group A (n=27)	Group B (n=27)	*p* value
Age (years): mean (± SD)	70.62±6.66	72.57±7.8	0.311
Sex (M:F)	12:15	19:8	0.098
Anti-*Hp* IgG, serum (mean ± SD) (U/mL)	30.44±33.94	16.24±5.77	0.041
Anti-Hp IgG, CSF (mean ± SD) (U/mL)	10.53±12.54	8.63±8.01	0.047

AD patients' performance in cognitive tests was as follows (mean score±SD): MMSE (18.03±6.56), CAMCOG (56.63±22.44), FRSSD (13.36±6.31), NPI (10.55±8.44), GDS (3.4±2.6). Controls' mean score in cognitive tests was 28.51±1.36 in MMSE and 1.74±1.63 in FRSSD. As expected, controls performed better than AD patients in MMSE ($p<0.001$) and FRSSD ($p<0.001$).

The mean concentration of anti-*H. pylori* IgG antibodies in the CSF of patients with AD was (10.53±12.54 U/mL), significantly higher than that observed in the CSF of age-matched control participants (8.63±8.01 U/mL; $p=0.047$).

As shown in table 2, the presence of anti-*H. pylori* IgG antibodies in the CSF of patients with AD was correlated with the degree of severity of the disease.

The mean concentration of anti-*H. pylori* IgG antibodies in the serum of patients with AD was 30.44±33.94 U/mL, significantly higher than that observed in the serum of age-matched control patients (16.24±5.77 U/mL; $p=0.041$).

Table 2. Mini-Mental State Examination (MMSE) score in Alzheimer's disease (AD) patients related to cerebrospinal fluid (CSF) anti-*Helicobacter pylori* IgG (>1.87 U/mL) positivity

MMSE	CSF Anti-*H. pylori* IgG >1.87 U/mL	CSF Anti-*H. pylori* IgG <1.87 U/mL	*p* value
Mean±SD	15.42±6.92	20.76±4.69	0.028
>20 (N=10)	2	8	0.018
<20 (N=17)	12	5	

DISCUSSION

The current series investigated for the first time the concentration of anti-*H. pylori* IgG antibodies in the CSF and serum of patients with AD and compared their levels with those of age-matched cognitively normal controls. Notably, the patients and control subjects were consecutive to eliminate the possibility of selection of groups, and if any bias in the selection may exist, this is universal for groups, thereby not affecting the results. The mean concentration of anti-*H. pylori* IgG in the CSF and serum of patients with AD was significantly greater than those found in the controls. Thus, the questions arising from these results are: what is the importance of the increased prevalence of *H. pylori* IgG antibodies in the CSF and serum of patients with AD and is there a role for this common infectious agent in the pathobiology of AD?

Apart from the cellular immune defective mechanisms playing an important role in the neurodegenerative process in AD [98], recent evidence also suggests that the possible presence of anti-neuronal antibodies and autoimmune mechanisms may be responsible for eliciting neuronal cell death in AD [43]. A key finding not only demonstrated the abnormal presence of anti-brain autoantibodies [99] and human Ig [43,100] in the brain parenchyma of AD tissues, but, most significantly, specific neurons that showed degenerative, apoptotic features contained these vascular-derived antibodies. In addition, subsequent studies detected classical complement components, C1q and C5b-9, in these Ig-positive neurons, which were also highly associated with reactive microglia over the Ig-negative neurons. It is possible that the mere presence of anti-neuronal autoantibodies in serum, whose importance had been previously dismissed, may be without pathological consequence (because of the "immunological privilege" of the brain, which excludes a direct access of Ig to the CNS under normal conditions) until there is a blood-brain barrier dysfunction to allow the deleterious effects of these autoantibodies access on their targets. These findings suggest autoimmunity-induced cell death in AD [43,100]. The evidence that autoantibodies may contribute to neuronal cell death in AD is also consistent with a wider literature in medicine implicating a causative role for autoantibodies in many peripheral neuropathies including Guillain-Barré syndrome [52] that shares pathogenetic similarities with AD, as well as glaucomatous optic neuropathy defined as "ocular AD"; the autoantibodies directed toward retinal antigens may be involved in facilitating apoptotic cell death in glaucoma patients [98,101].

The association between *H. pylori* infection and gastric autoimmunity is well established [102]. It is relevant to note that *H. pylori* infection is associated with the synthesis of parietal cell autoantibodies, that cross-react with the gastric mucosa and, after eradication of the infection, persist and contribute to recurrent antral chronic gastritis and intestinal metaplasia [52]. Moreover, serum parietal cell autoantibodies correlate with anti-*H. pylori* antibody titers [84]. Therefore, the serological titer of anti-*H. pylori* seems to reflect the autoimmunity status that correlates with gastric mucosal atrophy, thereby indirectly offering evidence of the severity of histologic inflammatory changes [85].

Importantly, patients with Guillain-Barré syndrome have the aforementioned specific IgG antibodies to VacA of *H. pylori* in the CSF, and the sequence homology found between VacA and human Na+/K+ ATPase A subunit suggests that antibodies to VacA involve ion channels in abaxonal Schwann cell plasmalemma resulting in the demyelination in some patients within the CSF [88].

Considering the above-mentioned data, it is possible to suggest that the increased titer of anti-*H. pylori* IgG antibodies observed in the CSF and serum samples of patients with AD may indirectly offer evidence for a role of this agent in the cascade events of neurodegenerative process in AD. A similar speculation also thought in glaucomatous optic neuropathy [52]. The most likely mechanism for the role of this organism is via molecular mimicry autoimmune sequelae. An interesting, although rather gross correlation, is the observation that the positivity status for *H. pylori* in the CSF appeared to correlate with the severity of clinical status in AD patients. Nevertheless, future studies in large AD cohorts throughout the clinical range and utilizing all AD parameters are needed to support the hypothesis that the presence of IgG antibodies to *H. pylori* may adversely influence progression of AD.

Notably, the possibility of the passive passage of IgG and antibodies through a normal blood-CSF barrier that might explain our findings should not be excluded. Moreover, theoretically, in case of advanced AD, with cerebral atrophy, the blood-CSF barrier might be frequently altered, with higher CSF protein content, and higher transudation of IgG and antibodies in the CSF, thereby again possibly explaining the correlation of the positivity status for *H. pylori* with the severity of clinical status in our AD patients. However, this consideration seems to be unlikely, because blood-brain barrier dysfunction is found early in the disease before the onset of clinical dementia [103], and moreover, the permeability of the blood-CSF barrier is not correlated to measures of dementia severity [104].

In this regard, some limitations of the present study may include the relatively small number of patients, and that the CSF antibody titers were not normalized to another protein to serve as control, such as IgG or albumin.

It is tempting to speculate that *H. pylori* infection may negatively influence the neurodegerative process in AD. Amongst the possible mechanisms involved may be molecular mimicry-related toxicity by *H. pylori* autoantibodies and various *H. pylori* toxic antigens to endothelium and neuron proteins, release in the circulation of *H. pylori*-related vasoactive substances, or increased susceptibility of neurons to *H. pylori* various substances. These hypotheses require future validation. In theory, *H. pylori* antibodies may circulate in the blood stream and enter the CSF via the blood-CSF barrier where they may reach a level sufficient to impact the development or progression of AD.

Extending our findings, we investigated 63 consecutive patients with amnestic mild cognitive impairment (MCI) and 35 anemic controls underwent upper gastrointestinal endoscopy, histologic and serological examinations [105]. The prevalence of *H. pylori* infection was 88.9% in MCI patients and 48.6% in controls, as confirmed by biopsy ($P<0.001$, odds ratio: 8.47, 95%CI: 3.03-23.67). Mean serum anti-*H. pylori* IgG concentration and plasma total homocysteine (Hcy) titer were also higher in MCI patients than controls. When compared with the anemic participants, MCI patients exhibited more often histologic multifocal (body and antral) gastritis. Interestingly, the positivity status for *H. pylori* serology appeared to correlate with cognitive deterioration in our *H. pylori* positive MCI patients [105]. Chronic gastritis, as a result of *H. pylori* infection, can lead to malabsorption of vitamins (B_{12}) and folate, which results in failure of methylation by 5-methyl-tetrahydrofolic acid and hence accumulation of Hcy [98]. The elevated Hcy, in turn, could trigger endothelial damage and result in atherothrombotic disorders and AD. In this respect, investigators reported that *H. pylori*–induced chronic atrophic gastritis or atrophic gastritis *per se* decreases serum vitamin B_{12} and folate concentrations, thereby increasing the Hcy, a potent contributor to vascular disorders; serum Hcy concentrations correlate inversely with serum vitamin B_{12} and folate levels and positively with atrophic scores [98]. Hcy appears to be an independent risk factor not only for dementia and AD, but also for vascular disease. It is thought to be implicated in endothelial damage and neurodegeneration via oxidative injury in these diseases [98]; oxidative damage has also been described in the brain of subjects MCI, suggesting that oxidative damage may be one of the earliest events in the onset and progression of AD. It has been shown that the serum Hcy concentration correlates with the severity of dementia, and it is a significant predictor of the severity of dementia [98]. From another interesting point, *H. pylori* infection is actually associated with vitamin B_{12}- and/or iron deficiency anemia, whereas eradication of *H. pylori* infection is associated with reversal of vitamin B_{12}- and/or iron deficiency and improvement of anemia [51].

Considering the above-mentioned data, we can speculate that *H. pylori* infection might contribute, at least in part, to the pathogenesis of MCI and AD through induction of chronic atrophic gastritis, vitamin B_{12}-folate deficiency and Hcy sequence [106].

CLOSING COMMENTS

Our data suggest that AD and MCI appear to have an infectious link related to *H. pylori* involved in the pathophysiology of these disease. *H. pylori* infection may influence the pathophysiology of MCI-AD sequence by:

1) promoting platelet and platelet–leukocyte aggregation, also proposed to play pathophysiologic roles in AD development [98,105]; platelets are a source of the major constituent of senile plaques Abeta, considered to be the primary and central event in the etiology and pathogenesis of AD or MCI [107], and both increased platelet activation and increased circulating Abeta have been identified in AD. Moreover, Abeta role may be to inflict vascular damage and hence, impair blood-brain barrier function; increased blood-brain barrier permeability, increased platelet aggregation and cerebral vasoconstriction predispose the AD brain to thrombotic and/or ischemic events [43,108,109];

2) releasing proinflammatory and vasoactive substances, such as cytokines (IL-1, IL-6, IL-8, IL-10, IL-12, TNF-α, IFN-γ), eicosanoids (leukotrienes, prostaglandins catalyzed by cyclo-oxygenase enzymes), and acute phase proteins (fibrinogen, C-reactive protein) [51,110] involved in a number of vascular disorders including MCI, AD [28,111-117] and other AD-related neuropathies such as glaucoma [98,105,118];

3) stimulating mononuclear cells to produce a tissue factor-like procoagulant that converts fibrinogen into fibrin [98];

4) causing the development of cross mimicry between endothelial and *H. pylori* antigens;

5) increasing the aforementioned Hcy, implicated in endothelial damage and neurodegeneration via oxidative injury in these neurodegenerative diseases [98];

6) producing reactive oxygen metabolites (ROMs) and circulating lipid peroxides also involved in the pathophysiology of AD [98]; accumulating evidence suggests that ROMs are potent deleterious agents causing cell death or other forms of irreversible cell damage, and oxidative stress in the neuronal loss in AD and MCI [119,120]. ROMs accumulation impairs endothelial barrier function and promotes leukocyte adhesion, induces alterations in normal vascular function and results in the development of AD [121], events that are also triggered in *H. pylori*-induced gastrointestinal injury [122]. Moreover, there is evidence for a role of oxidative damage in contributing to Abeta deposition in AD [123]; and

7)　　　　　　　　influencing the apoptotic process, an important form of cell death in many neurodegenerative diseases including AD, possibly MCI [98] or Down syndrome that predisposes to the early onset of the neurodegeneration of AD [113]. In particular, increased endothelin-1 (a potent constrictor of arterioles and venules), NO, and inducible nitric oxide synthase (iNOS) levels are associated with *H. pylori* infection [124,125]. Relative data in AD indicate that endothelin-1-like immunoreactivity in the AD brains is significantly increased in frontal and occipital cortex than those in the control brains thereby explaining the decreased cerebral blood flow in AD patients [126]. The immunoreactive cells are often located in small clusters close to blood vessels [127] and Abeta peptides potentiate endothelin-1 induced vasoconstriction [128]. Besides, recent evidence in humans indicates that the expression of nitrergic system, the synthesis of NO, the peroxynitrite reactive production and the protein tyrosine nitration are activated over the entire chronic course of AD, and that the presence of Abeta increases the presence of neuronal nitric oxide synthase (nNOS) and iNOS isoforms over the chronic course of AD in pyramidal-like neurons [80]; the overproduction of NO, the increase in both peroxynitrite and superoxide production, the mitochondrial membrane depolarization and the caspase activation contribute to neuronal death [80,119], mainly via apoptosis. Further supporting this concern, it has been shown that endothelin-1-induced vasoconstriction of the anterior optic nerve vessels and NO modulation of vascular tone in the ophthalmic artery may produce glaucomatous damage [129]. Notably, *H. pylori* is capable of inducing apoptotic effects through the mitochondrial apoptotic pathway involving activation of the proapoptotic proteins Bax and Bak, activation of certain caspases or through inducible NO [98]; NO as a rapidly diffusing gas and neurotoxin may facilitate retinal ganglion cells apoptosis in glaucomatous optic [81] and probably AD neuropathy [80]. Support for the consideration of NO neurotoxicity in glaucoma is provided by experimental evidence demonstrating that retinal ganglion cell apoptosis is attenuated by selective inhibitors of iNOS or neutralizing antibodies against TNF-α, thereby suggesting that inhibition of the inducible isoform NOS2 or TNF-α may provide novel therapeutic targets for neuroprotection in the treatment of glaucomatous optic neuropathy [80]; because, TNF-α induces apoptotic neuronal cell death in neurodegenerative diseases including AD or possibly MCI [26,29,129,130], further studies are needed to clarify if comparable inhibitions of TNF-α may also provide novel therapeutic targets for neuroprotection in the treatment of AD or MCI.

REFERENCES

[1]   Ferri CP, Prince M, Brayne C, et al. Global prevalence of dementia: a Delphi consensus study. *Lancet,* 2005 366, 2112-2117.

[2]   Blasko I, Grubeck-Loebenstein B. Role of the immune system in the pathogenesis, prevention and treatment of Alzheimer's disease. *Drugs Aging,* 2003 20, 101-113.

[3]   Aisen PS. The development of anti-amyloid therapy for Alzheimer's disease: from secretase modulators to polymerisation inhibitors. *CNS Drugs,* 2005 19, 989-996.

[4]   Buttini M, Masliah E, Barbour R, et al. Beta-amyloid immunotherapy prevents synaptic degeneration in a mouse model of Alzheimer's disease. *J. Neurosci,* 2005 25, 9096-9101.

[5]   Town T, Nikolic V, Tan J. The microglial "activation" continuum: from innate to adaptive responses. *J. Neuroinflammation,* 2005 2, 24.

[6]   Malm TM, Koistinaho M, Parepalo M, et al. Bone-marrow-derived cells contribute to the recruitment of microglial cells in response to beta-amyloid deposition in APP/PS1 double transgenic Alzheimer mice. *Neurobiol. Dis,* 2005 18, 134-142.

[7]   Blasko I, Grubeck-Loebenstein B. Role of the immune system in the pathogenesis, prevention and treatment of Alzheimer's disease. *Drugs Aging,* 2003 20, 101-113.

[8]   Rogers J, Lue LF. Microglial chemotaxis, activation, and phagocytosis of amyloid β-peptide as linked phenomena in Alzheimer's disease. *Neurochem. Int,* 2001 39, 333-340.

[9]   Hashioka S, Monji A, Ueda T, Kanba S, Nakanishi H. Amyloid-beta fibril formation is not necessarily required for microglial activation by the peptides. *Neurochem. Int,* 2005 47, 369-376.

[10] Tuppo EE, Arias HR. The role of inflammation in Alzheimer's disease. *Int. J. Biochem. Cell. Biol,* 2005 37, 289-305.

[11] Singh VK. Immune-activation model in Alzheimer disease. *Mol. Chem. Neuropathol,* 1996 28, 105-111.

[12] Mrak RE, Griffin WS. Glia and their cytokines in progression of neurodegeneration. *Neurobiol. Aging,* 2005 26, 349-354.

[13] Singh VK. Neuroautoimmunity: pathogenic implications for Alzheimer's disease. *Gerontology,* 1997 43, 79-94.

[14] Aarli JA. Role of cytokines in neurological disorders. *Curr. Med. Chem,* 2003 10, 1931-1937.

[15] Iribarren P, Cui YH, Le Y, Wang JM. The role of dendritic cells in neurodegenerative diseases. *Arch. Immunol. Ther. Exp. (Warsz),* 2002 50, 187-196.

[16] Minagar A, Shapshak P, Fujimura R, et al. The role of macrophage/microglia and astrocytes in the pathogenesis of three neurologic disorders: HIV-associated dementia, Alzheimer disease, and multiple sclerosis. *J. Neurol. Sci,* 2002 202, 13-23.

[17] Akiyama H, Barger S, Barnum S, et al. Inflammation and Alzheimer's disease. *Neurobiol. Aging,* 2000 21, 383–421.

[18] Nelson PT, Soma LA, Lavi E. Microglia in diseases of the central nervous system. *Ann. Med,* 2002 34, 491-500.

[19] Gordon MN. Microglia and immune activation in Alzheimer's disease. *J. Fla. Med. Assoc,* 1993 80, 267-270.

[20] Ulvestad E, Williams K, Bjerkvig R, et al. Human microglial cells have phenotypic and functional characteristics in common with both macrophages and dendritic antigen-presenting cells. *J. Leukoc. Biol,* 1994 56, 732-740.

[21] McGeer PL, Itagaki S, Tago H, McGeer EG. Reactive microglia in patients with senile dementia of the Alzheimer type are positive for the histocompatibility glycoprotein HLA-DR. *Neurosci. Lett,* 1987 79, 195-200.

[22] Williams K Jr, Ulvestad E, Cragg L, et al. Induction of primary T cell responses by human glial cells. *J. Neurosci. Res,* 1993 36, 382-390.

[23] Takuma K, Yan SS, Stern DM, Yamada K. Mitochondrial dysfunction, endoplasmic reticulum stress, and apoptosis in Alzheimer's disease. *J. Pharmacol. Sci,* 2005 97, 312-316.

[24] LeBlanc AC. The role of apoptotic pathways in Alzheimer's disease neurodegeneration and cell death. *Curr. Alzheimer Res,* 2005 2, 389-402.

[25] Chong ZZ, Li F, Maiese K. Stress in the brain: novel cellular mechanisms of injury linked to Alzheimer's disease. *Brain Res. Brain Res. Rev,* 2005 49, 1-21.

[26] Huang Y, Erdmann N, Peng H, et al. The role of TNF related apoptosis-inducing ligand in neurodegenerative diseases. *Cell. Mol. Immunol,* 2005 2, 113-122.

[27] Giuliani F, Hader W, Yong VW. Minocycline attenuates T cell and microglia activity to impair cytokine production in T cell-microglia interaction. *J. Leukoc. Biol,* 2005 78, 135-143.

[28] Lee EO, Shin YJ, Chong YH. Mechanisms involved in prostaglandin E2-mediated neuroprotection against TNF-alpha: possible involvement of multiple signal transduction and beta-catenin/T-cell factor. *J. Neuroimmunol,* 2004 155, 21-31.

[29] Zhao M, Cribbs DH, Anderson AJ, et al. The induction of the TNFalpha death domain signaling pathway in Alzheimer's disease brain. *Neurochem. Res,* 2003 28, 307-318.

[30] Su JH, Anderson AJ, Cribbs DH, et al. Fas and Fas ligand are associated with neuritic degeneration in the Alzheimer's disease brain and participate in beta-amyloid-induced neuronal death. *Neurobiol. Dis,* 2003 12, 182-193.

[31] Lombardi VR, Fernandez-Novoa L, Etcheverria I, et al. Association between APOE epsilon4 allele and increased expression of CD95 on T cells from patients with Alzheimer's disease. *Methods Find Exp. Clin. Pharmacol,* 2004 26, 523-529.

[32] Ethell DW, Buhler LA. Fas ligand-mediated apoptosis in degenerative disorders of the brain. *J. Clin. Immunol,* 2003 23, 439-446.

[33] Morishima Y, Gotoh Y, Zieg J, et al. Beta-amyloid induces neuronal apoptosis via a mechanism that involves the c-Jun N-terminal kinase pathway and the induction of Fas ligand. *J. Neurosci,* 2001 21, 7551-7560.

[34] Yao M, Nguyen TV, Pike CJ. Beta-amyloid-induced neuronal apoptosis involves c-Jun N-terminal kinase-dependent downregulation of Bcl-w. *J. Neurosci,* 2005 25, 1149-1158.

[35] Marx F, Blasko I, Grubeck-Loebenstein B. Mechanisms of immune regulation in Alzheimer's disease: a viewpoint. *Arch Immunol Ther Exp (Warsz),* 1999 47, 205-209.

[36] Monsonego A, Weiner HL. Immunotherapeutic approaches to Alzheimer's disease. *Science,* 2003 302, 834-838.

[37] Tatton WG, Chalmers-Redman RM, Ju WY, et al. transcription. Apoptosis in neurodegenerative disorders: potential for therapy by modifying gene. *J. Neural Transm. Suppl,* 1997 49, 245-268.

[38] Siao CJ, Tsirka SE. Extracellular proteases and neuronal cell death. Extracellular proteases and neuronal cell death. *Cell. Mol. Biol. (Noisy-le-grand),* 2002 48, 151-161.

[39] Bayer AU, Keller ON, Ferrari F, Maag KP. Association of glaucoma with neurodegenerative diseases with apoptotic cell death: Alzheimer's disease and Parkinson's disease. *Am. J. Ophthalmol,* 2002 133, 135-137.

[40] McKinnon SJ. Glaucoma: ocular Alzheimer's disease? *Front. Biosci,* 2003 8, s1140-s1156.

[41] Kountouras J, Zavos C, Chatzopoulos D. Induction of apoptosis as a proposed pathophysiological link between glaucoma and *Helicobacter pylori* infection. *Med. Hypotheses,* 2004 62, 378-381.

[42] Okuda Y, Apatoff BR, Posnett DN. Apoptosis of T cells in peripheral blood and cerebrospinal fluid is associated with disease activity of multiple sclerosis. *J. Neuroimmunol,* 2006 171, 163-170.

[43] D'Andrea MR. Add Alzheimer's disease to the list of autoimmune diseases. *Med. Hypotheses,* 2005 64, 458-463.

[44] Kinoshita J. Pathogens as a cause of Alzheimer's disease. *Neurobiol. Aging,* 2004 25, 639-640.

[45] Itzhaki RF, Wozniak MA, Appelt DM, Balin BJ. Infiltration of the brain by pathogens causes Alzheimer's disease. *Neurobiol. Aging,* 2004 25, 619-627.

[46] Robinson SR, Dobson C, Lyons J. Challenges and directions for the pathogen hypothesis of Alzheimer's disease. *Neurobiol. Aging,* 2004 25, 629-637.

[47] NIH Consensus Conference. *Helicobacter pylori* in peptic ulcer disease. NIH Consensus Development Panel on *Helicobacter pylori* in Peptic Ulcer Disease. *JAMA,* 1994 272, 65-69.

[48] Blaser MJ. *Helicobacter pylori* and the pathogenesis of gastroduodenal inflammation. *J. Infect. Dis,* 1990 161, 626-633.

[49] Mendall MA, Goggin PM, Molineaux N, et al. Relation of *Helicobacter pylori* infection and coronary heart disease. *Br. Heart J,* 1994 71, 437-439.

[50] McColl KE. What remaining questions regarding *Helicobacter pylori* and associated diseases should be addressed by future research? View from Europe. *Gastroenterology,* 1997 113, s158-s162.

[51] Kountouras J, Mylopoulos N, Chatzopoulos D, et al. Eradication of *Helicobacter pylori* may be beneficial in the management of chronic open-angle glaucoma. *Arch. Intern. Med,* 2002 162, 1237-1244.

[52] Kountouras J, Deretzi G, Zavos C, et al. Association between *Helicobacter pylori* infection and acute inflammatory demyelinating polyradiculoneuropathy. *Eur. J. Neurol.* 2005 12, 139-143.

[53] Xu Q, Schett G, Perschinka H, et al. Serum soluble heat shock protein 60 is elevated in subjects with atherosclerosis in a general population. *Circulation,* 2000 102, 14-20.

[54] Sawayama Y, Ariyama I, Hamada M, et al. Association between chronic *Helicobacter pylori* infection and acute ischemic stroke: Fukuoka Harasanshin Atherosclerosis Trial (FHAT). *Atherosclerosis,* 2005 178, 303-309.

[55] De la Torre JC, Stefano GB. Evidence that Alzheimer's disease is a microvascular disorder: the role of constitutive nitric oxide. *Brain Res. Brain Res. Rev,* 2000 34, 119-136.

[56] Hofman A, Ott A, Breteler MM, et al. Atherosclerosis, apolipoprotein E, and prevalence of dementia and Alzheimer's disease in the Rotterdam Study. *Lancet,* 1997 349, 151-154.

[57] Mecocci P, Parnetti L, Reboldi GP, et al. Blood-brain-barrier in a geriatric population: barrier function in degenerative and vascular dementias. *Acta Neurol. Scand,* 1991 84, 210-213.

[58] Wardlaw JM, Sandercock PA, Dennis MS, Starr J. Is breakdown of the blood-brain barrier responsible for lacunar stroke, leukoaraiosis, and dementia? *Stroke,* 2003 34, 806-812.

[59] Pasquier F, Leys D. Why are stroke patients prone to develop dementia? *J. Neurol,* 1997 244, 135-142.

[60] Kranzer K, Sollner L, Aigner M, et al. Impact of *Helicobacter pylori* virulence factors and compounds on activation and maturation of human dendritic cells. *Infect Immun,* 2005 73, 4180-4189.

[61] Enarsson K, Brisslert M, Backert S, Quiding-Jarbrink M. *Helicobacter pylori* induces transendothelial migration of activated memory T cells. *Infect. Immun,* 2005 73, 761-769.

[62] D'Elios MM, Amedei A, Benagiano M, et al. *Helicobacter pylori*, T cells and cytokines: the "dangerous liaisons". *FEMS Immunol Med. Microbiol.* 2005 44, 113-119.

[63] Hafsi N, Voland P, Schwendy S, et al. Human dendritic cells respond to *Helicobacter pylori*, promoting NK cell and Th1-effector responses in vitro. *J. Immunol,* 2004 173, 1249-1257.

[64] Suzuki T, Kato K, Ohara S, et al. Localization of antigen-presenting cells in *Helicobacter pylori*-infected gastric mucosa. *Pathol. Int,* 2002 52, 265-271.

[65] Rathinavelu S, Kao JY, Zavros Y, Merchant JL. *Helicobacter pylori* outer membrane protein 18 (Hp1125) induces dendritic cell maturation and function. *Helicobacter,* 2005 10, 424-432.

[66] Voland P, Hafsi N, Zeitner M, et al. Antigenic properties of HpaA and Omp18, two outer membrane proteins of *Helicobacter pylori. Infect. Immun,* 2003 71, 3837-3843.

[67] Archimandritis A, Sougioultzis S, Foukas PG, et al. Expression of HLA-DR, costimulatory molecules B7-1, B7-2, intercellular adhesion molecule-1 (ICAM-1) and Fas ligand (FasL) on gastric epithelial cells in *Helicobacter pylori* gastritis; influence of *H. pylori* eradication. *Clin. Exp. Immunol,* 2000 119, 464-467.

[68] Krauss-Etschmann S, Gruber R, Plikat K, Antoni I, et al. Increase of antigen-presenting cells in the gastric mucosa of *Helicobacter pylori*-infected children. *Helicobacter,* 2005 10, 214-222.

[69] D'Elios MM, Amedei A, Azzurri A, et al. Molecular specificity and functional properties of autoreactive T-cell response in human gastric autoimmunity. *Int. Rev. Immunol,* 2005 24, 111-122.

[70] Jones NL, Day AS, Jennings H, et al. Enhanced disease severity in *Helicobacter pylori*-infected mice deficient in Fas signaling. *Infect. Immun,* 2002 70, 2591-2597.

[71] Hasumi K, Tanaka K, Saitoh S, et al. Roles of tumor necrosis factor-alpha-receptor type 1 and Fas in the *Helicobacter pylori*-induced apoptosis of gastric epithelial cells. *J. Gastroenterol. Hepatol,* 2002 17, 651-658.

[72] Wu YY, Tsai HF, Lin WC, et al. *Helicobacter pylori* enhances tumor necrosis factor-related apoptosis-inducing ligand-mediated apoptosis in human gastric epithelial cells. *World J. Gastroenterol,* 2004 10, 2334-2339.

[73] Neu B, Puschmann AJ, Mayerhofer A, et al. TNF-alpha induces apoptosis of parietal cells. *Biochem. Pharmacol,* 2003 65, 1755-1760.

[74] Watanabe S, Takagi A, Koga Y, et al. *Helicobacter pylori* induces apoptosis in gastric epithelial cells through inducible nitric oxide. *J. Gastroenterol. Hepatol,* 2000 15, 168-174.

[75] Potthoff A, Ledig S, Martin J, et al. Significance of the caspase family in *Helicobacter pylori* induced gastric epithelial apoptosis. *Helicobacter,* 2002 7, 367-777.

[76] Maeda S, Yoshida H, Mitsuno Y, et al. Analysis of apoptotic and antiapoptotic signalling pathways induced by *Helicobacter pylori. Gut,* 2002 50, 771-778.

[77] Chang CS, Chen WN, Lin HH, et al. Increased oxidative DNA damage, inducible nitric oxide synthase, nuclear factor kappaB expression and enhanced antiapoptosis-related proteins in *Helicobacter pylori*-infected non-cardiac gastric adenocarcinoma. *World J. Gastroenterol,* 2004 10, 2232-2240.

[78] Liu HF, Liu WW, Wang GA, Teng XC. Effect of *Helicobacter pylori* infection on Bax protein expression in patients with gastric precancerous lesions. *World J. Gastroenterol,* 2005 11, 5899-5901.

[79] Yamasaki E, Wada A, Kumatori A, et al. *Helicobacter pylori* vacuolating cytotoxin induces activation of the proapoptotic protein Bax and Bak, leading to cytochrome c release and cell death, independent of vacuolation. *J. Biol. Chem,* 2006 281, 11250-11259.

[80] Fernandez-Vizarra P, Fernandez AP, Castro-Blanco S, et al. Expression of nitric oxide system in clinically evaluated cases of Alzheimer's disease. *Neurobiol. Dis,* 2004 15, 287-305.

[81] Tezel G, Wax MB. The mechanisms of hsp27 antibody-mediated apoptosis in retinal neuronal cells. *J. Neurosci,* 2000 20, 3552-3562.

[82] Vorobjova T, Faller G, Maaroos HI, et al. Significant increase in antigastric autoantibodies in a long-term follow-up study of *H. pylori* gastritis. *Virchows Arch,* 2000 437, 37-45.

[83] Negrini R, Savio A, Poiesi C, et al. Antigenic mimicry between *Helicobacter pylori* and gastric mucosa in the pathogenesis of body atrophic gastritis. *Gastroenterology,* 1996 111, 655-665.

[84] Basso D, Gallo N, Zambon CF, et al. Antigastric autoantibodies in *Helicobacter pylori* infection: role in gastric mucosal inflammation. *Int. J. Clin. Lab. Res,* 2000 30, 173-178.

[85] Sheu BS, Shiesh SC, Yang HB, et al. Implications of *Helicobacter pylori* serological titer for the histological severity of antral gastritis. *Endoscopy,* 1997 29, 27-30.

[86] Moran AP, Prendergast MM. Molecular mimicry in *Campylobacter jejuni* and *Helicobacter pylori* lipopolysaccharides: contribution of gastrointestinal infections to autoimmunity. *J. Autoimmun,* 2001 16, 241-256.

[87] Chiba S, Sugiyama T, Matsumoto H, et al. Antibodies against *Helicobacter pylori* were detected in the cerebrospinal fluid obtained from patients with Guillain-Barre syndrome. *Ann. Neurol,* 1998 44, 686-688.

[88] Chiba S, Sugiyama T, Yonekura K, et al. An antibody to VacA of *Helicobacter pylori* in cerebrospinal fluid from patients with Guillain-Barre syndrome. *J. Neurol. Neurosurg. Psychiatry,* 2002 73, 76-78.

[89] Gavalas E, Kountouras J, Deretzi G, et al. *Helicobacter pylori* and multiple sclerosis. *J. Neuroimmunol,* 2007 188, 187-189.

[90] Kountouras J, Zavos C, Chatzopoulos D. Apoptosis and autoimmunity as proposed pathogenetic links between *Helicobacter pylori* infection and idiopathic achalasia. *Med. Hypotheses,* 2004 63, 624-629.

[91] Kountouras J, Mylopoulos N, Konstas AG, et al. Increased levels of *Helicobacter pylori* IgG antibodies in aqueous humor of patients with primary open-angle and exfoliation glaucoma. *Graefes Arch. Clin. Exp. Ophthalmol,* 2003 241, 884-890.

[92] Malaguarnera M, Bella R, Alagona G, et al. *Helicobacter pylori* and Alzheimer's disease: a possible link. *Eur. J. Intern. Med,* 2004 15, 381-386.

[93] Kountouras J, Tsolaki M, Gavalas E, et al. Relationship between *Helicobacter pylori* and Alzheimer disease. *Neurology,* 2006 66, 938-940.

[94] Fennerty MB. Helicobacter pylori. Arch. Intern. Med, 1994 154, 721-727.

[95] McKhann G, Drachman D, Folstein M, et al. Clinical diagnosis of Alzheimer's disease: report of the NINCDS-ADRDA Work Group under the auspices of Department of Health and Human Services Task Force on Alzheimer's Disease. *Neurology,* 1984 34, 939-944.

[96] Kountouras J, Mylopoulos N, Boura P, et al. Relationship between *Helicobacter pylori* infection and glaucoma. *Ophthalmology*, 2001 108, 599-604.

[97] Mitchell HM, Mascord K, Hazell SL, Daskalopoulos G. Association between the IgG subclass response, inflammation and disease status in *Helicobacter pylori* infection. *Scand. J. Gastroenterol*, 2001 36, 149-155.

[98] Kountouras J, Gavalas E, Zavos C, et al. Alzheimer's disease and *Helicobacter pylori* infection: defective immune regulation and apoptosis as proposed common links. *Med. Hypotheses*, 2007 68, 378-388.

[99] Fernandez-Shaw C, Marina A, Cazorla P, et al. Anti-brain spectrin immunoreactivity in Alzheimer's disease: degradation of spectrin in an animal model of cholinergic degeneration. *J. Neuroimmunol*, 1997 77, 91-98.

[100] Bouras C, Riederer BM, Kovari E, et al. Humoral immunity in brain aging and Alzheimer's disease. *Brain Res. Brain Res. Rev,* 2005 48, 477-487.

[101] Maruyama I, Nakazawa M, Ohguro H. [Autoimmune mechanisms in molecular pathology of glaucomatous optic neuropathy]. *Nippon Ganka Gakkai Zasshi,* 2001 105, 205-212.

[102] Parente F, Negrini R, Imbesi V, et al. Presence of gastric autoantibodies impairs gastric secretory function in patients with *Helicobacter pylori*-positive duodenal ulcer. *Scand. J. Gastroenterol,* 2001 36, 474-478.

[103] Skoog I, Wallin A, Fredman P, et al. A population study on blood-brain barrier function in 85-year-olds: relation to Alzheimer's disease and vascular dementia. *Neurology*, 1998 50, 966-971.

[104] Hampel H, Kotter HU, Moller HJ. Blood-cerebrospinal fluid barrier dysfunction for high molecular weight proteins in Alzheimer disease and major depression: indication for disease subsets. *Alzheimer Dis. Assoc. Disord,* 1997 11, 78-87.

[105] Kountouras J, Tsolaki M, Boziki M, et al. Association between *Helicobacter pylori* infection and mild cognitive impairment. *Eur. J. Neurol,* 2007 14, 976-982.

[106] Kountouras J, Gavalas E, Boziki M, Zavos C. *Helicobacter pylori* may be involved in cognitive impairment and dementia development through induction of atrophic gastritis, vitamin B12-folate deficiency, and hyperhomocysteine sequence. *Am. J. Clin. Nutr,* 2007 86, 805-809.

[107] Pike KE, Savage G, Villemagne VL, et al. Beta-amyloid imaging and memory in non-demented individuals: evidence for preclinical Alzheimer's disease. *Brain,* 2007 130, 2837-2844.

[108] Hasitz M, Racz Z, Nagy A, Lipcsey A. Importance of platelet functions in Alzheimer's disease. *Arch. Gerontol. Geriatr,* 1995 21, 53-61.

[109] Halliday G, Robinson SR, Shepherd C, Kril J. Alzheimer's disease and inflammation: a review of cellular and therapeutic mechanisms. *Clin. Exp. Pharmacol. Physiol,* 2000 27, 1-8.

[110] Kountouras J, Zavos C, Chatzopoulos D. A concept on the role of *Helicobacter pylori* infection in autoimmune pancreatitis. *J. Cell Mol. Med,* 2005 9, 196-207.

[111] Cacquevel M, Lebeurrier N, Cheenne S, Vivien D. Cytokines in neuroinflammation and Alzheimer's disease. *Curr. Drug Targets,* 2004 5, 529-534.

[112] Finch CE. Developmental origins of aging in brain and blood vessels: an overview. *Neurobiol. Aging,* 2005 26, 281-291.

[113] Hallam DM, Capps NL, Travelstead AL, et al. Evidence for an interferon-related inflammatory reaction in the trisomy 16 mouse brain leading to caspase-1-mediated neuronal apoptosis. *J. Neuroimmunol,* 2000 110, 66-75.

[114] Ma SL, Tang NL, Lam LC, Chiu HF. The association between promoter polymorphism of the interleukin-10 gene and Alzheimer's disease. *Neurobiol. Aging,* 2005 26, 1005-1010.

[115] Sugaya K, Uz T, Kumar V, Manev H. New anti-inflammatory treatment strategy in Alzheimer's disease. *Jpn. J. Pharmacol,* 2000 82, 85-94.

[116] Xia M, Qin S, McNamara M, et al. Interleukin-8 receptor B immunoreactivity in brain and neuritic plaques of Alzheimer's disease. *Am. J. Pathol,* 1997 150, 1267-1274.

[117] Singh VK, Guthikonda P. Circulating cytokines in Alzheimer's disease. *J. Psychiatr. Res,* 1997 31, 657-660.

[118] Kountouras J, Zavos C, Chatzopoulos D. Primary open-angle glaucoma: pathophysiology and treatment. *Lancet,* 2004 364, 1311-1312.

[119] Kawamoto EM, Munhoz CD, Glezer I, et al. Oxidative state in platelets and erythrocytes in aging and Alzheimer's disease. *Neurobiol. Aging,* 2005 26, 857-864.

[120] Butterfield DA, Sultana R. Redox proteomics identification of oxidatively modified brain proteins in Alzheimer's disease and mild cognitive impairment: insights into the progression of this dementing disorder. *J. Alzheimers Dis,* 2007 12, 61-72.

[121] Aliyev A, Chen SG, Seyidova D, et al. Mitochondria DNA deletions in atherosclerotic hypoperfused brain microvessels as a primary target for the development of Alzheimer's disease. *J. Neurol. Sci,* 2005 229-230, 285-292.

[122] Kountouras J, Chatzopoulos D, Zavos C. Reactive oxygen metabolites and upper gastrointestinal diseases. *Hepatogastroenterology,* 2001 48, 743-751.

[123] Beal MF. Mitochondrial dysfunction and oxidative damage in Alzheimer's and Parkinson's diseases and coenzyme Q10 as a potential treatment. *J. Bioenerg. Biomembr,* 2004 36, 381-386.

[124] Akimoto M, Hashimoto H, Shigemoto M, Yokoyama I. Relationship between recurrence of gastric ulcer and the microcirculation. *J. Cardiovasc. Pharmacol,* 1998 31, s507-s508.

[125] Slomiany BL, Piotrowski J, Slomiany A. Up-regulation of endothelin-converting enzyme-1 in gastric mucosal inflammatory responses to *Helicobacter pylori* lipopolysaccharide. *Biochem. Biophys. Res. Commun,* 2000 267, 801-805.

[126] Minami M, Kimura M, Iwamoto N, Arai H. Endothelin-1-like immunoreactivity in cerebral cortex of Alzheimer-type dementia. *Prog. Neuropsychopharmacol. Biol. Psychiatry,* 1995 19, 509-513.

[127] Zhang WW, Badonic T, Hoog A, et al. Astrocytes in Alzheimer's disease express immunoreactivity to the vaso-constrictor endothelin-1. *J. Neurol. Sci,* 1994 122, 90-96.

[128] Shin YJ, Chong YH. Mechanisms involved in prostaglandin E2-mediated neuroprotection against TNF-alpha: possible involvement of multiple signal transduction and beta-catenin/T-cell factor. *J. Neuroimmunol,* 2004 155, 21-31.

[129] Tezel G, Kass MA, Kolker AE, et al. Plasma and aqueous humor endothelin levels in primary open-angle glaucoma. *J. Glaucoma,* 1997 6, 83-89.

[130] Guerreiro RJ, Santana I, Brás JM, et al. Peripheral inflammatory cytokines as biomarkers in Alzheimer's disease and mild cognitive impairment. *Neurodegener.Dis,* 2007 4, 406-412.

In: Alzheimer's Disease in the Middle-Aged
Editor: Hyun Sil Jeong, pp. 137-153

ISBN: 978-1-60456-480-8
© 2008 Nova Science Publishers, Inc.

Chapter 5

SPATIAL CORRELATIONS BETWEEN β-AMYLOID (Aβ) DEPOSITS AND BLOOD VESSELS IN EARLY-ONSET ALZHEIMER'S DISEASE

R.A. Armstrong[*]

Vision Sciences, Aston University, Birmingham B4 7ET, UK.

ABSTRACT

In cases of late-onset Alzheimer's disease (AD), there is a spatial correlation between the classsic 'cored' type of β-amyloid (Aβ) deposit and the large vertically penetrating arterioles in the cerebral cortex suggesting that blood vessels are involved in the pathogenesis of the classic deposits. In this chapter, the spatial correlations between the diffuse, primitive, and classic Aβ deposits and blood vessels were studied in 10 cases of early-onset AD in the age range 40 – 65 years. Sections of frontal cortex were immunostained with antibodies against Aβ and with collagen IV to reveal the Aβ deposits and blood vessel profiles. In the early-onset cases as a whole, all types of Aβ deposit and blood vessel profiles were distributed in clusters. There was a positive spatial correlation between the clusters of the diffuse Aβ deposits and the larger (>10μm) and smaller diameter (<10μm) blood vessel profiles in one and three cases respectively. The primitive and classic Aβ deposits were spatially correlated with larger and smaller blood vessels both in three and four cases respectively. Spatial correlations between the Aβ deposits and blood vessels may be more prevalent in cases expressing amyloid precursor protein (APP) than presenilin 1 (PSEN1) mutations. Apolipoprotein E (Apo E) genotype of the patient did not appear to influence the spatial correlation with blood vessel profiles. The data suggest that the larger diameter blood vessels are less important in the pathogenesis of the classic Aβ deposits in early-onset compared with late-onset AD.

[*] Dr. R.A. Armstrong, Vision Sciences, Aston University, Birmingham B4 7ET, UK. Tel: 0121-359-3611; Fax 0121-333-4220; EMail R.A.Armstrong@aston.ac.uk

KeyWords: Clustering, frontal cortex, blood vessels, diffusion, perivascular clearance, spatial correlation.

INTRODUCTION

The incidence of Alzheimer's disease (AD) in the population over 65 years of age has been estimated to be 1.3 - 6.2% (Mortimer, 1983). The incidence in younger patients is more difficult to estimate, but from death certificate data and assuming average disease duration of 7 years, AD is believed to affect approximately 0.5% of the population between 40 and 70 years of age (Mortimer, 1983). Approximately 60% of individuals with dementia are ultimately diagnosed with AD (Tomlinson et al., 1972) and about 1% of the elderly population develops senile dementia each year. Hence, there is a marked increase in the prevalence of senile dementia with age with evidence that some individuals that live into their 9th and 10th decades have a reduced risk of AD (Tomlinson et al., 1972; Peress et al., 1978). This chapter is largely concerned with AD in the middle-aged population, i.e., in those individuals with a disease onset less than 65 years of age, more often referred to as early-onset AD.

PATHOLOGY OF AD

Since the first descriptions of pre-senile dementia by Alois Alzheimer in 1907 (Alzheimer, 1907), the formation of senile plaques (SP) (also known as β-amyloid or Aβ deposits) and neurofibrillary tangles (NFT) have been regarded as the defining lesions of Alzheimer's disease (AD) (Mirra et al., 1991). SP are classified into a number of morphological subtypes, viz., diffuse, primitive, and classic deposits (Delaere et al., 1991; Armstrong, 1998,). A unique combination of histological features appears to be associated with the formation of each type of deposit (Armstrong, 1998). Hence, diffuse deposits have a close spatial association with neuronal perikarya (Allsop et al., 1989), primitive deposits with synapto-axonal degeneration not involving the cell body (Giaccone et al., 1989), and classic deposits with blood vessels (Armstrong, 1998). Hence, degeneration of a particular cell type or anatomical structure could result in the formation of a plaque with a specific morphology. The discovery of β-amyloid (Aβ) as the most important molecular constituent of the SP (Glenner and Wong, 1984) led ultimately to the 'Amyloid Cascade Hypothesis', the most important model of the molecular pathology of AD developed over the last 15 years (Hardy and Higgins, 1992). This hypothesis proposes that the deposition of Aβ is the initial pathological event in AD leading to the formation of NFT, cell death, and ultimately dementia. The molecular composition of Aβ deposits, however, is complex and includes in addition to Aβ, apolipoprotein E (Apo E) (Yamaguchi et al., 1994), α_1-antichymotrypsin, sulphated glycosaminoglycans, and complement factors (Verga et al., 1989). Moreover, the mature primitive and classic deposits also contain dystrophic neurites immunoreactive to the protein tau. The classic deposits are especially complex and contain a variety of molecular constituents within the amyloid 'core' and the surrounding 'ring' (Armstrong, 1998). Hence, chromogranin A and paired helical filament (PHF) antigens appear to be localised to the 'ring' while complement factors and immunoglobulins are found in the plaque 'core'. The presence of immune system factors within the 'core' has suggested that blood proteins and more specifically immunological factors (McGeer *et al.*, 1991) may be involved in the pathogenesis of the Aβ deposits.

One of the most important molecular markers of NFT is tau and in AD, all six isoforms of tau are abnormally phosphorylated and aggregated into PHF. In addition, NFT may acquire a variety of molecular determinants as tau undergoes various post-translational modifications (Chen *et al.*, 2004). These include hyperphosphorylation and glycosylation crucial to the development of mature NFT, as well as ubiquitination, glycation, polyamination, nitration, and proteolysis, which may represent mechanisms within neurons to remove damaged, misfolded, or aggregated proteins.

EARLY-ONSET AD AND GENETICS

Genetic factors are more directly involved in the pathogenesis of early-onset than late-onset AD and a number of different genes have been implicated. Rare cases are linked to mutations of the amyloid precursor protein (APP) gene (Chartier-Harlin et al., 1991; Goate *et al.*, 1991) and a larger group to the presenilin (PSEN) genes PSEN1 (Sherrington *et al.*, 1993) and PSEN2 (Levy-Lahad *et al.*, 1995). In addition, the apolipoprotein E (Apo E) gene is an important risk factor associated with late-onset FAD (Strittmater *et al.*, 1993); possession of one or more ε4 alleles significantly increasing the risk of the disease and is also likely to be a factor in early-onset AD. APP. PSEN mutations and Apo E genotype, however, do not explain all familial cases of AD (Cruts *et al.*, 1998; Grazini *et al.*, 2006). Linkage studies show the presence of additional AD susceptibility genes on chromosomes 9, 10, and 12 (Sillen *et al.*, 2006) with the most compelling case for a gene on chromosome 12 (Panja *et al.*, 2006).

AD PATHOGENESIS AND CEREBRAL BLOOD VESSELS

The involvement of the cerebral blood vessels in the pathogenesis of the Aβ deposits in Alzheimer's disease (AD) is controversial (Attems *et al.*, 2004). Some studies have found spatial correlations between Aβ deposits and blood vessels suggesting that degeneration of the blood vessels themselves (Yamaguchi *et al.*, 1992; Wisniewski and Wegiel, 1994) or diffusion of substances from the blood vessels may be involved in the pathogenesis of Aβ deposits (Perlmutter and Chui, 1990; Perlmutter *et al.*, 1990; Miyakawa *et al.*, 1992). By contrast, other studies have reported that the spatial correlations observed between Aβ deposits and blood vessels are fortuitous and arise because of the high densities of capillary profiles and Aβ deposits in histological sections of the AD brain (Kawai *et al.*, 1991; Luthert and Williams, 1991).

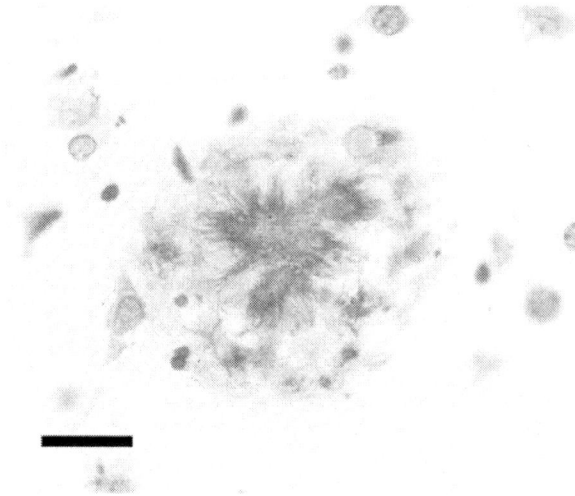

Figure 1. A classic β-amyloid (Aβ) deposit (Aβ, Cresyl violet) (Bar = 20μm).

In the cerebral cortex of cases of late-onset AD, however, the diffuse, primitive, and classic types of Aβ deposit occur in clusters that often exhibit a regular periodicity parallel to the pia mater (Armstrong et al., 1993). Of the three morphological subtypes of Aβ deposit common in AD (Delaere et al., 1991; Armstrong, 1998), the classic ('cored') deposits, which consist of a solid amyloid core surrounded by a 'corona' of dystrophic neurites (Fig 1) (Armstrong, 1998), is the only subtype to exhibit a consistent spatial relationship with blood vessels (Armstrong et al., 1998; Armstrong, 2006a). In the cerebral cortex in late-onset AD, the classic deposits are often clustered around the larger diameter (>10μm) blood vessels and especially the vertically penetrating arterioles in the upper laminae (Fig 2) (Armstrong, 2006a).

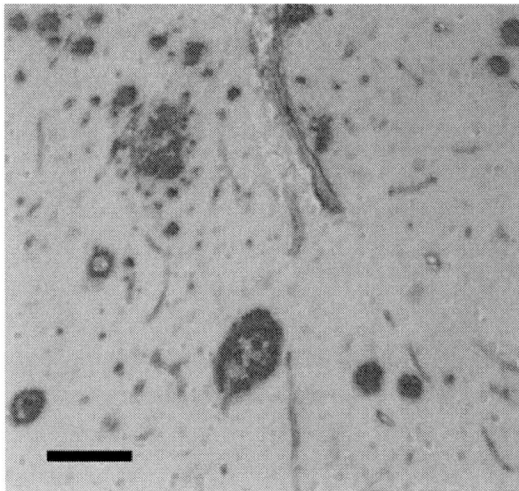

Figure 2. β-amyloid (Aβ) deposits and blood vessels in a triple-stained section (Aβ, Collagen IV, Cresyl violet) of the frontal cortex in a patient with late-onset Alzheimer's disease (Bar = 50μm).

DIFFERENCES IN PATHOLOGICAL PHENOTYPE BETWEEN EARLY AND LATE-ONSET AD

The pathological phenotype of late-onset sporadic AD (SAD) closely resembles that of early-onset familial cases (FAD) (Haupt *et al.*, 1992; Nochlin *et al.*, 1993). In a study of 90 outpatients with AD, the hypothesis was tested that cognitive impairment was different in FAD and SAD (Haupt et al 1992). The results did not yield any statistically significant differences between groups for any of the neuropsychological variables investigated. In addition, Nochlin et al (1993) compared the density of NFT and SP in various brain areas in 60 cases of AD. No significant differences in severity scores of NFT or SP were found between the FAD and SAD cases. However, there was an inverse correlation between age of onset of dementia and density of NFT and SP in all regions when the FAD and SAD data were combined. Hence, with the exception of the severity of pathological change, it is normally concluded that there are no essential differences in the pathological phenotype of FAD and SAD. Nevertheless, some differences in Aβ deposition have been reported between familial and sporadic cases (Gomez-Isla *et al.*, 1999; Ishii *et al.*, 2001) and hence, there could be differences in the spatial relationships between Aβ deposits and the vasculature in early and late-onset AD.

AIMS AND OBJECTIVES

The present study examined the spatial correlations between the diffuse, primitive, and classic Aβ deposits and the blood vessel profiles in ten cases of early-onset AD including FAD cases linked to APP and PSEN1 mutations, cases expressing Apo E genotype 3/4, and cases not linked to any of these genes. The principle objective was to test the hypothesis that the spatial relationships between the Aβ deposits and blood vessels in early-onset cases were essentially similar to those previously reported in late-onset AD (Armstrong *et al.*, 1998; Armstrong 2006a).

MATERIALS AND METHODS

Cases

Ten cases of early-onset AD (Table 1) were obtained from the Brain Bank, Department of Neuropathology, Institute of Psychiatry, King's College, London, UK. Informed consent was given for the removal of all brain tissue according to the 1996 Declaration of Helsinki (as modified Edinburgh, 2000).

Table 1. Details of early-onset Alzheimer disease (AD) cases studied

Case	Gender	Onset	Cause of death	Genetic link	Apo E
A	M	61	Bronchopneumonia	APP_{717}	3/3
B	F	52	Bronchopneumonia	APP_{717}	3/3
C	F	37	Bronchopneumonia	PSEN1	3/3
D	F	57	Intestinal obstruction	PSEN1	2/3
E	F	65	Ischaemic heart disease	ND	3/4
F	F	64	Bronchopneumonia	ND	3/4
G	F	59	Bronchopneumonia	ND	3/3
H	F	62	Bronchopneumonia	ND	2/3
I	F	58	Bronchopneumonia	ND	3/3
J	F	63	Ischaemic heart disease	ND	3/3

Abbreviations: M = Male, F = Female, APP = Amyloid precursor protein, PSEN1 = Presenilin 1, Apo E = Apolipoprotein E genotype, ND = AD cases not linked to any of the known genes.

Patients were clinically assessed and all fulfilled the 'National Institute of Neurological and Communicative Disorders and Stroke and the Alzheimer Disease and Related Disorders Association' (NINCDS/ADRDA) criteria for probable AD (Tierney *et al.*, 1988). The histological diagnosis of AD was established by the presence of widespread neocortical SP consistent with the 'Consortium to Establish a Registry of Alzheimer Disease' (CERAD) criteria (Mirra *et al.*, 1991). Four of the cases were linked to specific gene mutations, two linked to the APP_{717} mutation and two to PSEN1 mutations (G209V, E280A). All of these cases also expressed Apo E genotypes 2/3 or 3/3. The remaining cases were not linked to any of the known genes. However, two of the cases expressed the ε4 allele (Apo E genotype 3/4). The remaining cases had Apo E genotypes 2/3 or 3/3.

Histological Methods

A block of the superior frontal cortex was removed from each case at the level of the genu of the corpus callosum. Coronal sections, 7μm in thickness, were stained with a rabbit polyclonal antibody (Gift of Prof. B.H. Anderton) raised against the 12-28 amino acid sequence of the Aβ protein (Spargo *et al.*, 1990) to reveal the deposits. The antibody was used at a dilution of 1 in 1200 and incubated at 4° overnight. Sections were pretreated with 98% formic acid for 6 min to enhance immunoreactivity. Aβ was visualised using the streptavidin-biotin horseradish peroxidase procedure with diaminobenzidine as the chromogen. Sections were also immunostained with collagen type IV antiserum (Europath Ltd, U.K.) to reveal the microvessels (Kawai *et al.*,1990; Luthert and Williams, 1991; Armstrong, 2006a). The antiserum was used at 1:500 dilution following protease digestion of the section with a solution of 0.04% pepsin. Collagen type IV stains a component of the cerebrovascular basement membrane (Yurchenko and Schittny, 1990) and hence, reveals arterioles, venules, precapillaries, and capillaries (Armstrong, 2006a) (Fig 2). The three most common morphological types of Aβ deposit were identified using previously published criteria (Delaere *et al.*, 1991; Armstrong, 1998). Hence, diffuse deposits were 10 - 200μm in diameter, irregular in shape with diffuse boundaries and lightly stained, primitive deposits were 20 - 60μm well demarcated, more symmetrical in shape, and strongly stained, and classic deposits were 20 - 60μm had a distinct central core surrounded by a 'corona' of dystrophic neurites (figure 1).

Clustering of Aβ Deposits and Blood Vessels

The spatial patterns of the Aβ deposits and blood vessels were studied parallel to the pia mater in the upper 1mm of the cortex (which includes laminae I, II and III) using a magnification of x100. Aβ deposits occur at high density and the vertically penetrating arterioles are especially prominent in this region (Bell and Ball, 1990; Armstrong, 2006a). A strip of cortex 17600 to 25600μm in length, and which included a sulcus and a gyrus, was studied using 1000 x 200μm contiguous sample fields, the short dimension of the field being aligned with the surface of the pia mater. Between 64 and 128 contiguous sample fields were used to sample each gyrus. A micrometer grid with grid lines at intervals of 10μm was used as the sample field. The number of Aβ deposits was counted manually in each field. The frequency of the larger diameter (>10μm) and smaller diameter (<10μm) blood vessels in a field was estimated by 'lattice sampling', i.e., by counting the number of times a vessel profile intersected the grid lines of the field (Armstrong, 2003a).

Statistical Analysis

The data were analysed by spatial pattern analysis described in detail in previous studies (Armstrong, 1993; 2006a; 2006b). Essentially, the variance/mean (V/M) ratio is used as an index of non-randomness and determines whether the Aβ deposits and blood vessel profiles were distributed randomly (V/M = 1), regularly (V/M < 1), or in clusters (V/M > 1) along the strip of cortex parallel to the pia mater. V/M ratio is calculated at various field sizes, e.g., 200 x 1000μm (the original field size) and then at 400 x 1000μm, 800 x 1000μm etc., up to a size limited by the length of cortex sampled. The V/M ratio is plotted against the increasing field size to reveal the spatial pattern. If the deposits or blood vessels are clustered, then the analysis indicates whether the clusters themselves are randomly or regularly distributed and provides an estimate of the mean dimension of the clusters in a plane parallel to the pia mater. To test possible differences between genetic subtypes, cases were divided into four groups, viz., APP, PSEN1, Apo E 3/4, and cases not linked to any of the known genes. Cluster sizes of Aβ deposits and blood vessels, assuming a maximum size of 6400μm, were compared between groups using analysis of variance (ANOVA), chi-square (χ^2) contingency tests, and Fisher's 2 x 2 exact test (STATISTICA software, Statsoft Inc., 2300 East 14th St, Tulsa Ok, 74104, USA). Cases expressing apo E 3/4 were also compared with those expressing Apo E 2/3 and 3/3.

The degree of correlation between the density of Aβ deposits and the frequency of contacts with the blood vessel profiles was tested at each field size using Pearson's correlation coefficient (Armstrong, 2003b). Correlations at small field sizes (≤400μm) indicate a close spatial relationship between individual blood vessels and Aβ deposits while correlation at larger field sizes only (≥1600μm) is probably due to the general abundance of blood vessels and deposits in the tissue (Kawai *et al.*,1990; Luthert and Williams, 1991; Armstrong, 2003b).

SPATIAL PATTERNS OF Aβ DEPOSITS AND BLOOD VESSELS

Examples of the spatial patterns exhibited by the Aβ deposits in the upper laminae of the superior frontal cortex are shown in Fig 3. The diffuse deposits in the APP_{717} case exhibited a V/M peak at a field size of 3200μm suggesting the presence of clusters of deposits 3200μm in diameter, regularly distributed parallel to the pia mater.

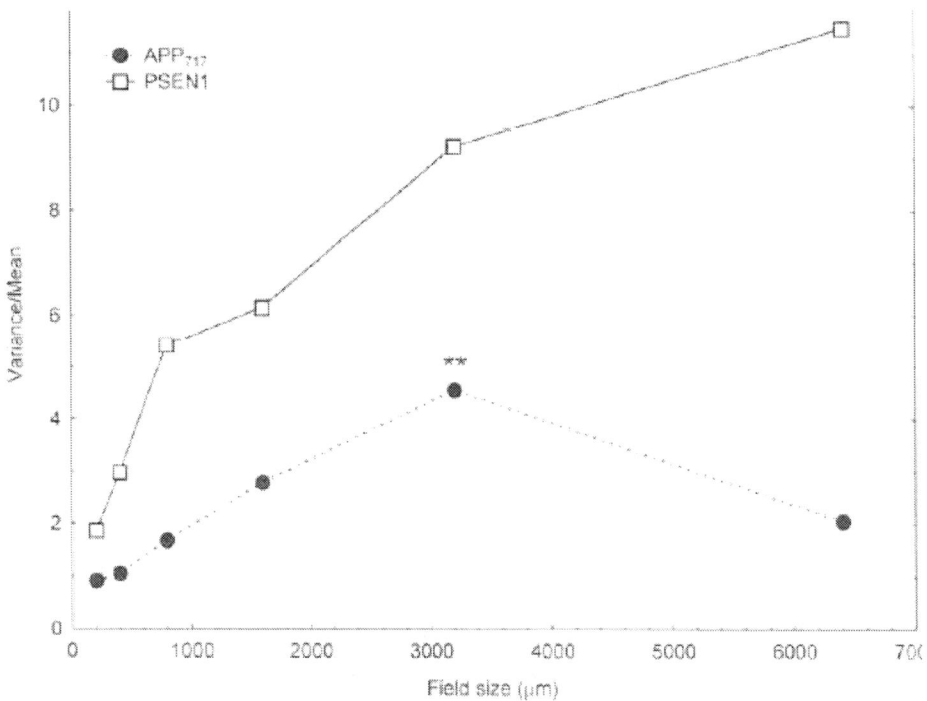

Figure 3. The spatial distribution of the diffuse-type β-amyloid deposits along the upper laminae of the frontal cortex of a patient (Case A) with familial Alzheimer disease (FAD, APP_{717}) and of the classic deposits in a case linked to a PSEN1 mutation as revealed by spatial pattern analysis. Asterisks indicate significant V/M peaks.

In the PSEN1 case, the V/M ratio increased with field size without reaching a peak suggesting large scale clustering of the classic deposits (≥6400μm in diameter). The spatial patterns of the Aβ deposits and blood vessel profiles in each of the ten cases are summarized in table 2.

Table 2. Mean cluster sizes (μm) of the diffuse, primitive, and classic β-amyloid (Aβ) deposits and the larger diameter (>10μm) and smaller diameter (<10μm) blood vessels in 10 cases of early-onset Alzheimer's disease

Aβ deposits			Blood vessels		
Case	Diffuse	Primitive	Classic	>10μm	<10μm
A	3200	3200	≥6400	≥6400	3200
B	3200	≥6400	3200	400	≥6400
C	400	≥6400	≥6400	≥6400	200
D	≥6400	3200	≥6400	200	400
E	3200	≥6400	1600	1600	≥6400
F	≥6400	≥6400	≥6400	400	≥6400
G	≥6400	3200	1600	400	≥6400
H	3200	6400	3200	800	400,3200
I	1600	≥6400	1600	200	≥6400
J	≥6400	≥6400	≥6400	400	≥6400

Data preceded by ≥ indicate large scale clustering of Aβ deposits or blood vessel profiles of at least 6400μm. Data not preceded by ≥ indicate clusters that are regularly distributed parallel to the pia mater. (-) density of classic deposits too low to determine spatial pattern. Comparison of cluster sizes: Analysis of variance (ANOVA): Aβ deposits, Genetic group, $F = 0.19$ ($P > 0.05$), Deposit type $F = 0.95$ ($P > 0.05$), Interaction $F = 0.62$ ($P > 0.05$); Blood vessels, Genetic group $F = 1.17$ ($P > 0.05$), Blood vessel type $F = 2.46$ ($P > 0.05$), Interaction $F = 2.00$ ($P > 0.05$).

The diffuse, primitive, and classic Aβ deposits occurred in clusters; the diffuse deposit clusters being regularly distributed along the cortex parallel to the pia mater in six cases, and the primitive and classic deposits each in four and five cases respectively. In the remaining cases, the Aβ deposits occurred in larger clusters (diameter ≥6400μm) without evidence of regular spacing. The large and small diameter blood vessels were also clustered; the larger vessels being regularly distributed parallel to the pia mater in eight cases and the smaller blood vessels in four cases. There were no significant differences in the mean cluster sizes of the Aβ deposits in the different genetic subtypes ($F = 0.19$, $P > 0.05$). In addition, cluster sizes of the Aβ deposits were similar in cases expressing different Apo E genotypes ($F = 0.19$, $P > 0.05$).

SPATIAL CORRELATIONS BETWEEN Aβ DEPOSITS AND BLOOD VESSELS

Correlations between the diffuse Aβ deposits and blood vessel profiles for a single case (Case A, APP_{717}) are shown in figure 4.

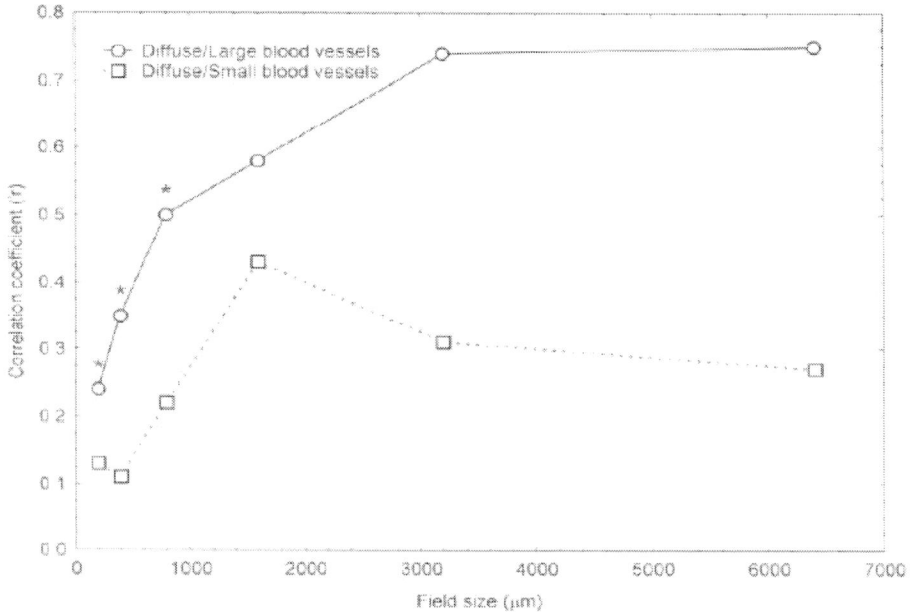

Figure 4. Spatial correlations (Pearson's 'r') between the diffuse-type β-amyloid deposits and blood vessels along the upper laminae of the frontal cortex of a patient (Case A) with familial Alzheimer disease (FAD, APP$_{717}$). Asterisks indicate significant positive spatial correlations.

The diffuse deposits were positively correlated with the larger diameter blood vessels at field sizes 200-800μm inclusive but there were no significant correlations with the smaller blood vessels at any field size. Spatial correlations between the densities of the Aβ deposits and blood vessel profiles in the data as a whole are shown in table 3.

Table 3. Spatial correlations between the diffuse (D), primitive (P), and classic (C) 'cored' β-amyloid (Aβ) deposits and the larger diameter (>10μm) and smaller diameter (<10μm) blood vessels in 10 cases of early-onset Alzheimer's disease

Case	Large blood vessels (>10μm)			Small blood vessels (<10μm)		
	D	P	C	D	P	C
A	1*,2*,4*	NS	2*,4*,8*	NS	NS	2*,4*,8*
B	NS	2*,4*	NS	NS	1***,2**,4**	1**,2**,4*
C	NS	1*,4*	NS	NS	NS	NS
D	NS	NS	NS	NS	NS	NS
E	NS	NS	NS	NS	1*,2**	NS
F	NS	NS	NS	NS	NS	NS
G	NS	NS	NS	1*,2*	NS	NS
H	NS	NS	1*,2*,4*	NS	NS	16*
I	NS	NS	1*,4*	1**	1*,2*,4*,8*	NS
J	NS	1*,2*	NS	1*,2*,4**	2*,4*,8**	1***,2**

Data show the field size (1 = 200μm, 2 = 400μm, 4 = 800μm, 8 = 1600μm) at which a significant spatial correlation occurred (*P<0.05, **P<0.01), NS = no significant correlations at any field size.

There was a positive spatial correlation between the clusters of the diffuse Aβ deposits and the larger (>10μm) and smaller diameter (<10μm) blood vessel profiles in one and three cases respectively. The primitive Aβ deposits were spatially correlated with larger and smaller blood vessels in three and four cases and the classic deposits in three and four cases respectively. Spatial correlations between Aβ deposits and blood vessels were more frequent in cases linked to APP_{717} than PSEN1 mutations, APP_{717} cases exhibiting positive spatial correlations in 6/12 analyses and PSEN1 mutations in 1/12 analyses (Fisher's exact test, one tail, P = 0.034). There were no differences in the frequency of spatial correlation in cases expressing different Apo E genotypes ($\chi^2 = 3.73$, 2DF, P > 0.05).

HYPOTHESES TO EXPLAIN DIFFERENCES BETWEEN EARLY AND LATE-ONSET AD

Spatial correlations between the Aβ deposits and the blood vessels were present in only a small number of the early-onset AD cases. The frequency of significant spatial correlations between the diffuse and primitive deposits and blood vessel profiles was similar in early-onset compared with previously published data from late-onset cases (Armstrong et al., 1998); the most striking differences affecting the classic deposits and the larger diameter vessels. In early-onset AD, three cases showed a significant correlation (P < 0.05) while in late-onset AD, all 11 cases studied showed a highly significant spatial correlation with the larger diameter blood vessels ($\chi^2 = 8.61$, P < 0.01) (Armstrong, 2006a).

Differences in the Pattern of Vasculature

A number of hypotheses could explain the differences in spatial correlation between the classic Aβ deposits and larger diameter blood vessels in early and late-onset AD. First, spatial correlations might reflect differences in the pattern of vasculature in the two groups of patients. However, neither the mean cluster size (t = 1.57, P > 0.05) nor the spatial pattern of the large or small diameter blood vessels differed between the early-onset cases compared with the late-onset cases (Armstrong, 2006a). Hence, if amyloid deposition limits or reduces capillary density leading to the observation of less amyloid deposition in relation to capillaries but more in relation to the larger vessels (Armstrong, 2006a), then the effect would be similar in both groups.

Differences in Density and Cluster Size of Aβ Deposits

Second, the pattern of spatial correlation could depend on density and the cluster size of the classic Aβ deposits; cases with more diffuse, less dense clusters of deposits being less likely to exhibit a spatial correlation. There were no significant differences in the mean densities of the classic deposits in the present cases and the previously reported older cases (t = 1.27, P > 0.05) (Armstrong, 2006a). The mean cluster size of the classic Aβ deposits, however, was greater in early compared with late-onset AD (t = 3.56, P < 0.01). Hence, in early-onset AD, clusters of classic deposits were larger but less dense than in older cases and therefore, may be less likely to exhibit a significant spatial correlation with blood vessels.

Age Differences

Third, variations in the pattern of spatial correlation could result from differences in patient age. Haem rich deposits <200µm in diameter associated with blood vessels and with Aβ deposits are more common in individuals older than 50 years (Cullen et al 2005). In addition, Aβ deposition around the larger blood vessels could reflect impaired drainage since extracellular fluid is drained from the brain to the cervical lymph nodes via the perivascular channels (Weller and Nicoll, 2003). Hence, increased resistance to this drainage in older patients could result in the increased aggregation of Aβ around the vessels and the formation of classic deposits.

Damage to the Blood Brain Barrier

Fourth, there may be differences in the degree of damage to the blood brain barrier in early and late-onset AD. Blood vessels with collapsed or degenerated endothelia are evident in many AD cases (Kalaria and Hedera, 1995) and occur concurrently with Aβ deposition. A number of plasma proteins could therefore leak from damaged vessels including amyloid P, α-antichymotrypsin, antitrypsin, antithrombin III, and complement factors (Kalaria, 1992; Kalaria, et al., 1993) and Apo E (Saunders et al.,1993) and become incorporated into Aβ deposits. Diffusion of substances from vessels could be a possible explanation for the distribution of the classic deposits since the number of classic deposits in older patients decline exponentially with distance from the vessel consistent with a diffusional process (Armstrong, 2006a). The most likely protein to originate from blood vessels is amyloid-P, since the liver is the only tissue of the body which exhibits its mRNA (Kalaria, et al.,1991). Plasma proteins such as amyloid-P may act as 'molecular chaperones' and be involved in the aggregation of Aβ to form plaque amyloid. Hence, in older AD patients, Aβ deposits associated with vessels may acquire a molecular chaperone originating in the plasma resulting in the condensation of Aβ to form the plaque core. By contrast, there may be less age-related damage to the blood brain barrier in younger patients resulting in a distribution of the classic deposits less dependent on the spatial location of blood vessels. The data also imply that different factors may be involved in the pathogenesis of the classic deposits in cases of early onset AD.

Influence of Genetic Subtype on the Pattern of Correlation

Although numbers of cases are small, the data suggest that the relationship between Aβ deposits and blood vessels was similar in cases expressing different Apo E genotypes. However, the relationship may differ in APP$_{717}$ and PSEN1 cases. Cluster size and density of

Aβ deposits did not differ between the various genetic subtypes. However, increased density of Aβ$_{42}$ containing deposits has been demonstrated in APP and PSEN cases compared with SAD (Ishii *et al.*, 2001). It is possible that APP and PSEN1 mutations directly influence the pathogenesis of Aβ deposits in and around the blood vessels resulting in different patterns of spatial correlation. For example, Aβ has a marked toxic effect on cultured vascular endothelial cells, Aβ$_{42}$ being the more toxic species (Folin *et al.*, 2005). Hence, there may be variations in the proportion of different Aβ peptides formed around blood vessels associated with the different gene mutations that could affect the degree of vascular damage, leakage of plasma proteins, and result in different patterns of vascular pathology in FAD.

CONCLUSION

The data suggest that the classic Aβ deposits are less frequently spatially correlated with the larger blood vessels in early-onset AD compared with late-onset AD and therefore whether or not such a correlation is observed may depend on the age of the patient. Possible explanations for this difference include variations in the pattern of drainage via the perivascular channels (Weller and Nicoll, 2003), differences in the spatial pattern of Aβ deposits, and variations in the degree of damage to the blood brain barrier between early-onset and late-onset cases. Greater damage to the blood brain barrier in older patients could result in increased diffusion of substances from the blood vessels that influence the growth and development of the classic deposits. Different factors are likely to be involved in the formation of the classic Aβ deposits in early-onset compared with late-onset AD.

ACKNOWLEDGEMENTS

Brain tissue sections for this study were kindly provided by the Brain Bank, Dept. of Neuropathology, Institute of Psychiatry, King's College London, UK.

REFERENCES

Alzheimer, A. (1907) On a peculiar disease of the cerebral cortex. *Allgemeine Zeitschrift für Psychiatrie und Psychish-Gerichtlich Medicin.* 64, 146-148.

Allsop, D., Haga, S., Haga, C., Ikeda, S.I., Mann, D.M.A., Ishii, T. (1989) Early senile plaques in Down's syndrome brains show a close relationship with cell bodies of neurons. *Neuropath. Appl. Neurobiol* 15, 531-542.

Armstrong, R. (1993) The usefulness of spatial pattern analysis in understanding the pathogenesis of neurodegenerative disorders, with particular reference to plaque formation in Alzheimer's disease. *Neurodegen.* 2, 73-80.

Armstrong, R. (1998) β-amyloid plaques: stages in life history or independent origin? *Dement. Geriatr. Cogn. Disord.* 9, 227-238.

Armstrong, R. (2003a) Quantifying the pathology of neurodegenerative disorders: quantitative measurements, sampling strategies, and data analysis. *Histopathol.* 42, 521-529.

Armstrong, R. (2003b) Measuring the degree of spatial correlation between histological features in thin sections of brain tissue. *Neuropathol.* 23, 245-253.

Armstrong R. (2006a) Classic β-amyloid deposits cluster around large diameter blood vessels rather than capillaries in sporadic Alzheimer's disease. *Curr. Neurovasc. Res.* 3, 289-294.

Armstrong, R. (2006b) Methods of studying the planar distribution of objects in histological sections of brain tissue. *J. Microsc.* 221, 153-158.

Armstrong, R, Myers, D, Smith, C. (1993) The spatial patterns of β/A4 deposit subtypes in Alzheimer's disease. *Acta Neuropathol.* 86, 36-41.

Armstrong, R, Cairns, N, Lantos, P. (1998) Spatial distribution of diffuse, primitive, and classic amyloid-β deposits and blood vessels in the upper laminae of the frontal cortex in Alzheimer's disease. *Alz. Dis. Assoc. Disord.* 12, 378-383.

Attems, J, Lintner, F, Jellinger, K. (2004) Amyloid beta peptide 1-42 highly correlates with capillary cerebral amyloid angiopathy and Alzheimer disease pathology. *Acta Neuropathol.* 107, 283-291.

Bell, M, Ball, M. (1990) Neuritic plaques and vessels of visual cortex in ageing and Alzheimer's dementia. *Neurobio. Ageing.* 11, 359-370.

Chartier-Harlin, M, Crawford, F, Houlden, H, Warren, A, Hughes, D, Fidani, L, Goate, A, Rossor, M, Rocques, P, Hardy, J, Mullan, M. (1991) Early onset Alzheimer's disease caused by mutations at codon 717 of the β-amyloid precursor protein gene. *Nature* 353, 844-846.

Chen, F., David, D., Ferrari, A., Gotz, J. (2004) Posttranslational modifications of tau: role in human tauopathies and modelling in transgenic animals. *Curr. Drug. Targets* 5, 503-515.

Cruts, M, van Duijn, C, Backhovens, H, van den Broeck, M, Wehnert, A, Serneels, S, Sherrington, R, Hutton, M, Hardy, J, St George-Hyslop, P, Hofman, A, von Broeckhoven, C. (1998) Estimates of the genetic contribution of presenilin-1 and -2 mutations in a population based study of presenile Alzheimer's disease. *Hum. Mole. Biol.* 7, 43-51.

Cullen, K, Kocsi, Z, Stone, J. (2005) Pericapillary haem-rich deposits: evidence for microhaemorrhages in aging human cerebral cortex. *J. Cer. Blood Flow Met.* 25, 1656-1667.

Delaere, P, Duyckaerts, C, He, Y, Piette, F, Hauw, J. (1991) Subtypes and differential laminar distributions of β/A4 deposits in Alzheimer's disease: relationship with the intellectual status of 26 cases *Acta Neuropathol.* 81, 328-335.

Folin, M, Baiguera, S, Tommasini, M, Guidolin, D, Conconi, M, de Carlo, E, Nussdorfer, G, Parnigotto, P. (2005) Effects of beta-amyloid on rat neuromicro vascular endothelial cells cultured in vitro. *Int. J. Mole Med.* 15, 929-935.

Giaccone, G., Tagliavini, F., Linol, G., Bouras, C., Frigerio, L. (1989) Down's patients: Extracellular preamyloid deposits precede neuritic degeneration and senile plaques. *Neurosci. Lett.* 97, 232-238.

Glenner, G.G., Wong, C.W. (1984) Alzheimer's disease and Down's syndrome: sharing of a unique cerebrovascular amyloid fibril protein. *Biochem. Biophys. Res. Commun.* 122, 1131-1135.

Goate, R, Chartier-Harlin, M, Mullan, M, Brown, J, Crawford, F, Fidani, L, Giuffra, L, Haynes, A, Irving, N, James, L, Mant, R, Newton, P, Rooke, K, Roques, P, Talbot, C, Pericak-Vance, M, Roses, A, Williamson, R, Rossor, M, Owen, M, Hardy, J. (1991) Segregation of a missense mutation in the amyloid precursor protein gene with familial Alzheimer's disease. *Nature* 349, 704-706.

Gomez-Isla, T, Growdon, W, McNamara, M, Nochlin, D, Bird, T, Arango, J, Lopera, F, Kosik, K, Lantos, P, Cairns, N, Hyman, B. (1999) The impact of different presenilin 1 and presenilin 2 mutations on amyloid deposition, neurofibrillary tangle changes, and neuronal loss in the familial Alzheimer's disease brain: evidence for other phenotype-modifying factors. *Brain* 122, 1709-1719.

Grazini, M, Prabas, J, Silva, F, Oliveira, S, Santana, I, Oliveira, C. (2006) Genetic basis of Alzheimer's dementia: role of mitochondrial DNA mutations. *Genes, Brain, and Behaviour* 5 (supp 2), 92-107.

Hardy, J.A., Higgins, G.A. (1992) Alzheimer's disease: The amyloid cascade hypothesis. *Science* 256, 184-185.

Haupt, M, Kurz, A, Pollman, S, Romero, B. (1992) Alzheimer's disease: identical phenotype of familial and non-familial cases. *J. Neurol.* 239, 248-250.

Ishii, K, Lippa, C, Tomiyama, T, Miyatake, F, Ozawa, K, Tamaoka, A, Hasegawa, T, Fraser, P, Shoji, S, Nee, L, Pollen, D, St George-Hyslop, P, Ii K, Ohtake, T, Kalaria, R, Rossor, M, Lantos, P, Cairns, N, Farrer, L, Mori, H. (2001) Distinguishable effects of Presenilin-1 and APP717 mutations on amyloid plaque deposition. *Neurobiol. Aging.* 22, 367-376.

Kalaria, R, Golde, T, Cohen, M, Younkin, S, Younkin, S. (1991) Absence of detectable mRNA of serum amyloid P (SAP) in human brain, choroid plexus, and meninges suggests that the presence of SAP in CSF is due to transport across the blood-brain barrier. *J. Neuropathol. Exp. Neurol.* 50, 339.

Kalaria, R. (1992) The blood-brain barrier and cerebral microcirculation in Alzheimer disease. *Cerebrovasc Brain Met. Rev.* 4, 226-260.

Kalaria, R, Kroon, S, Perry, G. (1993) Serum proteins and the blood-brain barrier in the pathogenesis of Alzheimer's disease. In: M. Nicolini, P.F. Zatta, B. Corain, eds. Alzheimer's disease and related disorders, *Advances in Biosciences* 87, Pergamon Press, UK, 281-282.

Kalaria, R, Hedera, P. (1995) Differential degeneration of the cerebral microvasculature in Alzheimer's disease. *NeuroReport* 6, 477-480.

Kawai, M, Kalaria, R, Harik, S, Perry, G. (1990) The relationship of amyloid plaques to cerebral capillaries in Alzheimer's disease. *Am .J. Pathol.* 137, 1435-1446.

Levy-Lahad, E, Wasco, W, Poorkaj, P, Romano, D, Oshima, J, Pettingell, W, Yu, C, Jondro, P, Schmidt, S, Wang, K, Crowley, A, Fu, Y, Guenette, S, Galas, D, Nemens, E, Wijsman, E, Bird, T, Schellenberg, G, Tanzi, R. (1995) Candidate gene for chromosome 1 familial Alzheimer's disease locus. *Science* 269, 973-977.

Luthert, P, Williams, J. (1991) A quantitative study of the coincidence of blood vessels and A4 protein deposits in Alzheimer's disease. *Neurosci. Lett.* 126, 110-112.

McGeer, P.L., McGeer, E.G., Kawamata, T., Yamada, T., Akiyama, H. (1991) Reactions of the immune system in chronic degenerative neurological diseases. *Can. J. Neurol. Sci.*18, 376-379.

Mirra, S, Heyman, A, McKeel, D, Sumi, S, Crain, B, Brownlee, L, Vogel, F, Hughes, J, van Belle, G, Berg, L. (1991) The consortium to establish a registry for Alzheimer's disease

(CERAD). II. Standardisation of the neuropathological assessment of Alzheimer's disease. *Neurol.*41, 479-486.

Miyakawa, T, Katsuragi, S, Yamashita, K, Ohuchi, K. (1992) Morphological study of amyloid fibrils and preamyloid deposits in the brain with Alzheimer's disease. *Acta Neuropathol.*83, 340-346.

Mortimer, J.A. (1983) Alzheimer's disease and senile dementia: Prevalence and incidence. In: Reisberg, B. Ed. *Alzheimer's disease: The Standard reference.* McMillan, London and New York, pp141-148.

Nochlin, D, Van Belle, G, Bird, T, Sumi, S. (1993) Comparison of the severity of neuropathologic changes in familial and sporadic Alzheimer's disease. *Alz Dis.Assoc.Dis.*7: 212-222

Panja, F, Colacicco, A, D'Introno, A, Capurso, C, Liaci, M, Capurso, S, Capurso, A, Solfrizzi, V (2006) Candidate genes for late-onset Alzheimer's disease: Focus on chromosome 12. *Mech Age Dev* 127, 36-47.

Peress, N.S., Kane, W.C., Kitchener, D. (1978) Central nervous system findings in the tenth decade autopsy population. *Prog.Brain Res.*40, 473-483.

Perlmutter, L, Chui, C. (1990) Microangiopathy, the vascular basement membrane and Alzheimer's disease: A review. *Brain Res.Bull* 24, 677-686.

Perlmutter, L, Chui, C, Saperia, D, Athanikar, J. (1990) Microangiopathy and the colocalisation of heparan sulfate proteoglycan with amyloid in senile plaques of Alzheimer's disease. *Brain Res.*508, 9-11.

Saunders, A, Strittmatter, W, Schmechel, D, St. George-Hyslop, P, Pericak-Vance, M, Joo, S, Rose, B, Gasella, J, Crapper-MacLachan, D, Albersts, M, Hulette, C, Crain, B, Goldgaber, D, Roses, A. (1993) Association of apolipoprotein E allele e4 with late-onset familial and sporadic Alzheimer's disease. *Neurology* 43, 1467-1472.

Sherrington, R, Rogaev, E, Liang, Y, Rogaeva, E, Levesque, G, Ikeda, M, Chi, H, Lin, C, Li, G, Holman, K, Tsuda, T, Mar, L, Foncin, J, Bruni, A, Moulese, M, Sorbi, S, Rainero, I, Pinessi, L, Nee, L, Chumakov, I, Pollen, D, Brookes, A, Sauseau, P, Polinski, R, Wasco, R, Dasilva, H, Haines, J, Pericak-Vance, M, Tanzi, R, Roses, A, Fraser, P, Rommens, J, St George-Hyslop, P. (1993) Cloning of a gene bearing missense mutations in early onset familial Alzheimer's disease. *Nature* 375, 754-760.

Sillen, A, Forsell, C, Lilius, L, Axwlman, K, Bjork, B, Onkamo, P, Kere, J, Winblad, B, Graff C. (2006) Genome scan on Swedish Alzheimer disease families. *Mole Psy.*11, 182-186.

Spargo, E, Luthert, P, Anderton, B, Bruce, M, Smith, D, Lantos, P. (1990) Antibodies raised against different proteins of the A4 protein identify a subset of plaques in Down's syndrome. *Neurosci.Lett.*115, 345-350.

Strittmatter, W, Wiesgraber, K, Huang, D, Dong, L, Salvesan, G, Pericak-Vance, M, Schmachel, D, Saunders, A, Goldgaber, D, Roses, A. (1993) Binding of human apolipoprotein E to synthetic amyloid-β peptide: isoform specific effects and implications for late-onset Alzheimer's disease. *Proc.Natl.Acad.Sci.USA* 90, 8098-8102.

Tierney, M, Fisher, R, Lewis, A, Zorzitto, M, Snow, W, Reid, D, Nieuwstraten, P. (1988) The NINCDS-ADRDA work group criteria for the clinical diagnosis of probable Alzheimer's disease. *Neuro.*38: 359-364.

Tomlinson BE, Kitchener D (1972) Granulovacuolar degeneration of hippocampal pyramidal cells. J.Pathol.106: 165-185.

Verga, L., Frangione, B., Tagliavini, F., Giaccone, G., Migheli, A., Bugiani, O.(1989) Alzheimer's and Down's patients: cerebral preamyloid deposits differ ultrastructurally and histochemically from the amyloid of senile plaques. *Neurosci.Lett.*105, 294-299.

Weller, R, Nicoll, J. (2003) Cerebral amyloid angiopathy; Pathogenesis and effects on the ageing and Alzheimer brain. *Neurol Res* 25, 611-616.

Wisniewski, H, Wegiel, J. (1994) β-amyloid formation by myocytes of leptomeningeal vessels. *Acta Neuropathol.*87, 223-241.

Yamaguchi, H, Yamazaki, T, Lemere, C, Frosch, M, Selkoe, D. (1992) Beta-amyloid is focally deposited within the outer basement membrane in the amyloid angiopathy of Alzheimer's disease. *Am.J.Pathol.*141, 249-259.

Yamaguchi, H., Ishiguro, K., Sugihara, S., Nakazato. Y., Kawarabayashi, T., Sun, Y., Hirai, S. (1994) Presence of apolipoprotein ε on extracellular neurofibrillary tangles and on meningeal blood vessels precedes the Alzheimer β-amyloid deposition. *Acta Neuropathol.*88, 413-419.

Yurchenco, P, Schittny, J, (1990) Molecular architexture of basement membranes. *FASEB J.*4, 1577-1590.

In: Alzheimer's Disease in the Middle-Aged
Editor: Hyun Sil Jeong, pp. 155-168

ISBN: 978-1-60456-480-8
© 2008 Nova Science Publishers, Inc.

Chapter 6

Aß IMMUNIZATION IN THE TREATMENT OF ALZHEIMER'S DISEASE

*I. Ferrer**

Institut Neuropatologia, Servei Anatomia Patològica, IDIBELL-Hospital Universitari de Bellvitge, Universitat de Barcelona, Hospitalet de Llobregat, Spain
Prof. Isidro Ferrer Institut Neuropatologia Servei Anatomia Patològica
IDIBELL-Hospital Universitari de Bellvitge carrer Feixa Llarga sn
08907 Hospitalet de Llobregat Spain

ABSTRACT

Passive and active Aβ immunization were tested in Alzheimer's disease (AD) murine models in an attempt to provoke immune responses geared to reducing β-amyloid aggregation and cerebral β-amyloid burden. Positive results in terms of improved behavior and reduced plaque formation were found following active and passive Aβ immunization in AD transgenic mice. Pioneering trials in moderate AD cases showed variable clinical improvement and decreased β-amyloid plaques, but maintained β-amyloid angiopathy and hyperphosphorylated tau pathology. However, the trial was stopped because of the appearance of meningoencephalitis in a subset of patients. This was due to T-cell-mediated immune responses in addition to the expected antibody-related immune response. These results have prompted the development of new approaches aimed to reducing side-effects such as encephalitis and microhemorrhages, and to optimizing immunization. Together, experimental designs have delineated Aβ immunization as a potent therapeutic tool at early stages of the disease, either administered alone, or more probably, in combination with other drugs.

INTRODUCTION

Alzheimer's disease (AD) is characterized by β-amyloid (Aβ) deposition (a product of the amyloid precursor protein: APP) in the form of senile (diffuse and neuritic) plaques, and

---

* tel. lab.: +34 93 4035808 tel. secretary: +34 93 2607452 e-mail:8082ifa@comb.cat

β-amyloid angiopathy, together with tau hyperphosphorylation in neurofibrillary tangles, neuropil threads and dystrophic neurites surrounding β-amyloid deposits; there is also synaptic dropping and nerve cell loss [1, 2] Progression of AD in the cerebral cortex has been categorized into stages depending on neurofibrillary tangle and tau pathology as entorhinal and transentorhinal (I and II), hippocampal and limbic (III and IV), and neocortical (V and VI) stages; regarding β-amyloid burden, AD has been categorized as stage A, B and C [3]. Importantly, clinical and pathological correlations point to the appearance of mental impairment at stage III or IV, and the development of Alzheimer dementia at stages V and VI. This is a crucial point: once the disease is diagnosed there is already significant brain degeneration.

AD is a typical human disease, although AD-like pathology occurs in a reduced number of species including primates and canines. In addition, certain aspects of the disease can be reproduced in transgenic mice bearing the homologous pathogenic AD mutations responsible for familial AD cases, namely mutations in the genes encoding APP, preseniline 1 and preseniline 2, which are involved in the metabolism of APP and in the production of β-amyloid [4]. It is worth stressing that old transgenic mice show impaired behavior and amyloid plaques surrounded by aberrant neurites, but they do not develop neurofibrillary tangles as occurs in sporadic and in familial AD [5]. In spite of these limitations, APP and related transgenic mice are currently used as models of AD.

It is clear that β-amyloid, as the main component of senile plaques and β-amyloid angiopathy, plays a pivotal role in AD. However, included under the term β-amyloid are several molecules, including small peptides together with Aβ1-40 and Aβ1-42. In addition, β-amyloid is present in the form of soluble oligomers and fibrillar compounds that misfold and comprise protein aggregates [6-8].

Aβ AS A THERAPEUTIC TARGET FOR AD

A major focus in the treatment of AD is the prevention of Aβ misfolding and the disruption of Aβ aggregation by using distinct approaches including selective small molecules, synthetic peptides, chaperones and Aβ binding proteins, as well as Aβ immunization [9, 10].

Immunization with Aβ peptides and vaccination with anti-Aβ antibodies have emerged as important strategies for AD, both aimed at reducing Aβ aggregation and β-amyloid plaque burden [11-17].

ACTIVE IMMUNIZATION IN MICE

Shenk et al. [18] first reported that intraperitoneal injections of Aβ1-42 peptide and adjuvant prevented amyloid-β deposition in young mice and decreased the plaque burden when administered to old PDAPP transgenic mice. Importantly, Aβ immunization also reduced behavioral impairment and memory loss in other AD murine models [19-20]. Similar results were obtained by using different routes, including nasal administration [21 22], and methods, such as encapsulation of biodegradable particles[23].

Active immunization induces humoral immune responses, but also cellular immune responses mediated by T lymphocytes, mainly directed to the C-terminal domain (Aβ16-42) [24-26].

Cellular responses mediated by T-cells may cause encephalitis. In addition, peripheral injection of Aβ peptides also leads to cerebral microhemorrhages in aged transgenic mice [26-28].

For these reasons, several adjuvants have been applied in an attempt to optimize sensitization, and to reduce side-effects [29-32]. Furthermore, modification of the immunogens may reduce deleterious effects. For example, immunization with short β-amyloid immunogens, either tandem repeat of two lysine-linked Aβ1-15 sequences or the Aβ1-15 sequence synthesized to an active T1 T-helper-cell epitope, each with the addition of three Arg-Gly-Asp motifs, reduces cerebral load and learning deficits in the absence of Aβ-specific T-cell immune responses [33].

PASSIVE IMMUNIZATION IN MICE

Passive immunization has been conducted after administration of specific antibodies to determined Aβ sequences. The effects are different depending on the sequence recognized by the antibody, plaque-binding and time of administration [34]. Likewise, distinct morphological types of plaques are differentially cleared depending on the type of antibody [35]. As an example, antibodies to Aβ1-40, Aβ1-42 and Aβ1-16 prevent the appearance of later plaques when administered to young Tg2576 mice at a time when no plaques are present. Yet Aβ1-40 and Aβ1-42 did not attenuate the number of plaques and did not clear β-amyloid deposits in old transgenic mice [36].

The reasons for the variable efficiency of different antibodies are little known. Antibodies directed to the amino-terminal of Aβ reduce amyloid plaque burden in transgenic mice [37]. Likewise, antibodies directed against residues 4-10 of β42 inhibit fibrillogenesis and cytotoxicity [38]. Yet passive immunization with monoclonal antibodies directed to the mid-region of Aβ (amino acids 13-28: m266) also decreased amyloid plaque burden and rapidly increased Aβ plasma levels in a mouse model of AD [39, 40]. A single dose of this monoclonal antibody in old transgenic mice improved memory deficits but did not reduce β-amyloid burden [41]. Immunization with antibodies to the Aβ42/43 C-terminal domain also reduced amyloid plaques, and increased brain soluble Aβ and plasma levels of Aβ [42]. Therefore, although antibodies directed to the N-terminal region of Aβ have been proposed as the only ones capable of reducing plaque pathology [34, 36], later studies have shown that certain antibodies raised against the C-terminus can also be beneficial.

In spite of these achievements, meningoencephalitis has also been observed following passive immunization in a transgenic murine model of AD [43].

Regarding antibody administration, several routes have been proposed, including intracerebral infusion. A single intracerebroventricular injection of anti-fibrillar Aβ antibody in Tg2576 APP transgenic mice reduced cerebral plaques, reversed depletion of SNAP-25, abolished astroglial activation, and reduced inflammation, as revealed by reduced interleukin-1β-positive microglia surrounding congophilic plaques. Furthermore, no brain micro-hemorrhages or systemic toxicity were observed in these mice [44-46]. Improved results were even found in transgenic mice following intracerebroventricular injection of anti-oligo Aβ antibody [47].

The use of monoclonal antibodies to Aβ oligomers (amyloid beta-derived diffusible ligands, ADDLs) has proved beneficial without increasing side-effects. Antibodies to Aβ oligomers reduce binding and fibrillization, and decrease synaptic attachment [48]. Single-chain antibodies to oligomeric Aβ reduce deposits in APP transgenic mice following intracerebral injection [49]. Finally, passive immunization with monoclonal antibodies that recognize Aβ conformational epitopes in dimeric, small oligomeric and higher Aβ structures has been shown to improve learning and memory, but not to reduce β-amyloid plaques a few days after immunization [50].

IMMUNIZATION IN OTHER SPECIES

In addition to murine models, immunization with Aβ has been assayed in other animals. Immunization with fibrillar Aβ1-42 in aged dogs resulted in specific IgM and IgG responses directed to Aβ, together with a non-significant CSF increase in Aβ1-40, and a decrease in Aβ1-42 in cortex [51].

Immunization with Aβ peptide in old Caribbean vervet monkeys generates antibodies, which are present in plasma and CSF, and which label Aβ-amyloid plaques in humans, AD transgenic mice and old vervet brains; bind Aβ1-7; and recognize monomeric and oligomeric Aβ. Amyloid plaques were detected in the brains of 11 of the 13 control animals, but not in the four of the five immunized monkeys that survived 10 months after the immunization. None of these animals suffered from encephalitis after immunization [52]. In a similar line, rhesus monkeys immunized with aggregated Aβ1-42 developed high anti-Aβ titers and increased levels of Aβ in plasma [53].

Aß IMMUNIZATION IN HUMANS

Aβ immunization in humans was carried out by using human aggregated Aβ42 (AN1792) and QS-21 adjuvant with mild-to-moderate AD patients. Phase 1 study revealed a positive antibody response in more than a half of the patients; five deaths occurred during the study follow-up but none of them was related to the treatment; one patient had suffered from meningoencephalitis that was discovered after death [54]. Phase 2 study was conducted in 300 immunized patients and 72 patients treated with adjuvant alone. Of the 300 treated cases, 19.7% developed antibody responses; discrete cognitive differences and decreased CSF tau were also observed among antibody responders. However, meningoencephalitis appeared in 18 cases (6%) [55]. Because of this complication, immunization was stopped after one (two patients), two (274 patients), and three (24 patients) injections [56]. Interestingly, increased loss of brain volume did not parallel impaired cognitive function; this dissociation was attributed to reduced β-amyloid content and associated fluids in responders over placebo [57].

Aβ immunization generated Aβ N-terminal antibodies to Aβ1-8 peptide that were not dependent on Aβ conformation or aggregation [58], but meningoencephalitis was attributed to the presence of T-cells [59].

Neuropathological studies of the first cases of post-immunization meningoencepahiltis (figure) revealed crucial aspects that can be summarized as follows: 1. focal reduced burden of parenchymal amyloid deposits (amyloid plaques) when compared with conventional AD cases; 2. lack of differences in relation to vascular deposits (cerebral amyloid angiopathy); 3. no apparent effects on neurofibrillary tangles or neuropil threads, but reduced tau deposits in relation to plaques; 4. marked infiltration of microglia and occasional multinucleated giant cells filled with β-amyloid in places with reduced plaques; 5. residual, very dense and compact plaques; 6. meningoencephalitis with predominant T lymphocytes; and 7. demyelination of the cerebral white matter and macrophage infiltration [60, 61]. Microhemorrhages were found in one case[61].

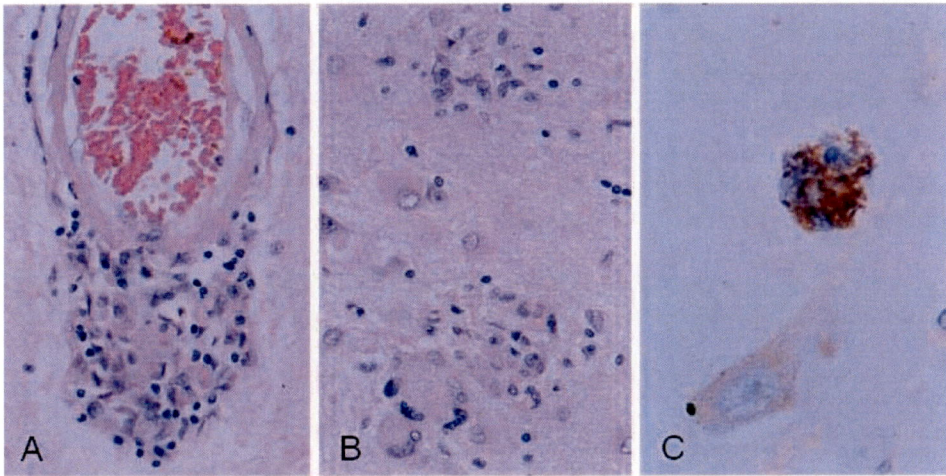

Figure. Side-effects of Aβ immunization in human brain after the AN1792-QS-21 trial. A. Perivascular inflammatory infiltrates; B. Microglial activation and formation of multinucleated giant cells; C. Phagocytosis of compact β-amyloid in microglia and multinucleated giant cells. Paraffin sections x200.

Additionally, proteasome and immunoproteasome activation, together with local presentation of MHC class I molecules, were found in microglial and multinucleated giant cells. Finally, reduced SOD-1 expression and local inhibition of stress kinases involved in tau phosphorylation were consistent with reduced tau hyper-phosphorylation of aberrant neurites [61]. Neuropathological studies in another immunized patient without encephalitis revealed reduced β-amyloid plaques but also the presence of neurofibrillary tangles and amyloid angiopathy in the frontal cortex [62]. Although most antibodies generated by immunization were directed to the N-terminus, immunohistochemistry in the post-mortem AD brains showed clearance of all major species of Aβ (Aβ40, Aβ42 and N-terminus truncated Aβ) [63].

In parallel with the reduced fibrillar amyloid aggregates in senile plaques, biochemical studies have shown a marked increase of total soluble brain β-amyloid levels following Aβ immunization [64]. Since soluble Aβ peptides produce reactive species, impair normal metabolism, reduce blood flow and induce mitochondrial apoptotic toxicity [65], the deleterious effects of solubilized amyloid peptides must be seen as putative complications of Aβ immunotherapy.

OTHER APPROACHES: PHAGES, VIRAL AND NON-VIRAL AB DNA VACCINES

Other approaches geared to optimizing immunization have been conducted, following engineering phages expressing peptide and EFRH [66]. In an attempt to reduce adverse effects, recombinant adeno-associated virus Aβ vaccine expressing a fusion protein containing Aβ1-42 and cholera toxin B subunit was assayed in a mouse model of AD [67]. Immunization resulted in reduced behavioral impairment and a reduction in the number of Aβ cortical plaques in transgenic mice [67]. Similarly, adenovirus vectors encoding the Aβ1-42 or the 99 carboxyl terminal of APP, and granulocyte-macrophage colony stimulating factor (GM-CSF), induced an immune response that reduced Aβ deposits in AD transgenic mice [68, 69]. Effects were more pronounced following immune response by adenovirus vectors encoding 11 tandem repeats of Aβ1-6 and GM-CSF [70]. Also, in the search for safe anti-Aβ-amyloid vaccines, virus particles or virus-like particles bound to Qβ phage linked to twelve amino acid peptides containing the N-terminal and nine amino acids of Aβ produced high IgG responses in the absence of T-cell proliferation, thus minimizing the possibility of encephalitis following immunization [71].

Non-viral Aβ DNA vaccines have also been developed [72]. Reduced plaque formation has been found at 18 months following vaccination starting after Aβ deposition [73]. Combined approaches have also been developed, using plasmid DNA coding for the human Aβ42 peptide together with low doses of pre-aggregated peptides [74].

ADDITIONAL MECHANISTIC ASPECTS OF ACTIVE AND PASSIVE Aß IMMUNIZATION

T-cell-mediated responses following immunization are largely dependent on the dosage of IFN-γ, as transient meningoencephalitis following single immunization with Aβ10-24 occurs only in APP-transgenic mice expressing limited amounts of IFN-γ [75]. Moreover, IFN-γ enhances clearance of Aβ microglia and T-cell motility in vitro, thus together suggesting that limited IFN-γ expression in the brain is crucial to produce T-cell-mediated immune infiltrates following Aβ immunization [75]. On the other hand, transforming growth factor-β1 (TGF-β1) is also involved in the modulation of immunization responses, as increased T-cell responses are found following Aβ1-42 immunization in mice overproducing TGF-β1 [76].

Microglia have primary roles in the clearance of β-amyloid after passive immunization. In the first 24 h, clearance of diffuse plaques occurs without microglial activation. However, compact amyloid deposits are cleared between 1 and 3 days after intracranial administration of anti-Aβ antibodies in Tg2576 mice, and the clearance of compact amyloid deposits is associated with microglial activation [77]. As a complement to these findings, high affinity of the anti-Aβ antibodies for Fc receptors on microglial cells appears to be more important than high affinity for Aβ itself [34].

Additional aspects of Aβ immunization are related to other brain compartments. Studies in humans have shown no effects of immunization on neuropil threads or neurofibrillary tangles but there is a decrease of dystrophic neurites associated with amyloid deposits [60-

62]. In this line, clearance of early hyperphosphorylated tau in triple AD transgenic model occurs via de?? proteasome [78]. Yet no significant clearance of hyperphosphorylated tau aggregates occurs at later stages [78]. The limited efficiency of Aβ immunization in the treatment of associated tau pathology is further supported by the lack of effects on tau phosphorylation after active immunization in P301L transgenic mice [79].

Improvement of behavior and prevention of memory loss have been observed in mice models of AD and in human AD cases following Aβ immunization [80]. Interestingly, β-amyloid immunotherapy has been shown to prevent synaptic degeneration in a mouse model of AD [81]. Moreover, intracerebroventricular injection of Aβ inhibits long-term potentiation in rat hippocampus, and this effect is prevented following the injection of a monoclonal antibody to Aβ [82]. Aβ oligomers are responsible for impaired long-term potentiation in these rats, and are therefore also implicated in Aβ-related memory impairment. In consequence, these observations show that Aβ immunotherapy may yield direct benefits in synaptic function.

Finally, immunization restores blood brain barrier integrity in Tg2576 APP transgenic mice [83].

FUTURE PROSPECTS

It seems clear that active or passive Aβ immunization may be beneficial in AD provided that no risk of vascular complications or encephalitis is associated with the new immunotherapies. Novel immunogens encompassing B-cell epitopes but lacking T-cell reactive sites seem promising [84, 85].

However, several points have to be addressed in the future. Both active and passive immunizations in murine models of AD are less effective when treatment is initiated after the onset of clinical symptoms [36, 86]. This fact, together with the observation of increased brain levels of potentially harmful soluble amyloid peptides in human cases following Aβ immunization [64], suggests that anti-β-amyloid immunization may be most effective as a prophylactic measure when deposition is minimal and degradation of toxic peptides is still efficient [64]. Furthermore, antibodies raised to small peptides target to Aβ B cell epitopes (Aβ 1-15) seem to be useful and eliminate side-effects linked to T cell responses [87]. Moreover, treatments focused on the neutralization of oligomers [88] either alone or in combination with procedures to disassemble β-amyloid should probably be used in the near future. Alternative immunotherapies directed to the β- secretase cleavage site of APP are also promising [89]. Finally, since immunization has little effect on tau hyperphosphorylation, combined measures to reduce hyper-phosphorylation of tau will be needed.

ACKNOWLEDGEMENTS

This work was funded by the Spanish Ministry of Health, Instituto de Salud Carlos III: grants PI05/1570 and PI040184. We thank T. Yohannan for editorial help.

REFERENCES

[1]   Mirra SS, Hyman BT. Ageing and dementia. In: Greenfield's Neuropathology. Graham DI, Lantos PL. Arnold, London, New York, *New Delhi*, 2002; pp: 195-271.

[2]   Duyckaerts C, Dickson DW. Neuropathology of Alzheimer's disease. In: Neurodegeneration: The molecular pathology of dementia and movement disorders. Dickson D (ed), ISN *Neuropath Press*, Basel 2003; pp 47-65.

[3]   Braak H, Braak E. Temporal sequence of Alzheimer's disease-related pathology. In Cerebral cortex vol 14: Neurodegenerative and age-related changes in structure and function of cerebral cortex. Peters A, Morrison JH (eds), *Kluwer Academic/Plenum Press:* New York, Boston, Dordrecht, London, Moscow, 1999; pp 475-512.

[4]   McKeon-O'Malley C, Tanzi R. Etiology, genetics, and pathogenesis of Alzheimer's disease. In: Functional neurobiology of aging. Hof PR, Mobbs Cv (eds), Academic Press: san Diego, San Francisco, New York, Boston, London, Sydney, Tokyo, 2001; pp: 333-348.

[5]   McGowan E, Pickford F, Dickson DW. Alzheimer animal models: models of deposition in transgenic mice. In: Neurodegeneration: The molecular pathology of dementia and movement disorders. Dickson D (ed), *ISN Neuropath Press*, Basel 2003; pp: 74-79.

[6]   Lacor PN, Buniel MC, Furlow PW, Clemente AS, Velasco PT, Wood M, Viola KL, Klein WL. Aβ oligomer-induced aberrations in synapse composition, shape, and density provide a molecular basis for loss of connectivity in Alzheimer's disease. *J. Neurosci.* 2007;27:796-807.

[7]   Haass C, Selkoe DJ. Soluble protein oligomers in neurodegeneration: lessons from the Alzheimer's amyloid β-peptide. *Nat. Rev. Mol. Cell Biol.* 2007;8:101-112.

[8]   Walsh DM, Selkoe DJ. Aβ oligomers -- a decade of discovery. *J. Neurochem.* 2007; Feb 5 Epub ahead of print.

[9]   Ono K, Naiki H, Yamada M. The development of preventives and therapeutics for Alzheimer's disease that inhibit the formation of Aβ amyloid fibrils (fAβ), as well as destabilized preformed fAβ. *Curr. Pharm. Des.* 2006;12:4357-4375.

[10]   Estrada LD, Soto C. Disrupting β-amyloid aggregation for Alzheimer disease treatment. *Curr. Top Med. Chem.* 2007;7:115-126.

[11]   Schenk D, Hagen M, Seubert P. Current progress in β-amyloid immunotherapy.*Curr. Opin. Immunol.* 2004;16:599-606.

[12]   Gelinas DS, DaSilva K, Fenili D, St George-Hyslop P, McLaurin J. Immunotherapy for Alzheimer's disease. *Proc. Natl. Acad. Sci.* USA 2004;101, suppl 2:14657-14662.

[13]   Nitsch RM. Immunotherapy of Alzheimer disease. Alzheimer *Dis. Assoc. Disord.*2004;18:185-189.

[14]   McGeer EG, McGeer PL. Aβ immunotherapy and other means to remove amyloid. Curr Drug Targets CNS *Neurol Disord* 2005;4:569-573.

[15]   Goni F, Sigurdson EM. New directions towards safer and effective vaccines for Alzheimer's disease. *Curr. Opin. Mol. Ther.* 2005;7:17-23.

[16]   Solomon B. Alzheimer's disease immunotherapy: from in vitro amyloid immunomodulation to in vivo vaccination. *J. Alzheimers. Dis.* 2006;9:433-438.

[17] Brendza RP, Holtzman DM. Amyloid-β immunotherapies in mice and men. Alzheimer *Dis. Assoc. Disord.* 2006;20:118-123.

[18] Schenk D, Barbour R, Dunn W, Gordon G, Grajeda H, Guido T, Hu K, Huang J, Johnson-Wood K, Khan K, Kholodenko D, Lee M, Liao Z, Lieberburg I, Motter R, Mutter L, Soriano F, Shopp G, Vasquez N, Vandevert C, Walker S, Wogulis M, Yednock T, Games D, Seubert P. Immunization with amyloid-β attenuates Alzheimer-disease-like pathology in the PDAPP mouse. *Nature* 1999;400:173-177.

[19] Morgan D, Diamond DM, Gottschall PE, Ugen KE, Dickey C, Hardy J, Duff K, Jantzen P, DiCarlo G, Wilcock D, Connor K, Hatcher J, Hope C, Gordon M, Arendash GW. Aβ peptide vaccination prevents memory loss in an animal model of Alzheimer's disease. *Nature* 2000;408:982-985.

[20] Janus C, Pearson J, McLaurin J, Mathews PM, Jiang Y, Schmidt SD, Chishti MA, Horne P, Heslin D, French J, Mount HT, Nixon RA, Mercken M, Bergeron C, Fraser PE, St George-Hyslop P, Westaway D. Aβ peptide immunization reduces behavioral impairment and plaques in a model of Alzheimer's disease. *Nature* 2000;408:979-982.

[21] Weiner HL, Lemere CA, Maron R, Spooner ET, Grenfell TJ, Mori C, Issazadeh S, Hancock WW, Selkoe DJ. Nasal administration of amyloid-β peptide decreases cerebral amyloid burden in a mouse model of Alzheimer's disease. *Ann. Neurol* 2000;48:567-579.

[22] Lemere CA, Maron R, Spooner ET, Grefell TJ, Mori C, Desai R, Hancock WW, Weiner HL, Selkoe DJ. Nasal treatment induces anti-Aβ antibody production and decreases cerebral amyloid burden in PD-APP mice. *Ann. NY. Acad. Sc.i* 2000;920:328-331.

[23] Brayden DJ, Templeton L, McClean S, Barbour R, Huang J, Nguyen M, Ahern D, Motter R, Johnson-Wood K, Vasquez N, Schenk D, Seubert P. Encapsulation in biodegradable microparticles enhances serum antibody response to parenterally-delivered β-amyloid in mice. *Vaccine* 2001;19:4185-4193.

[24] Monsonego A, Maron R, Zota V, Selkoe DJ, Weiner HL. Immune hyporesponsiveness to β-amyloid peptide in amyloid precursor protein transgenic mice: implications for the pathogenesis and treatment of Alzheimer's disease. *Proc. Natl. Acad. Sci.* USA 2001;98:10273-10278.

[25] Town T, Jan J, Sansone N, Obregon D, Klein T, Mullan M. Characterization of murine immunoglobulin G antibodies against human amyloid- β1-42. *Neurosci.* Lett 2001;307:101-104.

[26] Cribbs D, Ghochikkyan A, Vasilevko V, Tran M, Petrushina I, Sadzikava N, Babikyan D, Kesslak P, Kieber-Emmons T, Cotman C, Agadjanyan M,. Adjuvant-dependent modulation of Th1 and Th2 responses to immunization with β-amyloid. In *J. Immunol.* 2003;15:505-514.

[27] Pfeifer M, Boncristiano S, Bondolfi L, Stalder A, Deller T, Staufenbiel M, Mathews PM, Jucker M. Cerebral hemorrhage after passive anti-Aβ immunotherapy. *Science* 2002;298:1379.

[28] Racke MM, Boone LI, Hepburn DL, Parsadainian M, Bryan MT, Ness DK, Piroozi KS, Jordan WH, Brown DD, Hoffman WP, Holtzman DM, Bales KR, Gitter BD, May PC, Paul SM, DeMattos RB. Exacerbation of cerebral amyloid angiopathy-associated microhemorrhage in amyloid precursor protein transgenic mice by immunotherapy is

dependent on antibody recognition of deposited forms of amyloid-β. *J. Neurosci.* *2005;25:629-636.*

[29] Lemere C, Spooner E, Leverone J, Mori C, Clements J. Intranasal immunotherapy for the treatment of Alzheimer's disease: Escherichia coli LT and LT(R192G) as mucosal adjuvants. *Neurobiol Aging* 2002;23:991-1000.

[30] Maier MN, Seabrook TJ, Lemere CA. Modulation of the humoral and cellular immune response in immunotherapy by the adjuvants monophosphoryl lipid A (MPL), cholera toxin B subunit (CTB) and E. coli enterotoxin LT(R192G). *Vaccine* 2005;23:5149-5159.

[31] Frenkel D, Maron R, Burt DS, Weiner HL. Nasal vaccination with a proteosome-based adjuvant and glatiramer acetate clears β-amyloid in a mouse model of Alzheimer disease. *J. Clin. Invest.* 2005;115:2423-2433.

[32] Asuni AA, Boutajangout A, Scholtzova H, Knudsen E, Li YS, Quartermain D, Frangione B, Wisniewski T, Sigurdson EM. Vaccination of Alzheimer's model mice with Aβ derivative in alum adjuvant reduces Aβ burden without microhemorrhages. Eur *J. Neurosci.* 2006;24:2530-2542.

[33] Maier M, Seabrook TJ, Lazo ND, Jiang L, Janus C, Lemere CA. Short amyloid-β (Aβ) immunogens reduce Aβ cerebral load and learning deficits in an Alzheimer's disease mouse model in the absence of an Aβ-specific cellular immune response. *J. Neurosci.* 2006;26:4717-4728.

[34] Bard F, Barbour R, Cannon C, Carretto R, Fox M, Games D, Guido T, Hoenow K, Hu K, Johnson-Wood K, Khan K, Khodolenko D, Lee C, Lee M, Motter R, Nguyen M, Reed A, Schenk D, Tang P, Vasquez N, Seubert P, Yednock T. Epitope and isotype specificities of antibodies to β-amyloid peptide for protection against Alzheimer's disease-like neuropathology. *Proc. Natl. Acad. Sci.* USA 2003; 100;2023-2028.

[35] Bussiere T Bard F, Barbour R, Grajeda H, Guido T, Khan K, Schenk D, Games D, Seubert P, Buttini M. Morphological characterization of Thioflavine-S-positive amyloid plaques in transgenic Alzheimer mice and effect of passive A β immunotherapy on their clearance. Am *J. Pathol.* 2004;165:987-995.

[36] Levites Y, Das P, Price RW, Rochette MJ, Kostura LA, McGowan EM, Murphy MP, Golde TE. Anti-Aβ42- and anti-Aβ40-specific mAbs attenuate amyloid deposition in an Alzheimer disease mouse model. *J. Clin. Invest.* 2006; 116: 193-201.

[37] Bard F, Cannon C, Barbour R, Burke RL, Games D, Grajeda H, Guido T, Hu K, Huang J, Johnson-Wood K, Klan K, Kholodenko D, Lee M, Lieberburg I, Motter R, Nguyen M, Soriano F, Vasquez N, Weiss K, Welch B, Seubert P, Shenk D, Yednock T. Peripherally administered antibodies against amyloid β-peptide enter the central nervous system and reduce pathology in a mouse model of Alzheimer disease. *Nat. Med.* 2000;6:916-919

[38] McLaurin J, Cecal R, Kierstead ME, Tian X, Phinney AL, Manea M, French JE, Lambermon MH, Darabie AA, Brown ME, Janus C, Chishti MA, Horne P, Westaway D, Fraser PE, Mount HT, Przybylski M, St George-Hyslop P. Therapeutically effective antibodies against amyloid-β peptide target amyloid-β residues 1-40 and inhibit cytotoxicity and fibrillogenesis. *Nat. Med.* 2002;8:1263-1269.

[39] DeMattos R, Bales K, Cummins D, Dodart JC, Paul S, Holtzman D. Peripheral anti-Aβ antibody alters CNS and plasma clearance and decreases brain Aβ burden in a mouse model of Alzheimer's disease. *Proc. Natl. Acad. Sci.* USA 2001;98:8850-8855.

[40] DeMattos R, Bales K, Cummins D, Paul S, Holtzman D. Brain to plasma amyloid-beta efflux: a measure of brain amyloid burden in a mouse model of Alzheimer's disease. *Science* 2002;295:2264-2267.

[41] Dodart JC, Bales K, Gannon K, Greene S, DeMattos R, Mathis C, DeLong C, Wu S, Wu X, Holtzman D, Paul S. Immunization reverses memory deficits without reducing brain Aβ burden in Alzheimer's disease model. *Nature Neurosci.* 2002;5:452-457.

[42] Asami-Odaka A, Obayashi-Adachi Y, Matsumoto Y, Takahashi H, Fukumoto H, Horiguchi T, Suzuki N, Shoji M. Passive immunization of the Abeta42(43) C-terminal-specific antibody BC05 in a mouse model of Alzheimer's disease. *Neurodegener Dis.* 2005;2:36-43.

[43] Lee EB, Leng LZ, Lee VM, Trojanowski JQ. Meningoencephalitis associated with passive immunization of a transgenic murine model of Alzheimer's amyloidosis. FEBS Lett 2005;579:2564-2568.

[44] Chauhan NB, Siegel GJ. Reversal of amyloid beta toxicity in Alzheimer's disease model Tg2576 by intraventricular anti-amyloid beta antibody. *J. Neurosci. Res.* 2002;69:10-23.

[45] Chauhan NB, Siegel GJ. Intracerebroventricular passive immunization with anti-Aβ antibody in Tg2576. *J. Neurosci. Res.* 2003;74:142-147.

[46] Chauhan NB, Siegel GJ. Intracerebroventricular passive immunization in transgenic mouse models of Alzheimer's disease. Expert Rev *Vaccines* 2004;3:717-725.

[47] Chauhan NB. Intracerebroventricular passive immunization with anti-oligo Aβ antibody in TgCRND8. *J. Neurosci. Res.* 2007;85:451-463.

[48] Lambert MP, Velasco PT, Chang L, Viola KL, Fernandez S, Lacor PN, Khuon D, Gong Y, Bigio EH, Shaw P, DeFelice FG, Krafft GA, Klein WL. Monoclonal antibodies that target pathological assemblies of Aβ. *J. Neurochem.* 2007;100:23-35.

[49] Fukuchi K, Accavitti-Loper MA, Kim HD, Tahara K, Cao Y, Lewis TL, Caughey RC, Kim H, Lalonde R. Amelioration of amyloid load by anti-Aβ single chain antibody in Alzheimer mouse model. Biochem Biophys Res Commun 2006;344:79-86.

[50] Lee EB, Leng LZ, Zhang B, Kwong L, Trojanowski JQ, Abel T, Lee VMY. Targeting amyloid-β peptide (Aβ) oligomers by passive immunization with a conformation-selective monoclonal antibody improves learning and memory in precursor protein(APP) transgenic mice. *J. Biol. Chem.* 2006;281:4292-4289.

[51] Head E, Barrett EG, Murphy MP, Das P, Nistor M, Sarsoza F, Glabe CC, Kayed R, Milton S, Vasilevko V, Milgram NW, Agadjanyan MG, Cribbs DH, Cotman CW. Immunization with fibrillar Aβ1-42 in young and aged canines: antibody generation and characteristics, and effects on CSF and brain Aβ. *Vaccine* 2006;24:2824-2834.

[52] Lemere CA, Beierschmitt A, Iglesias M, Spooner ET, Bloom JK, Leverone ET, Zheng JB, Seabrook TJ, Louard D, Li D, Selkoe DJ, Palmour RM, Ervin FR. Alzheimer's disease Aβ vaccine reduces central nervous system Aβ levels in a non-human primate, the Caribbean vervet. *Am. J. Pathol.* 2004;165: 283-297.

[53] Gandy S, DeMattos RB, Lemere CA, Heppner FL, Leverone J, Aguzzi A, Ershler WB, Dai J, Fraser P, Hyslop PS, Holtzman DM, Walker LC, Keller ET. Alzheimer Aβ vaccination of rhesus monkeys (Macaca mulatta). Alzheimer Dis Assoc *Disord* 2004;18:44-46.

[54] Bayer AJ, Bullock R, Jones RW, Wilkinson D, Paterson KR, Jenkins L, Millais SB, Donoghue S. Evaluation of the safety and immunogenicity of synthetic Aβ42 (AN1792) in patients with AD. *Neurology* 2005;64:94-101.

[55] Orgogozo JM, Gilman S, Dartigues JF, Laurent B, Puel M, Kirby LC, Jouanny P, Dubois B, Eisner L, Flitman S, Michel BF, Boada M, Frank A, Hock C. Subacute meningoencephalitis in a subset of patients with AD after Aβ42 immunization. *Neurology* 2003;61:46-54.

[56] Gilman S, Koller M, Black RS, Jenkins L, Griffith SG, Fox NC, Eisner L, Kirby L, Rovira MB, Forette F, Orgogozo JM, AN1792(QS-21)-201 Study team. Clinical effects of Aβ immunization (AN1792) in patients with AD in an interrupted trial. *Neurology* 2005;64:1553-1562.

[57] Fox NC, Black RS, Gilman S, Rossor MN, Griffith SG, Jenkins L, Koller M, AN1792(QS-21)-201 Study. Effects of Aβ immunization (AN1792) on MRI measures of cerebral volume in Alzheimer disease. *Neurology* 2005;64:1563-1572.

[58] Lee M, Bard F, Johnson-Wood K, Lee C, Hu K, Griffith SG, Black RS, Schenk D, Seubert P. Aβ42 immunization in Alzheimer's disease generates Aβ N-terminal antibodies. *Ann. Neurol.* 2005;58:430-435.

[59] Robinson SR, Bishop GM, Lee HG, Munch G. Lessons from the AN1792 Alzheimer vaccine: lest we forget. *Neurobiol. Aging* 2004;25:609-615.

[60] Nicoll JA, Wilkinson D, Holmes C, Steart P, Markham H, Weller RO. Neuropathology of human Alzheimer disease after immunization with amyloid-β peptide: a case report. *Nat. Med.* 2003;9:448-452.

[61] Ferrer I, Boada M, Sanchez Guerra ML, Rey MJ, Costa-Jussa F. Neuropathology and pathogenesis of encephalitis following amyloid-β immunization in Alzheimer's disease. *Brain Pathol.* 2004;14:11-20.

[62] Masliah E, Hansen L, Adame A, Crews L, Bard F, Lee C, Seubert P, Games D, Kirby L, Schenk D. Aβ vaccination effects on plaque pathology in the absence of encephalitis in Alzheimer disease. *Neurology* 2005;64:129-131.

[63] Nicoll JA, Barton E, Boche D, Neal JW, Ferrer I, Thompson P, Vlachouli C, Wilkinson D, Bayer A, Games D, Seubert P, Schjenk D, Holmes C. Aβ species removal after Aβ immunization. *J. Neuropathol. Exp. Neurol.* 2006;65:1040-1048.

[64] Patton RL, Kalbach WM, Esch CL, Kokjohn TA, Van Vickle GD, Luehrs DC, Kuo YM, Lopez J, Brune D, Ferrer I, Masliah E, Newel AJ, Beach TG, Castano EM, Roher AE. Aβ peptide remnants in AN-1792-immunized Alzheimer's disease patients: a biochemical analysis. *Am. J. Pathol.* 2006;169:1048-1063.

[65] Watson D, Castano E, Kokjohn TA, Kuo YM, Lyubchenko Y, Pinsky D, Connolly ES, Esh C, Luehrs DC, Stine WB, Rowse LM, Emmerling MR, Roher AE. Physiochemical characteristics of soluble oligomeric Aβ and their pathologic role in Alzheimer's disease. *Neurol. Res.* 2005;27:869-881.

[66] Frenkel D, Katz O, Solomon B. Immunization against Alzheimer's β-amyloid plaques via EFRH phage administration. *Proc. Natl. Acad. Sci.* USA 2000;97:11455-11459.

[67] Zhang J, Wu X, Qin C, Qi J, Ma S, Zhang KH, Kong Q, Chen D, Ba D, He W. A novel recombinant adeno-associated virus vaccine reduces behavioral impairment and β-amyloid plaques in a mouse model of Alzheimer's disease. *Neurobiol. Dis.* 2003;14:365-379.

[68] Kim HD, Kong FK, Cao Y, Lewis TL, Kim H, Tang DC, Fukuchi K. Immunization of Alzheimer model mice with adenovirus vectors encoding amyloid beta-protein and GM-CSF reduces amyloid load in the brain. *Neurosci. Lett.* 2004; 370: 218-223.

[69] Kim HD, Cao Y, Kong FK, van Kampen KR, Lewis TL, Ma Z, Tang DC, Fukuchi K. Induction of Th2 immune response by co-administration of recombinant adenovirus vectors encoding amyloid beta-protein and GM-CSF. *Vaccine* 2005; 23: 2977-2986.

[70] Kim HD, Maxwell JA, Kong FK, Tang DC, Fukuchi K. Induction of anti-inflammatory immune response by an adenovirus vector encoding 11 tandem repeats of 1-6: toward safer and effective vaccines against Alzheimer's disease. *Biochem. Biophys. Res. Commun.* 2005; 336: 84-92.

[71] Chackerian B, Rangel M, Hunter Z, Peabody DS. Virus and virus-like particle-based immunogens for Alzheimer's disease induce antibody responses against β-amyloid-without concomitant T cell responses. *Vaccine* 2006;24:6321-6331.

[72] He Y, Sun SH, Chen RW, Guo YJ, He XW, Huang L, Chen ZH, Shi K, Zhu WJ. Effects of epitope combinations and adjuvants on immune responses to anti-Alzheimer disease DNA vaccines in mice. Alzheimer Dis Assoc Disord 2005;19:171-177.

[73] Okura Y, Miyakoshi A, Kohyama K, Park I, Staufenbiel M, Matsumoto Y. Nonviral Aβ DNA vaccine therapy against Alzheimer's disease: long term effects and safety. PNAS 2006;103:9619-9624.

[74] Schultz JG, Saklzer U, Mohajeri MH, Franke D, Heinrich J, Pavolovic J, Wollmer MA, Nitsch R, Moelling K. Antibodies from DNA peptide vaccination decrease the brain amyloid burden in a mouse model of Alzheimer's disease. *J. Mol. Med.* 2004; 82:706-714.

[75] Monsonego A, Imitola J, Petrovic S, Zota V, Nemirovsky A, Baron R, Fisher Y, Owens T, Weiner HL. Aβ-induced meningoencephalitis is IFN-γ-dependent and is associated with T cell-mediated clearance of Aβ in a mouse model of Alzheimer's disease. *Proc. Natl. Acad. Sci.* USA 2006;103:5048-5053.

[76] Buckwalter MS, Coleman B, Buttini M, Barbour R, Schenk D, Games D, Seubert P, Wyss-Coray T. Increased T cell recruitment to the CNS after amyloid β1-42 immunization in Alzheimer's mice overproducing transforming growth factor-β1. *J. Neurosci.* 2006;26:11437-11441.

[77] Wilcock DM, DiCarlo G, Henderson D, Jackson J, Clarke K, Ugen KE, Gordon MN, Morgan D. Intracranially administered anti-β antibodies reduce amyloid-β deposition by a mechanism both independent of and associated with microglial activation. *J. Neurosci.* 2003;23:3745-3751.

[78] Oddo S, Billings L, Kesslak JP, Cribbs DH, LaFeria FM. Aβ immunotherapy leads to clearance of early, but not late, hyperphosphorylated tau aggregates via the proteasome. *Neuron.* 2004;43:321-332.

[79] Kulic L, Kurosinski P, Chen F, Mohajeri MH, Li H, Nitsch RM, Gotz J. Active immunization trial in Aβ42-injected P301L tau transgenic mice. *Neurobiol. Dis* 2006;22:50-56.

[80] Morgan D. Immunotherapy for Alzheimer's disease. *J. Alzheimers Dis.* 2006;9:425-432.

[81] Buttini M, Masliah E, Barbour R, Grajeda H, Motter R, Johnson-Wood K, Khan K, Seubert P, Freedman S, Shenk D, Games D. β-amyloid immunotherapy prevents

synaptic degeneration in a mouse model of Alzheimer's disease. *J. Neurosci.* 2005;25:9096-9101.

[82] Klyubin I, Walsh DM, Lemere CA, Cullen WK, Shankar GM, Betts V, Spooner ET, Jiang L, Anwyl R, Selkoe DJ, Rowan MJ. Amyloid-β protein immunotherapy neutralizes Aβ oligomers that disrupt synaptic plasticity in vivo. *Nat. Med.* 2005;11:556-561.

[83] Dickstein DL, Biron KE, Ujiie M, Pfeifer CG, Jeffries AR, Jefferies WA. Aβ peptide immunization restores blood-brain barrier integrity in Alzheimer disease. *FASEB J.* 2006;20:426-433.

[84] Shenk DB, Seubert P, Grundman M, Black R. Aβ immunotherapy: lessons learned for potential treatment of Alzheimer's disease. *Neurodegener. Dis.* 2005;2:255-260.

[85] Maier M, Seabrook TJ, Lemere CA. Developing novel immunogens for an effective, safe Alzheimer's disease vaccine. *Neurodegener. Dis.* 2005;2:267-272.

[86] Das P, Murphy MP, Younkin LH, Younkin SG, Golde TE. Reduced effectiveness of Aβ 1-42 immunization in APP transgenic mice with significant amyloid deposition. *Neurobiol. Aging* 2001;22:721-727.

[87] Lemere CA, Maier M, Peng Y, Jiang L, Seabroock TJ. Novel Aβ immunogens: is shorter better? *Curr. Alzheimer. Res.* 2007;4:427-436.

[88] Townsend M, Cleary JP, Mehta T, Hofmeister J, Lesne S, O'Hare E, Walsh DM, Selkoe DJ. Orally available compound prevents deficits in memory caused by the Alzheimer amyloid-β oligomers. *Ann. Neurol.* 2006;60:668-676.

[89] Arbel M, Solomon B. Novel immunotherapy for Alzheimer's disease: antibodies against the β-secretase cleavage site of APP. *Curr. Alzheimer. Res.* 2007;4:437-445.

In: Alzheimer's Disease in the Middle-Aged
Editor: Hyun Sil Jeong, pp. 169-190

ISBN: 978-1-60456-480-8
© 2008 Nova Science Publishers, Inc.

Chapter 7

ESTIMATED PREMORBID IQ USING JAPANESE VERSION OF NATIONAL ADULT READING TEST IN INDIVIDUALS WITH ALZHEIMER'S DISEASE

Keiko Matsuoka[1, 2] and Yoshiharu Kim[2]
[1] Kamata TERAKOYA
[2] Division of Adult Mental Health, National Institute of
Mental Health, National Center of Neurology and Psychiatry

ABSTRACT

A number of studies have shown that oral reading ability is relatively unimpaired in patients with Alzheimer's disease (AD). Further, oral reading ability of irregular words is known to be highly correlated to intellectual function, however, there is scant information regarding that in Japanese speaking individuals with AD. The National Adult Reading Test (NART) is a reading test of 50 irregularly spelled English words that was designed as a tool to assess premorbid intellectual function. We recently developed a Japanese version of the NART (Japanese Adult Reading Test, JART) that utilizes 50 *Kanji* (ideographic script) compound words as stimuli. In our initial JART development study, Mini-Mental State Examination (MMSE) scores in a group of AD patients varied from 11 to 29, suggesting that they had a very mild to moderate level of overall cognitive impairment. In the present study, we investigated JART-predicted IQ results in terms of overall cognitive impairment severity as measured by the MMSE. We divided a JART-standardized AD group into 3 sub-groups based on MMSE scores, as follows: very mild AD, comprised of those with MMSE scores of 24 or greater (n=11); mild AD, comprised of those with scores between 19 and 24 (n=32); and moderate AD, comprised of those with scores lower than 19 (n=27). Normal elderly (NE) individuals, examined in our previous JART development study, were utilized as the control group. Using a one-way analysis of variance (ANOVA) with a post-hoc Sheffe's test, we found that the very mild AD group had a higher level of education than the mild AD, moderate AD, and NE groups. In a comparison of the very mild AD and NE groups, the former had significantly higher JART-predicted IQ results, whereas the obtained IQ values were not significantly different. These results were considered to reflect different premorbid educational and intelligence levels. In contrast, the moderate AD group, which had the same educational level as the NE group, had lower obtained IQ values than the NE group, whereas the JART-predicted IQ results did not differ. As for the mild AD group, the JART-predicted and obtained IQ results were not significantly different from those of the NE group. However, the discrepancy between

JART-predicted and obtained IQ was large in the mild AD group as compared to the NE group (9.5 vs. 0.5). These results suggest that JART-predicted IQ is valid for individuals with very mild to moderate levels of AD.

INTRODUCTION

For clinical evaluation of dementia, assessment of patient premorbid intelligence level may be useful for the detection of cognitive decline. However, information regarding intellectual ability prior to the onset of dementia are rarely available, thus development of methods to estimate premorbid intelligence is important. Although no perfect method for estimating premorbid ability presently exists (O'Carroll, 1995), several approaches have been developed and are currently employed, including those based on reading ability, vocabulary score, demographic variables, and word decision tasks (table 1).

Among these approaches, one of the most popular methods for estimating premorbid intelligence utilizes oral reading of irregular words. We recently developed an oral reading test (Japanese Adult Reading Test, JART) (Matsuoka, Uno, Kasai, Koyama, and Kim, 2006) for estimation of premorbid intelligence in Japanese individuals with Alzheimer's disease (AD). In this study, we conducted additional investigations regarding the validity of JART for individuals with different levels of AD.

NATIONAL ADULT READING TEST (NART)

JART is a Japanese version of the National Adult Reading Test (NART) (Nelson, 1981; Nelson and Willison, 1991), which is a test of oral reading ability comprised of 50 irregular words that was developed in England about 30 years ago.

Word-reading ability is strongly correlated with general intelligence level (Nelson and McKenna, 1975; Nelson and O'Connell, 1978) and the ability to read aloud is known to remain relatively intact in patients with dementia (Appell, Kertesz, and Fisman, 1982; Blair, Marczinski, Davis-Faroqie, and Kertesz, 2007; Cummings, Houlihan, and Hill, 1986; Hart, 1988; Nelson and McKenna, 1975; Nelson and O'Connell, 1978; Raymer and Berndt, 1996; Vuorinen, Laine, and Rinne, 2000). Based on these findings, oral reading ability is considered able to reveal premorbid intelligence level in patients with dementia.

The NART consists of 50 irregular words that are phonetically irregular, thus guesswork from spelling will not provide the correct pronunciation. If the subject does not know the irregular word, correct pronunciation cannot be guessed. Therefore, NART performance is thought to depend more on previous verbal knowledge than on current cognitive capacity (Nelson et al., 1978).

Table 1. Methods for predicting premorbid intelligence level in neurologically relevant English-speaking patients

Authors	Name of method	Population	Characteristics of method
Nelson & McKenna, 1975	Schonell Graded Word Reading Test (GWRT)	United Kingdom	Regression of score of Schonell Graded Word Reading Test raw score on full scale IQ
Nelson & KcKenna, 1975	Vocabulary subtest score	United Kingdom	Regression of Vocabulary subscale of Wechsler Adult Intelligence Scale (WAIS) score on full scale IQ
Wilson, et al., 1978	Wilson Index	United States	Estimation of WAIS IQ from demographic variables (i.e., age, sex, race, education, and occupation) in sample used for 1955 WAIS standardization
Nelson & O'Connell, 1978; Nelson, 1981	National Adult Reading Test (NART)	United Kingdom	Estimation of WAIS IQ from error score of 50 irregular words
Barona, et al., 1984	Demographically based index of premorbid IQ for the WAIS-R	United Kingdom	Age, sex, race, education, occupation, region-based prediction of WAIS-R intelligence
Crawford, et al., 1989a	National Adult Reading Test (NART)	United Kingdom	New regression equation generated with combination of standardization sample and cross-validation sample
Crawford, et al., 1989b	Regression equations estimating IQ from demographic variables	United Kingdom	Regression equations for estimation of premorbid IQ from demographic variables in a UK population
Beardsall & Brayne, 1990	Shortened NART	United Kingdom	Using the first half of NART words
Nelson, et al., 1991	National Adult Reading Test (NART), second edition	United Kingdom	Re-standardization of NART against WAIS-R IQ
Baddeley, et al., 1993	Spot-the-Word Test (SWT)	United Kingdom	Identifying words from non-words (word decision task)
Beardsall, 1998	Cambridge Contextual Reading Test (CCRT)	United Kingdom	Setting NART words within semantic and syntactic contexts

NART is believed to be among the most reliable tests in clinical use (Spreen and Strauss, 1998) and it also has a relatively high degree of inter-rater reliability (O'Carroll, 1987). Many studies have shown its validity, for example, Hart, Smith, and Swash (1986) showed that performance on NART was the best indicator of premorbid level of functioning. Crawford, Besson, Parker, Sutherland, and Keen (1987) also noted apparent unimpaired NART performance in their AD patients, while Sharpe (1991) suggested that the ability to pronounce irregular words correctly remains relatively unimpaired in dementia. Later, Bright, Jaldow, and Kopelman (2002) offered reassurance regarding the continued use of NART as a valid estimate of premorbid intelligence in a number of conditions. In a longitudinal study of normal elderly subjects, NART scores did not decline over time (Gallacher, Elwood, Hopkinson, et al., 1999; Korten, Henderson, Christensen, et al., 1997) and NART-R scores obtained an average of 3.5 years following WAIS-R testing correlated well with earlier obtained IQ scores (Berry, Carpenter, and Campbell, 1994). Also, the correlations between IQ at age 11 and NART scores at age 80 were significant in groups with and without dementia (McGurn, Starr, Topfer, et al., 2004). In other studies, estimated premorbid IQ was utilized for predicting the results of other neuropsychological tests, such as the Trail Making Test (Knight, McMahon, Green, and Skeaff, 2006), and later life mortality (Batty, Deary, and Gottfredson, 2007).

NART PERFORMANCE AND SEVERITY OF DEMENTIA

In spite of evidence regarding the validity of NART, some studies have pointed out that NART performance remains preserved only in the early stages of dementia. Fromm, Holland, Nebes, and Oakley (1991) conducted a longitudinal study of reading ability in subjects with dementia and found that NART was sensitive to dementia level. Further, Paque and Warrington (1995) showed that NART performance declines gradually over time, though the deterioration of WAIS-R IQ scores was more rapid and more severe. O'Carroll, Prentice, Murray, et al. (1995) concluded that NART results seriously underestimated premorbid IQ in patients with an Mini-Mental State Examination (MMSE) of 13 or less. Also, Storandt, Stone, and LaBarge (1995) found significant deficits AMNART performance even in very mild AD groups, while Patterson, Graham, and Hodges (1994) showed NART decline in subjects with very mild AD whose MMSE score was greater than 23.

Paolo, Tröster, Ryan, and Koller (1997) suggested that, while NART is sensitive to dementia severity, the estimated IQ result provided relevant clinical information. Maddrey, Cullum, Weiner, and Filley (1996) concluded that, even though NART-R scores showed a decrement with dementia severity, the decline was relatively mild and they supported the use of NART-R for estimating premorbid intellectual ability. As for the possible slight decline in reading performance with dementia, one longitudinal study suggested an MMSE-based correction for estimating premorbid IQ with AMNART (Taylor, Salmon, Rice, et al. 1996). In addition, Carswell, Graves, Snow, and Tierney (1997) suggested that a combination of NART errors and WAIS-R vocabulary age-scaled score provided slightly improved postdiction accuracy.

In summary, though NART performance might decline in severe stages of dementia, it seems to be relatively preserved in mild to moderate stage, and is considered to be valid for such subjects.

ADAPTATION OF NART TEST FOR LANGUAGES OTHER THAN ENGLISH

The first NART was developed in England (Nelson, 1982) and designed to be read by a native speaker living in England, thus it might be invalid for adaptation for people living outside England. In other words, NART performance reflects the locality of the tested individual. Therefore, NART-like tests in languages other than English have been developed in several countries.

As noted in the former section, the basic idea of NART is as follows. By using a preserved intellectual ability, oral reading of irregular words, estimation of the premorbid intelligence level in an individual with neurological deficits such as dementia is possible.

As shown in table 2, the ideas that led to the development of NART have been utilized to produce tests in several languages for indicating premorbid intelligence, and most studies conducted have shown their validity. Direct adaptation of the ideas extracted from English tests into those of other languages is, however, a difficult challenge. Since some, including Spanish and Italian, have a completely regular grapheme-to-phoneme mapping, not all tests necessarily use irregular pronunciation as the core skill tested (Del Ser, Gonza´lez-Montalvo, Martı´nez-Espinosa, Delgado-Villapalos, and Bermejo, 1997). In the case of Italian, infrequent accentuation and irregular accentuation were used to determine premorbid intelligence.

DEVELOPMENT OF JAPANESE VERSION OF NART (JAPANESE ADULT READING TEST, JART)

We developed a Japanese version of NART. The Japanese language is characterized by its complicated system of letter reading, which consists of both a phonetic script (*Hiragana* and *Katakana*) and an ideographic script (*Kanji*). In most cases, *Hiragana* and *Katakana* scripts are phonologically regular, and reading them is relatively easier than an ideographic script such as *Kanji*.

Kanji words are ideograms. In Japanese standard academic training, more than 1000 *Kanji* characters are taught in elementary and junior high school. *Kanji* script is perceptually more complex and demanding than English script, in that the former is constructed from a much larger number of basic perceptual elements than the 26 letters of the alphabet used to construct English words. Since *Kanji* script is ideographic, it usually has its own meanings. Unlike alphabets, *Kanji* script generally contains fewer phonemic factors, therefore, reading it by guesswork is difficult if one has not learned the *Kanji* script.

Table 2. Adaptations of National Adult Reading Test (NART) and Spot-the-Word-Test (SWT) into languages other than UK English

Authors	Name of test	Language	Characteristics of test
Blair, et al., 1989	NART-R (or NAART)	US English	Validated by North American pronunciation defined by dictionary
Grober, et al., 1991	AMNART	US English	Evaluated verbal IQ from AMNART errors and years of education
Schmand, et al., 1991	DART	Dutch	Consisting of a series of words with irregular pronunciation
Ryan, et al., 1992	NART, US equation	US English	Developing NART based predictions for WAIS-R using an American sample
Del Ser, et al., 1997	Word Accentuation Test	Spanish	Assessing accentuation of 30 infrequent Spanish words
Burin, et al., 2000	Spanish Word Accentuation Test (WAT) Buenos Aires version	Argentina Spanish	Thirty low-frequency words read aloud with stress pattern evaluated
Colombo, et al., 2000	Test di intelligenza Breve (TIB, Italian version of NART)	Italian	Reading performance of words with regular and irregular stress patterns for estimating premorbid IQ
Mackinnon, et al., 2000	French version of National Adult Reading Test (fNART)	French	French adaptation of NART using pronunciation accuracy to estimate WAIS-R IQ
Matsuoka, et al., 2006	Japanese Adult Reading Test (JART)	Japanese	Reading performance of Japanese ideographic script (*Kanji*) compound words for estimating premorbid IQ
Almkvist, et al., 2007	Swedish Lexical Decision Test (SLDT)	Swedish	Word knowledge (decision of real/pseudo word task), which is strongly associated with global cognitive functioning

Kanji script was introduced to Japan from China. However, unlike that used in Chinese, a single Japanese *Kanji* character often has a number of different ways of pronunciation. We show an example of a single *Kanji* and *Kanji* compound words in figure 1. The single *Kanji* that appears at the top of figure 1 signifies "winter", but it can be read as either [*fuyu*] or [*tou*] according to the orthographic content, as seen in the second line in figure 1. Also, *Kanji* characters are often used as components of *Kanji* compound words, in which each *Kanji* symbol provides unique information about the pronunciation of its component characters and the orthography-phonology relationship is word-specific. As Patterson suggested, none of the various pronunciation of a *Kanji* could be called regular or rule-governed, and the correct pronunciation of a *Kanji* compound word must simply be learned as a specific instance (Patterson, 1990). This means that the successful translation from orthography to phonology of *Kanji* compound words requires word-specific lexical procedures, making them approximately comparable to irregular words in English.

A longitudinal case study showed relatively preserved ability to read *Kanji* words aloud until a very advanced stage of the disease process (Sasanuma, Sakuma, and Kitano, 1992) and the ability to read *Kanji* was expected to be correlated to intelligence level in normal individuals. Based on these reasons, we decided to employ *Kanji* compound words in our development of JART.

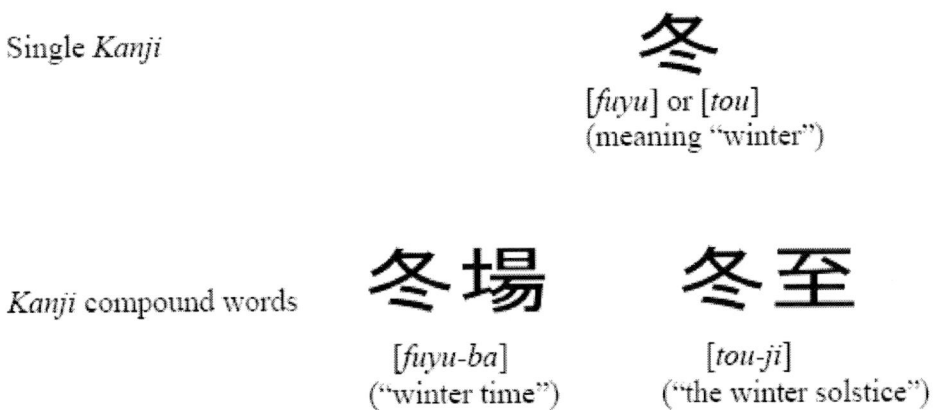

Single *Kanji*

冬

[*fuyu*] or [*tou*]
(meaning "winter")

Kanji compound words

冬場

[*fuyu-ba*]
("winter time")

冬至

[*tou-ji*]
("the winter solstice")

Figure 1. Examples of a single *Kanji* word (composed of one *Kanji* character) and *Kanji* compound words (composed of more than one character).

SELECTION OF 50 *KANJI* COMPOUND WORDS

Detailed information regarding our selection of *Kanji* compound words was previously described (Matsuoka, et al., 2006). First, we selected 100 *Kanji* compound words as a pool, from which 50 were selected for use in JART. For a preliminary study, we recruited 43 healthy elderly persons, who were native Japanese-language speakers and living in the community. In addition, none of them reported having suffered from a major psychiatric or neurological disorder. All subjects were subjected to a reading test of the 100 *Kanji* compound words, as well as 4 subtests of the Wechsler Adult Intelligence Scale-Revised (WAIS-R) (Shinagawa, Kobayashi, Fujita, and Maekawa, 1990; Wechsler, 1981) and the

MMSE (M.F. Folstein, S. E. Folstein, and McHugh, 1975; Mori, Mitani, and Yamadori, 1985). Two of the subjects received scores on the MMSE under 24 and were excluded from further study, leaving a total of 41 (mean age of 69.1 years, 11 females, 30 males). We then calculated a short form IQ from the results of the 4 WAIS-R subtests (Misawa, Kobayashi, Fujita, Maekawa, and Dairoku, 1993). Their mean MMSE score was 28.3, while the mean short-form IQ was 111.1, ranging from 86 to 134. In order to select the items that had the highest correlation with IQ, the correlation (Spearman's r) between a true/false score (true=1, false=0) for reading of each of the 100 *Kanji* compound words and the short-form IQ result was determined. Then, the 50 *Kanji* compound words that had the highest correlation with IQ were selected as the reading components to be included in JART, as shown in table 3.

Table 3. List of 50 *Kanji* compound words used in JART

Kanji Compound Word	Correct reading	Meaning	*Kanji* Compound Word	Correct reading	Meaning
冬至	tou-ji	the winter solstice	烏賊	i-ka	squid
秋刀魚	san-ma	saury fish	団扇	u-chi-wa	round fan
煙草	ta-ba-ko	tobacco	会釈	e-sha-ku	slight bow
水先	mi-zu-sa-ki	direction of a waterway	真似	ma-ne	imitation
不如帰	ho-to-to-gi-su	little cuckoo	抜擢	batteki	selection
委細	i-sa-i	details	案山子	ka-ka-shi	a scarecrow
挑発	chou-hatsu	provocation	雑魚	za-ko	small fry
応仁	ou-nin	name of Japanese era in 15th century	巫女	mi-ko	maiden in service of a shrine
詭弁	ki-ben	sophism	悪寒	o-kan	chills
親父	o-ya-ji	one's father	煩瑣	han-sa	be complicated
息吹	i-bu-ki	breath	呵責	ka-sha-ku	torture
担架	tan-ka	stretcher	流石	sa-su-ga	after all
家鴨	a-hi-ru	a duck	所以	yu-en	a reason
似非	e-se	pseudo	時宜	ji-gi	timing
呆気	akke	be astonished	耽溺	tan-de-ki	indulgence
皮相	hi-sou	an outward look	脆弱	zei-ja-ku	be fragile
何卒	na-ni-to-zo	please, kindly	向日葵	hi-ma-wa-ri	sunflower
甘受	kan-ju	submission	鷹揚	ou-you	be generous
自惚	u-nu-bo-re	self-conceit	紫陽花	a-ji-sa-i	hydrangea
黄昏	ta-so-ga-re	evening	暖簾	no-ren	split shop curtain
河豚	fu-gu	globefish	時化	shi-ke	stormy weather at sea
履行	ri-kou	fulfillment	捏造	ne-tsu-zou	concoction
傍系	bou-kei	collateral line	胡桃	ku-ru-mi	walnut
卓袱台	cha-bu-dai	low dining table	辣腕	ra-tsu-wan	outstanding ability
割愛	ka-tsu-ai	omission	贔屓	hi-i-ki	favoritism

SUBJECTS AND METHODS OF JART DEVELOPMENT

The subjects in our JART standardized study were 106 normal elderly (NE) individuals and 74 age-, education-, and sex-matched AD patients. Informed consent was obtained from all after explaining the aim of the study. The protocol was approved by the National Center of Neurology and Psychiatry Ethics Committee.

NE Group

The NE group was composed of healthy individuals who had registered with an out-placement office for elderly people in an urban area near Tokyo. All were native Japanese language speakers and living in the community. Exclusion criteria were: (1) past history of receiving any form of psychiatric treatment, (2) past history of head injury with loss of consciousness, (3) MMSE score less than 24, and (4) a Center for Epidemiologic Studies Depression (CES-D) Scale score over 15 (Radloff, 1977; Shima, Shikano, Kitamura, and Asai, 1985). Among the NE subjects, 1 reported a past history of medical treatment for depression, none had a history of head injury with loss of consciousness, 2 had an MMSE score less than 24, and 3 had a CES-D scale score over than 15. These 6 subjects were excluded from our further standardized analysis, leaving the NE group consisting of 100 individuals.

AD Group

We recruited AD patients from 4 different geriatric hospitals and clinics located in an urban area in Tokyo. All 74 patients underwent a clinical evaluation including computed tomography (CT) imaging, magnetic resonance imaging (MRI), and a neuropsychological assessment including MMSE. Following the diagnostic process, including a review of the history of each patient with both the patient and caregiver, the attending physician diagnosed AD according to the Diagnostic and Statistical Manual of Mental Disorders, 4th Edition (American Psychiatric Association, 1994). To exclude cases of mild cognitive impairment (MCI), patients whose MMSE score were over the cutoff of 23 were administrated a Wechsler Memory Scale-Revised (WMS-R) (Sugishita, 2001; Wechsler, 1987). We excluded patients whose scaled scores on delayed recall of WMS-R were over 70 points in further analysis, i.e., within 2 standard deviations from average. This procedure left an AD group of 70 individuals. MMSE scores in the group of AD patients varied from 11 to 29, suggesting they had very mild to moderate levels of overall cognitive impairment. We divided the AD group into 3 sub-groups based on MMSE scores, as follows: very mild AD, comprised of those with MMSE scores of 24 or greater (n=11); mild AD, comprised of those with scores between 19 and 24 (n=32); and moderate AD, comprised of those with scores lower than 19 (n=27).

The characteristics of the 3 AD groups and the NE group are presented in table 4. It was noted that the very mild AD group had a greater number of years of education than the other 3 groups, including NE.

Table 4. Demographic characteristics of subjects divided into groups based on dementia severity

	NE	AD			Statistics	Post hoc Sheffe's test
	n=100	Very mild (n=11)	Mild (n=32)	Moderate (n=27)		
Age, mean (SD)	69.6 (5.3)	72.7 (6.8)	70.1 (7.2)	71.7 (5.6)	$F_{(3,166)}$=1.174, P=0.32	
Male, %	37	64	38	15	χ^2=9.023, P=0.029	
Years of education, mean (SD)	11.5 (2.5)	13.7 (2.9)	12.2 (2.5)	11.0 (2.2)	$F_{(3,166)}$=3.95, P=0.009	Very mild > NE, Moderate
MMSE score, mean (SD)	28.0 (1.7)	25.0 (1.5)	20.8 (1.3)	16.0 (2.0)	$F_{(3,166)}$=436.2, P<0.001	NE > Very mild > Mild > Moderate

Note. NE=normal elderly; AD=Alzheimer's disease; SD=standard deviation; MMSE=Mini- Mental State Examination
Very mild, MMSE >23; mild, 18<MMSE<24; moderate, MMSE <19.

DEVELOPMENT AND VALIDATION REGRESSION EQUATION

Detailed results regarding the development of JART have been described (Matsuoka, et al., 2006). Briefly, a cross-validation method was used to assess the validity of the regression equation. To develop a regression equation, we randomly divided the NE group into the NE calculation (n=50) and NE validation (n=50) groups. We then regressed the estimated full-scale IQ (FSIQ), verbal IQ (VIQ), and performance IQ (PIQ) results, based on the number of errors on the JART in the NE calculation group. The obtained linear regression equations were as follows:

JART-predicted FSIQ = 124.1 − 0.964 x (number of errors on the JART)
(R^2 = 0.78, standard error = 6.27)
JART-predicted VIQ = 127.8 − 1.093 x (number of errors on the JART)
(R^2 = 0.84, standard error = 6.02)
JART-predicted PIQ = 117.0 − 0.708 x (number of errors on the JART)
(R^2 = 0.46, standard error = 9.06)

Then we used these equations to determine a predicted IQ for each individual in the NE validation group. In the NE validation group, JART-predicted FSIQ was significantly associated with years of education (Pearson's r = 0.34, p=0.015). Predicted FSIQ, VIQ, and PIQ accounted for 78%, 84%, and 46%, respectively, of the variance in observed FSIQ, VIQ, and PIQ, respectively. Using the FSIQ equation, we found that 96% (48/50) of the NE validation group showed their standard residual within ±2, while the standard errors of predicted FSIQ, VIQ, and PIQ were 6.27, 6.02, and 9.06, respectively.

When the equation was applied to the AD group, 84% (59/70) of the subjects had a higher predicted FSIQ than observed FSIQ (as seen in figure 2). We then examined group differences for JART-predicted IQs and observed IQs using independent t-tests. table 5 presents data from the AD group and the entire NE group. Independent t-tests showed that members of the AD group had lower scores than those in the NE group for observed FSIQ (t=4.75, p<0.001), VIQ (t=3.52, p<0.001), and PIQ (t=5.3, p>0.001). The JART-predicted IQs were not significantly different between the 2 groups (t=0.79, p=0.93). These results supported the clinical validity of JART to estimate premorbid IQ in individuals with AD.

Figure 3 presents a graph that visually shows the distribution of MMSE scores and JART-predicted IQ, while figure 4 shows those for MMSE scores and actually obtained WAIS-R IQ. As indicated in figure 3, the correlation between MMSE score and JART predicted IQ (Pearson's r) was moderately great in both groups (i.e., r=0.43 in NE group, p<0.01, and r= 0.49 in AD group, p<0.01, respectively). Further, the correlation between MMSE score and actually obtained IQ was slightly higher than that of predicted IQ (i.e., 0.54 in NE group, p<0.01, and 0.60 in AD group, p<0.01).

Table 5. JART-predicted IQs and actually obtained IQs

	NE (n=100)	AD (n=70)	t	P
JART- predicted FSIQ, mean (SD)	102.1 (12.1)	102.0 (12.0)	0.79	0.93
Actually obtained FSIQ, mean (SD)	102.0 (13.4)	90.8 (14.7)	4.75	<0.001
JART- predicted VIQ, mean (SD)	102.9 (13.7)	102.7 (13.5)	0.79	0.93
Actually obtained VIQ, mean (SD)	102.2 (14.9)	93.4 (14.0)	3.52	<0.001
JART- predicted PIQ, mean (SD)	100.9 (8.9)	100.8 (8.7)	0.79	0.93
Actually obtained PIQ, mean (SD)	101.4 (11.9)	88.5 (16.3)	5.23	<0.001

Note. NE=normal elderly; AD=Alzheimer's disease; SD=standard deviation; JART=Japanese Adult Reading Test; FSIQ=full scale IQ; VIQ=Verbal IQ; PIQ=Performance IQ.

From "Estimation of premorbid IQ in individuals with Alzheimer's disease using Japanese ideographic script (*Kanji*) compound words: Japanese version of National Adult Reading Test," By K. Matsuoka, et al. Psychiatry and Clinical Neurosciences, 60, p336. Copyright 2006 by the Folia Publishing Society. Reprinted with permission of the authors

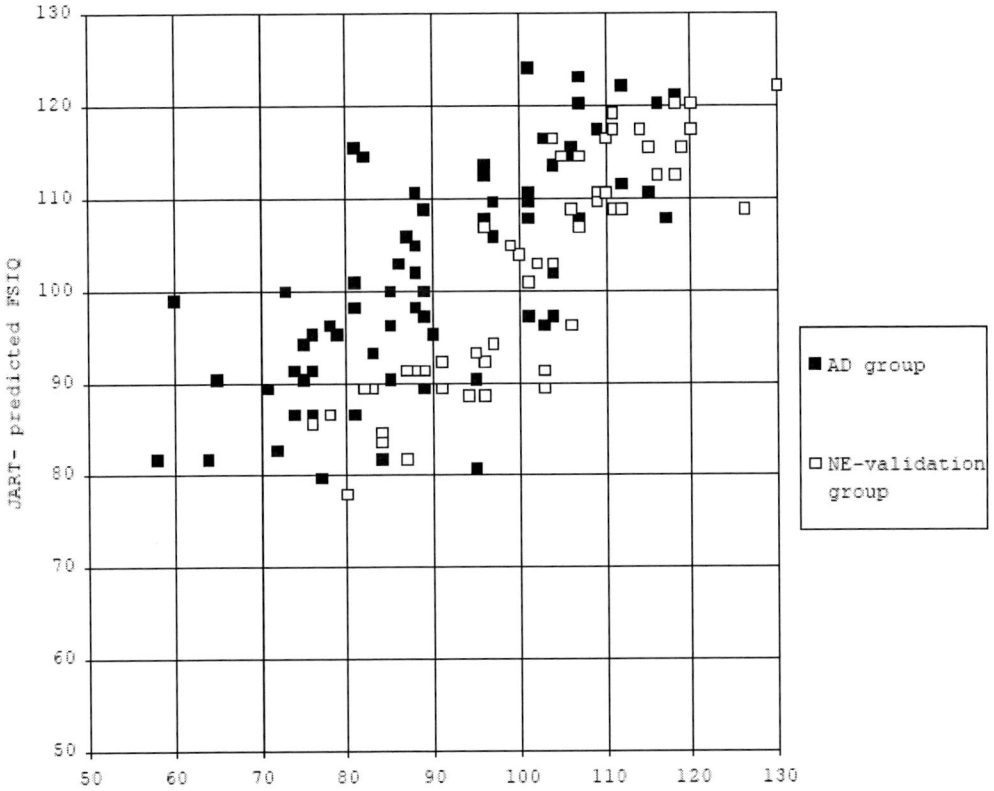

Note. NE=normal elderly; AD=Alzheimer's disease; JART=Japanese Adult Reading Test; FSIQ=full
scale IQ.
From "Estimation of premorbid IQ in individuals with Alzheimer's disease using Japanese ideographic
script (*Kanji*) compound words: Japanese version of National Adult Reading Test," By K.
Matsuoka, et al. Psychiatry and Clinical Neurosciences, 60, p336. Copyright 2006 by the Folia
Publishing Society. Reprinted with permission of the authors.

Figure 2. Distribution of JART-predicted FSIQ and actually obtained FSIQ scores.

The results of ANOVA and a post hoc Sheffe's test regarding group differences in JART-predicted IQs and actually obtained IQ are shown in table 6. Significant differences were observed in JART-predicted IQ between the groups. The post hoc test results revealed that the very mild AD group had a higher JART-predicted FSIQ than the NE group (112.2 vs. 102.1, p<0.05) and moderate group (112.2 vs. 96.0, p<0.05). In terms of obtained FSIQ, the very mild AD group did not differ significantly from the NE group (103.3 vs. 102.0, p>0.05). As for the mild AD group, JART-predicted FSIQ was equivalent to that of the NE group (103.5 vs. 102.1, p>0.05). Actually obtained FSIQ results were not significantly different between the 2 groups (94.0 vs. 102.0, p>0.05). However, the discrepancy between JART-predicted IQ and obtained IQ was greater in the mild AD group than in the NE group (9.5 vs. 0.1). In the moderate AD group, JART-predicted IQ did not differ statistically from that of the NE group (96.0 vs. 102.1, p>0.05), whereas actually obtained IQ was much lower than that of the NE group (81.9 vs. 102.0, p<0.05).

MMSE and JART predicted IQ

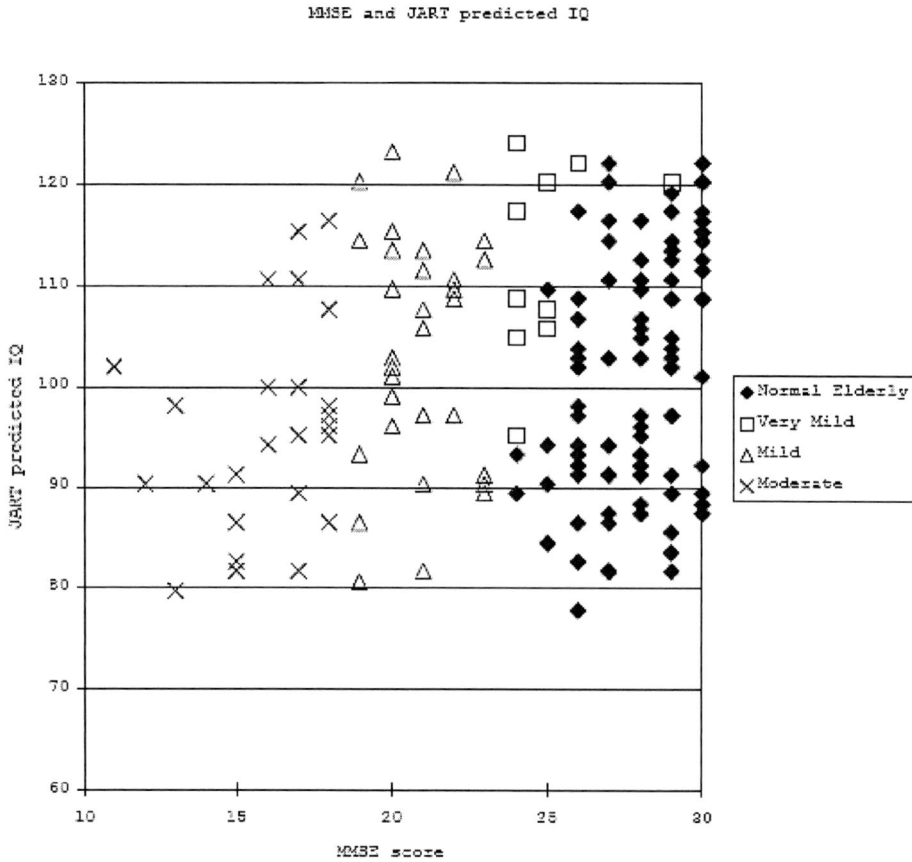

Note.   NE=normal   elderly;   AD=Alzheimer's   disease;   JART=Japanese   Adult   Reading   Test;
      MMSE=Mini-Mental State Examination; FSIQ=full scale IQ.
Very mild, MMSE>23; mild, 18<MMSE<24; moderate, MMSE<19.

Figure 3. Distribution of JART-predicted FSIQ scores in each severity group.

DISCUSSION

The aim of the present study was to examine the validity of JART for estimating premorbid IQ in individuals with mild to moderate levels of AD. We constructed a regression equation for estimating WAIS-R IQ from the number of errors on JART examinations given to a normal elderly group of individuals. Using a cross-validation process, our regression equation was shown valid to predict IQ in those normal elderly subjects. The JART-predicted IQ of the entire AD group in the present study was not different from that of the NE group, whereas obtained IQ was lower. Since the 2 groups were matched in terms of age, sex, and years of education, individuals in both were assumed to have similar levels of intelligence. Our results suggest that the equation is valid for estimating premorbid IQ in an entire population of individuals with AD.

Table 6. JART- predicted IQs and actually obtained IQs in each severity group

	NE	AD			$F_{(3, 166)}$	Post hoc Sheffe's test
		Very mild	Mild	Moderate		
	(n=100)	(n=11)	(n=32)	(n=27)		
JART-predicted FSIQ, mean	102.1	112.2	103.5	96.0	5.4	Very mild > NE, Moderate
(SD)	(12.1)	(9.1)	(11.6)	(10.0)		
Actually obtained FSIQ, mean	102.0	103.3	94.0	81.9	18.3	NE, Very mild, Mild > Moderate
(SD)	(13.4)	(11.3)	(13.6)	(11.8)		
JART-predicted VIQ, mean	102.9	114.3	104.4	96.0	5.4	Very mild > NE, Moderate
(SD)	(13.7)	(10.4)	(13.1)	(11.4)		
Actually obtained VIQ, mean	102.2	104.6	96.6	85.1	11.8	NE, Very mild, Mild > Moderate
(SD)	(14.9)	(14.4)	(12.4)	(10.7)		
JART-predicted PIQ, mean	100.9	108.2	101.9	96.4	5.4	Very mild > NE, Moderate
(SD)	(8.9)	(6.7)	(11.4)	(7.4)		
Actually obtained PIQ, mean	101.4	100.0	91.6	80.1	20.3	NE, Very mild, Mild > Moderate
(SD)	(11.9)	(8.8)	(16.0)	(15.1)		

Note. NE=normal elderly; AD=Alzheimer's disease; SD=standard deviation; JART=Japanese Adult Reading Test; NE=normal elderly; AD=Alzheimer's disease; FSIQ=full scale IQ; VIQ=Verbal IQ; PIQ=Performance IQ.
Very mild, MMSE>23; mild, 18<MMSE<24; moderate, MMSE<19

MMSE and obtained IQ

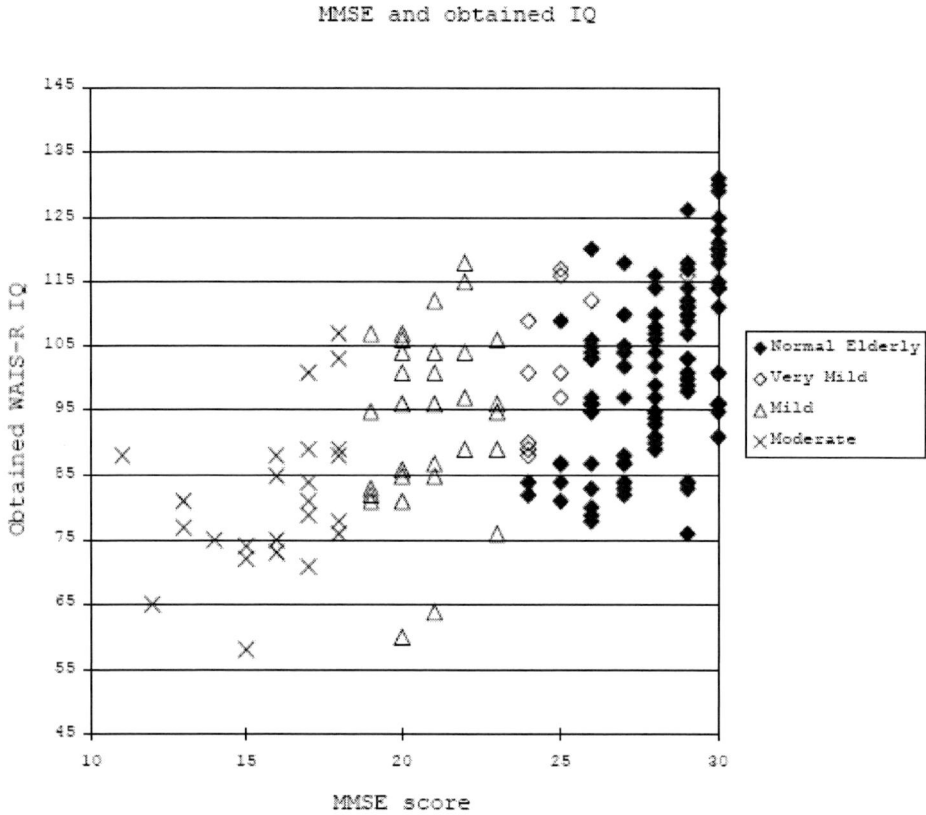

Note. NE=normal elderly; AD=Alzheimer's disease; JART=Japanese Adult Reading Test;
       MMSE=Mini-Mental State Examination; FSIQ=full scale IQ.
Very mild, MMSE>23; mild, 18<MMSE<24; moderate, MMSE<19.

Figure 4. Distribution of obtained FSIQ scores in each severity group.

We conducted a further investigation of JART validity by dividing the AD group into different levels of severity. In the entire AD group, the correlation between MMSE score and JART-predicted IQ was significant (Pearson's r = 0.49, p<0.01). That correlation might be interpreted to conclude that JART results are sensitive to dementia severity. However, it should also be noted that MMSE score reflects not only cognitive status but also education level, as a number of studies have shown that education and intelligence affects MMSE results (Almkvist and Bäckman, 1993; Butler, Ashford, and Snowdon, 1996; Farber, Schmitt, and Logue, 1988; Pavlik, Doody, Massman, and Chan, 2006). Thus, MMSE score may not always indicate only dementia severity, but also intellectual capacity, which is inevitably greater in well-educated individuals with higher intelligence than in those with lower levels of education and intelligence. Thus, a significant correlation between JART-predicted IQ and MMSE score might not indicate JART sensitivity to dementia severity, but rather intelligence level. In our post hoc analysis, the very mild AD group had a greater number of years of education than the moderate AD group. We speculated that these 2 groups were different populations in terms of premorbid IQ. If so, then our result showing that JART-predicted IQ was greater in the very mild AD group might support the validity of JART testing. However, we are unable to make a firm conclusion regarding this point from our cross-sectional data.

A comparison between the NE and very mild AD groups revealed that the very mild AD group had more years of education. This finding suggests that the 2 sample populations had different educational backgrounds, thus different premorbid IQs. Our results showed that the JART-estimated IQ in the very mild AD group was greater than that in the NE group, whereas obtained IQ was not different between these 2 groups. We concluded that the JART results correctly reflected the higher premorbid IQ in the very mild AD group.

As Grober et al. (1991) noted, intellectual decline may provide a better index of an early change in status indicative of very early dementia. Further, the present results indicate that individuals with very mild dementia do not always show a decline in intelligence scale score. By using a tool to assess premorbid IQ, it may be possible to determine if current intelligence has declined from the premorbid level. The discrepancy between the estimated- and obtained-IQ values was 8.9 in the very mild AD group, whereas it was 0.1 in the NE group. Thus, for individuals with very mild AD who do not display intelligence deterioration, the use of a premorbid IQ index may help in the detection of dementia and other cognitive changes.

In the mild AD group (MMSE score of 19 to 23), JART-predicted IQ was not significantly different from that of the NE group. However, though the difference between the mild AD and NE groups for actually obtained IQ was not significant, the difference between predicted-IQ and obtained IQ was greater in the mild AD group than in the NE group. This finding suggests that even when obtained intelligence level has declined slightly, oral reading performance as shown by JART results is well preserved. It also supports the validity of JART-predicted IQ for estimating premorbid intelligence, because the mild AD and NE groups were matched in age and education.

The moderate AD group (MMSE score of 11 to 18) showed a slight decline in JART-predicted IQ. However, a post hoc Sheffe's test revealed no significant difference for JART-predicted IQ between the moderate AD and NE groups. In contrast, actually obtained IQ in the moderate AD group was clearly lower. In addition to the suggestion regarding NART validity for mild to moderate AD individuals (Maddrey, et al., 1996; Paolo, et al., 1997), if the JART score shows a decline it will likely be relatively small, thus its use in estimating premorbid intellectual ability is supported by our results.

Our results also showed that oral reading of Japanese irregular words, represented by *Kanji* compounds, is relatively maintained in Japanese individuals with a mild to moderate level of AD, as has been reported for irregular English words. This result is in accord with previous studies that used Japanese *Kanji* for reading stimuli in examinations of AD patients. Sasanuma et al. (1992) reported 3 patients with dementia who demonstrated essentially perfect oral reading until a very advanced stage of the disease process. In another study of severe dementia, reading of *Kanji* was well preserved in patients with MMSE scores greater than 10, while it was declined in patients with MMSE scores lower than 10 (Nakamura, Meguro, Yamazaki, et al., 1997). Our results are in line with those studies and support the validity of JART for mild to moderate AD patients, i.e., those with MMSE scores greater than 11.

LIMITATIONS

Some caution must be used regarding the limitations of this study. First, our results showed that JART results were relatively poor for predicting performance IQ. This finding is similar to those seen in previous studies with NART. Second, our analysis concerning dementia severity was based on cross-sectional data, thus longitudinal changes of JART-predicted IQ were not evaluated in the present study. To conclude the longitudinal validity of JART-predicted IQ, a follow-up study is needed. Third, the 3 different AD severity groups were not matched in terms of education and sex distribution, which may make our conclusions preliminary.

CONCLUSION

A number of studies have shown that oral reading ability is relatively unimpaired in patients with AD. It is known that oral reading ability of irregular words is highly correlated to intellectual function, however, there is scant information regarding that in Japanese speaking individuals with AD. We developed a Japanese version of the NART (Japanese Adult Reading Test, JART) that utilizes 50 *Kanji* (ideographic script) compound words as stimuli. In this study, we investigated JART-predicted IQ results in terms of overall cognitive impairment severity as measured by the MMSE. Our results indicated that *Kanji* reading was relatively preserved in all of the tested groups, including individuals with moderate AD. We concluded that JART-predicted IQ is valid for individuals with very mild to moderate levels of AD.

ACKNOWLEDGMENTS

The authors thank Masatake Uno, Head of Yoshioka Rehabilitation Clinic, Kiyoto Kasai, Graduate School of Medicine, University of Tokyo, and Keiko Koyama, Tokyo Metropolitan Geriatric Hospital, for their cooperation with this study.

REFERENCES

[1]   Almkvist, O., Adveen, M., Henning, L., and Tallberg, I.M. (2007). Estimation of premorbid cognitive function based on word knowledge: The Swedish Lexical Decision Test (SLDT). *Scandinavian Journal of Psychology*, 48, 271-279.

[2]   Almkvist, O., and Bäckman, L. (1993). Detection and staging of early clinical dementia. *Acta Neurologica Scandinavica*, 88, 10-13.

[3]   American Psychiatric Association. (1994). Diagnostic and Statistical Manual of Mental Disorders, 4th edition. Washington DC: *American Psychiatric Association*.

[4]   Appell, J., Kertesz, A., and Fisman, M. (1982). A study of language functioning in Alzheimer patients. *Brain and Language*, 17, 71-91.

[5] Baddeley, A., Emslie, H., and Nimmo-Smith, I. (1993). The spot-the-word test: a robust estimate of verbal intelligence based on lexical decision. *British Journal of Clinical Psychology,* 32, 55-65.

[6] Barona, A., Reynolds, C.R., and Chastain, R. (1984). A demographically based index of premorbid intelligence for the WAIS-R. *Journal of Consulting and Clinical Psychology*, 52, 885-887.

[7] Batty, G.D., Deary, I.J., and Gottfredson, L.S. (2007). Premorbid (early life) IQ and later mortality risk: systematic review. *Annals of Epidemiology*, 17, 278-288.

[8] Beardsall, L. (1998). Development of the Cambridge Contextual Reading Test for improving the estimation of premorbid verbal intelligence in older persons with dementia. *British Journal of Clinical Psychology*, 37, 229-240.

[9] Beardsall, L. and Brayne, C. (1990). Estimation of verbal intelligence in an elderly community: An epidemiological study using NART. *British Journal of Clinical Psychology,* 29, 217-223.

[10] Berry, D.T.R., Carpenter, G.S., and Campbell, D.A. (1994). The New Adult Reading Test-Revised: Accuracy in estimating WAIS-R IQ scores obtained 3.5 years earlier from normal older persons. *Archives of Clinical Neuropsychology*, 9, 239-250.

[11] Blair, J.R., and Spreen, O. (1989). Predicting premorbid IQ: a revision of the National Adult Reading Test. *The Clinical Neuropsychologist*, 3, 129-136.

[12] Blair, M., Marczinski, C.A., Davis-Faroqie, N., and Kertesz, A. (2007). A longitudinal study of language decline in Alzheimer's disease and frontotemporal dementia. *Journal of the International Neuropsychological Society*, 13, 237-245.

[13] Bright, P., Jaldow, E., and Kopelman, M.D. (2002). The National Adult Reading Test as a measure of premorbid intelligence: a comparison with estimates derived from demographic variables. *Journal of the International Neuropsychological Society*, 8, 847-854.

[14] Burin, D.I., Jorge, R.E., Arizaga, R.A., and Paulsen, J.S. (2000). Estimation of premorbid intelligence: the word accentuation test- Buenos Aires version. *Journal of Clinical and Experimental Neuropsychology*, 22, 677-685.

[15] Butler, S. M., Ashford, J.W., and Snowdon, D. A. (1996). Age, education, and changes in the Mini-Mental State Exam scores of older women: findings from the num study. *Journal of the American Geriatric Society*, 44: 675-681.

[16] Carswell, L.M., Graves, R.E., Snow, W.G., and Tierney, M.C. (1997). Postdicting verbal IQ of elderly individuals. *Journal of Clinical and Experimental Neuropsychology,* 19, 914-921.

[17] Colombo, L., Brivio, C., Benaglio, I., Siri, S., and Cappa, S.F. (2000). Alzheimer patient's ability to read words with irregular stress. *Cortex*, 36, 703-714.

[18] Crawford, J.R., Besson, J.A.O., Parker, D.M., Sutherland, K.M., and Keen, P.L. (1987). Estimation of premorbid intellectual status in depression. *British Journal of Clinical Psychology,* 26, 313-314.

[19] Crawford, J. R., Parker, D. M., Stewart, L. E., and De Lacey, G. (1989a). Prediction of WAIS-R IQ with the National Adult Reading Test: Cross-validation and extension. *British Journal of Clinical Psychology*, 28, 267-273.

[20] Crawford, J.R., Stewart, L.E., Cochrane, R.H.B., Foulds, J.A., Besson, J.A.O., and Parker, D.M. (1989b). Estimating premorbid IQ from demographic variables:

regression equations derived from a UK sample. *British Journal of Clinical Psychology*, 28, 275-278.

[21]   Cummings, J.L., Houlihan, J.P., and Hill, M. (1986). The pattern of reading deterioration in dementia of the Alzheimer's type: observations and implications. *Brain and Language*, 29, 315-323.

[22]   Del Ser, T., Gonza´lez-Montalvo, J., Martı´nez-Espinosa, S., Delgado-Villapalos, C., and Bermejo, F. (1997). Estimation of premorbid intelligence in Spanish people with the Word Accentuation Test and its application to the diagnosis of dementia. *Brain and Cognition,* 33, 343–356.

[23]   Farber, J.F., Schmitt, F.A., and Logue, P.E. (1988). Predicting intellectual level from the Mini-Mental State Examination. *Journal of the American Geriatric Society* 36; 509-510, 1988.

[24]   Folstein, M.F., Folstein, S.E., and McHugh, P.R. (1975)'Mini-Mental State': a practical method for grading the cognitive state for the clinician. *Journal of Psychiatric Research*, 12, 189-198.

[25]   Fromm, D., Holland, A.L., Nebes, R.D., and Oakley, M.A. (1991). A longitudinal study of word-reading ability in Alzheimer's disease: evidence from the National Adult Reading Test. *Cortex,* 27, 367-376.

[26]   Gallacher, J.E.J., Elwood, P.C., Hopkinson, C., Rabbit, P.M.A., Stolley, B.T., Sweetnam, P.M., Brayne, C., and Huppert, F.A. (1999). Cognitive function in the Caerphilly study: association with age, social class, education and mood. *European Journal of Epidemiology*, 15, 161-169.

[27]   Grober, E., and Sliwinski, M. (1991). Development and validation of a model for estimating premorbid verbal intelligence in the elderly. *Journal of Clinical and Experimental Neuropsychology,* 13, 933-949.

[28]   Hart, S. (1988). Language and dementia: a review. Psychological Medicine, 18, 99-112.

[29]   Hart, S., Smith, C., and Swash, M. (1986). Assessing intellectual deterioration. *British Journal of Clinical Psychology*, 25, 119-124.

[30]   Knight, R.G., McMahon, J., Green, T.J., and Skeaff, C.M. (2006). Regression equations for predicting scores of persons over 65 on the Rey Auditory Verbal Learning Test, the mini-mental state examination, the trail making test and semantic fluency measures. *British Journal of Clinical Psychology*, 45, 393-402.

[31]   Korten, A.E., Henderson, A.S., Christensen, H., Jorm, A.F., Rodgers, B., Jacomb, P., and Mackinnon, A.J. (1997). A prospective study of cognitive function in the elderly. *Psychological Medicine*, 27, 919-930.

[32]   Mackinnon, A., Mulligan, R. (2005). The estimation of premorbid intelligence in French speakers. *Encephale*, 31, 31-43. (in French).

[33]   Maddrey, A.M., Cullum, C.M., Weiner, M.F., and Filley, C.M. (1996). Premorbid intelligence estimation and level of dementia in Alzheimer's disease. *Journal of the International Neuropsychological Society*, 2, 551-555.

[34]   Matsuoka, K., Uno, M., Kasai, K., Koyama, K., and Kim, Y. (2006). Estimation of premorbid IQ in individuals with Alzheimer's disease using Japanese ideographic script (*Kanji*) compound words: Japanese version of National Adult Reading Test. *Psychiatry and Clinical Neurosciences,* 60, 332-339.

[35] McGurn, B., Starr, J.M., Topfer, J.A., Pattie, A., Whiteman, M.C., and Lemmon, H.A. (2004). Pronunciation of irregular words is preserved in dementia, validating premorbid IQ estimation. *Neurology*, 62, 1184-1186.

[36] Misawa, G., Kobayashi, S., Fujita, K., Maekawa, H., and Dairoku, H. (1993). Japanese Wechsler Adult Intelligence Scale-Revised, short forms. Tokyo: *Nihon Bunka Kagakusha*. (in Japanese).

[37] Mori, E., Mitani, Y., and Yamadori, A. (1985). The validity of Japanese version of Mini-Mental State Examination in patients with nervous disorder. *Shinkei Shinri*, 1, 2-10. (in Japanese).

[38] Nakamura, K., Meguro, K., Yamazaki, H., Ishizaki, J., Saito, H., Saito, N., Shimada, M., Yamaguchi, S., Shimada, Y., and Yamadori, A. (1998). *Kanji*-predominant alexia in advanced Alzheimer's disease. *Acta Neurologica Scandinavica*, 97, 237-243.

[39] Nelson, H.E. (1981). National adult reading test (NART). Windsor: *NFER*-Nelson.

[40] Nelson, H.E., and McKenna, P. (1975). The use of current reading ability in the assessment of dementia. *The British Journal of Social and Clinical Psychology*, 14, 259-267.

[41] Nelson, H.E., and O'Connell, A. (1978). Dementia: the estimation of premorbid intelligence levels using the new adult reading test. *Cortex,* 14, 234-244.

[42] Nelson, H.E., and Willison, J.R. (1991). National adult reading test (NART). 2nd ed. Windsor: NFER-Nelson.

[43] O'Carroll, R.E. (1987). The inter-rater reliability of the National Adult Reading Test (NART): a pilot study. *British Journal of Clinical Psychology*, 26, 229-230.

[44] O'Carroll, R. E. (1995a). The assessment of premorbid ability: a critical review. *Neurocase,* 1, 83-89.

[45] O'Carroll, R.E., Prentice, N., Murray, C., Van Beck, M., Ebmeier, K.P., and Goodwin, G.M. (1995b). Further evidence that reading ability is not preserved in Alzheher's disease. *British Journal of Psychiary*, 167, 759-662.

[46] Paolo, A.M., Tröster, A.I., Ryan, J.J., and Koller, W.C. (1997). Comparison of NART and Barona demographic equation premorbid IQ estimates in Alzheimer's disease. *Journal of Clinical Psychology*, 53, 713-722.

[47] Paque, L., and Warrington, E.K. (1995). A longitudinal study of reading ability in patients suffering from dementia. *Journal of the International Neuropsychological Society*, 1, 517-524.

[48] Patterson, K.E. (1990). Basic process of reading: Do they differ in Japanese and English? Shinkei Shinrigaku (*Japanese Journal of Neuropsychology*), 6, 4-14.

[49] Patterson, K., Graham, N., and Hodges, J.(1994). Reading ability of the Alzheimer's type: A preserved ability? *Neuropsychology*, 8, 395-407.

[50] Pavlik, V.N., Doody, R.S., Massman, P.J., and Chan, W. (2006). Influence of premorbid IQ and education on progression of Alzheimer's disease. *Dementia and Geriatric Cognitive Disorders*, 26, 367-377.

[51] Radloff, L.S. (1977). The CES-D scale: a self-report depression scale for research in the general population. *Applied Psychological Measurement*, 1, 385-401.

[52] Raymer, A.M., and Berndt, R.S. (1996). Reading lexically without semantics: Evidence from patients with probable Alzheimer's disease. *Journal of the International Neuropsychological Society*, 2, 340-349.

[53] Ryan, J., and Paolo, A.M. (1992). A screening procedure for estimating premirbid intelligence in the elderly. *The Clinical Neuropsychologist*, 6, 53-62.

[54] Sasanuma, S., Sakuma, N., and Kitano, K. (1992). Reading *Kanji* without semantics: Evidence from a longitudinal study of dementia. *Cognitive Neuropsychology*, 9, 465-486.

[55] Schmand, B., Bakker, D., Saan, R., and Louman, J. (1991).The Dutch Reading Test for adults: a measure of premorbid intelligence level. *Tijdschrift voor Gerontologie Geriatrie,* 22, 15-19. (in Dutch).

[56] Sharpe, K. (1991). Estimation premorbid intellectual level in dementia using the National Adult Reading Test: a Canadian study. *British Journal of Clinical Psychology*, 30, 381-384.

[57] Shima, S., Shikano, T., Kitamura, T., and Asai, M. (1985). A new self-rating scale for depression. Seishin Igaku (*Japanese Journal of Clinical Psyshiatry*), 27, 717-723. (in Japanese).

[58] Shinagawa, F., Kobayashi, S., Fujita, K., and Maekawa, H. (1990). Japanese Wechsler Adult Intelligence Scale- Revised. Tokyo: *Nihon Bunka Kagakusha.* (in Japanese).

[59] Spreen, O., and Strauss, E. (1998). National Adult Reading Test (NART). In O. Spreen, and E. Strauss (Eds), A compendium of neuropsychological tests: administration, norms, and commentary. NY: *Oxford University Press.*

[60] Storandt, M., Stone, S., and LaBarge, E. (1995). Deficits in reading performance in very mild dementia of the Alzheimer type. *Neuropsychology*, 9, 174-176.

[61] Sugishita, M. (2001). Japanese version of Wechsler Memory Scale-Revised. Tokyo: *Nihon Bunka Kagakusha.* (in Japanese).

[62] Taylor, K.I., Salmon, D.P., Rice, V.A., Bondi, M.W., Hill, L.R., Ernesto, C.R., and Butters, N. (1996). Longitudinal examination of American National Adult Reading Test (AMNART) performance in dementia of the Alzheimer Type (DAT): validation and correction based on degree of cognitive decline. *Journal of Clinical and Experimental Neuropsychology*, 18, 883-891.

[63] Vuorinen, E., Laine, M., and Rinne, J. (2000). Common pattern of language impairment in vascular dementia and in Alzheimer disease. *Alzheimer Disease and Associated Disorders,* 14, 81-86.

[64] Wilson, R.S., Rosenbaum, G., Brown, G., Rourke, D., Whitman, D., and Grissell, J. (1978). An index of premorbid intelligence. *Journal of Consulting and Clinical Psychology,* 46, 1554-1555.

[65] Wechsler, D. (1981). Manual for the Wechsler Adult Intelligence Scale-Revised. New York: *The Psychological Corporation.*

[66] Wechsler, D. (1987). Manual for the Wechsler Memory Scale-Revised. New York: *The Psychological Corporation.*

In: Alzheimer's Disease in the Middle-Aged
Editor: Hyun Sil Jeong, pp. 191-207

ISBN: 978-1-60456-480-8
© 2008 Nova Science Publishers, Inc.

Chapter 8

THE LONGITUDINAL NEURODEGENERATIVE IMPACT OF ALZHEIMER'S DISEASE ON PICTURE NAMING

Francisco Javier Moreno-Martínez[1], Keith R Laws[2], Miguel Goñi-Imízcoz[3] and Alicia Sánchez-Martínez[1]

[1] Departamento de Psicología Básica I, U.N.E.D. Madrid, Spain
[2] School of Psychology, University of Hertfordshire, UK
[3] Servicio de Neurología, Hospital Divino Vallés, Burgos, Spain

ABSTRACT

Although semantic memory impairment is well-documented in patients with Alzheimer's disease (AD), it remains unclear if this neurodegenerative disease differentially affects semantic domains. Most studies have found that AD patients show differential impairments in their knowledge for living things (e.g. animals), a minority have also reported nonliving thing deficits (e.g. tools), while some have also found no evidence of category-specific effects at all in AD patients. In a longitudinal study, we observed the naming performance of a group of AD patients twice across an interval of one year. We investigated whether categorical effects or intrinsic variables (such as age of acquisition, familiarity, name agreement or visual complexity of the items) have a greater impact on naming performance. We conclude that intrinsic variables are better predictors of naming performance in both, AD and healthy participants, rather than the categorical status of the items.

Keywords: Dementia of the Alzheimer type. Categorical effects. Longitudinal study. Connnectionist models. Intrinsic variables.

INTRODUCTION

Alzheimer Disease (AD) is an entity that causes a progressive neurodegenerative process. At the histological level, AD is characterized by the presence of neuritis senile plaques and neurofibillar tangles. These histological changes concentrate in the cortical regions implicated in high-level cognitive processing and are especially associated with memory impairments. Indeed, one of the principal characteristics of AD is the impairment in semantic-conceptual knowledge or semantic memory: "the component of long-term memory which contains the permanent mental representation of our knowledge of objects, concepts, words, and their meanings" (Fung, Chertkow, and Templeman, 2000, p. 200).

One of the first markers of Alzheimer's disease (AD) is anomia, an impairment in the ability to name items (Bowles, Obler, and Albert, 1987; Gainotti, Daniele, Nocentini, and Silveri, 1989; Hodges, Patterson, Graham, and Dawson, 1996). Despite the fact that the relationship between anomia and semantic deficit in AD is well documented (Chertkow and Bub, 1990; Daum, Riesch, Sartori, and Birbaumer, 1996; Hodges, Salmon, and Butters, 1992; Mauri, Daum, Sartori, Riesch, and Birbaumer, 1994), some doubt remains as to whether impairment in naming differentially affects items from different categories.

A general agreement exists with respect to notion that AD is strongly associated to the impairment of conceptual knowledge and that the semantic impairment in AD is progressive as pathological changes accrue in the brain. Hence, some researchers have proposed a relationship between the degree of brain damage and the impairment of the semantic domains (i.e. living and nonliving things: Durrant-Peatfield, Tyler, Moss, and Levy, 1997; Gonnerman, Andersen, Devlin, Kempler, and Seidenberg, 1997). Connectionist models of semantic memory have proposed an interaction or crossover in the ability of patients to name items of living (i.e. animals) or nonliving (i.e. tools) domains, as the disease extends throughout the neocortex. Nonetheless, while Gonnerman et al.'s model (1997) predicts a better performance of the patients with living things at the beginning of the disease, and a worse performance with nonliving things at final stages, Tyler et al.'s model (1997, 2000) predicts exactly the opposite: a better performance with nonliving things at the beginning of the disease and an alteration of living things at final stages (see figure 1). These models are, of course, mutually incompatible.

Another approach suggests that concepts pertaining to the living thing domain may require a greater degree of processing or "cognitive effort" because of the fact that intrinsic variables such as age of acquisition, familiarity, visual complexity, and so on benefit nonliving things (Funnell and Sheridan, 1992; Moreno-Martínez, Tallón-Barranco, and Frank-García, 2007; Stewart, Parkin, and Hunking, 1992; Tippett, Grossman, and Farah, 1996). As general a rule, these variables are detrimental to the identification of living thing items, since the latter have less familiarity and greater visual complexity than nonliving things. It has therefore been proposed that the normal pattern in neuropsychological studies would be to find more cases of living thing impairments (Laws, Crawford, Gnoato and Sartori, 2007; Tippett, Meier, Blackwood, and Diaz-Asper, 2007). A study by Cuetos, Dobarro, and Martínez (2005) did not find evidence of a significant influence of domain in AD patients. On the contrary, Cuetos and collaborators found that intrinsic variables such as the age of acquisition, familiarity and lexical frequency were the significant factors underlying naming success. Similarly, Tippett et al. (2007) recently reported that the determining factor in finding category-specific impairment in AD was the degree of experimental control over such intrinsic variables. Finally, a meta-analytic study of category-specific impairment in AD by Laws, Adlington, Gale, Moreno-Martínez, and Sartori (2007) examined over 500 AD and 500 controls. They found that although the majority of studies report larger living than nonliving impairments, the effect sizes across the living and nonliving domains do not significantly differ.

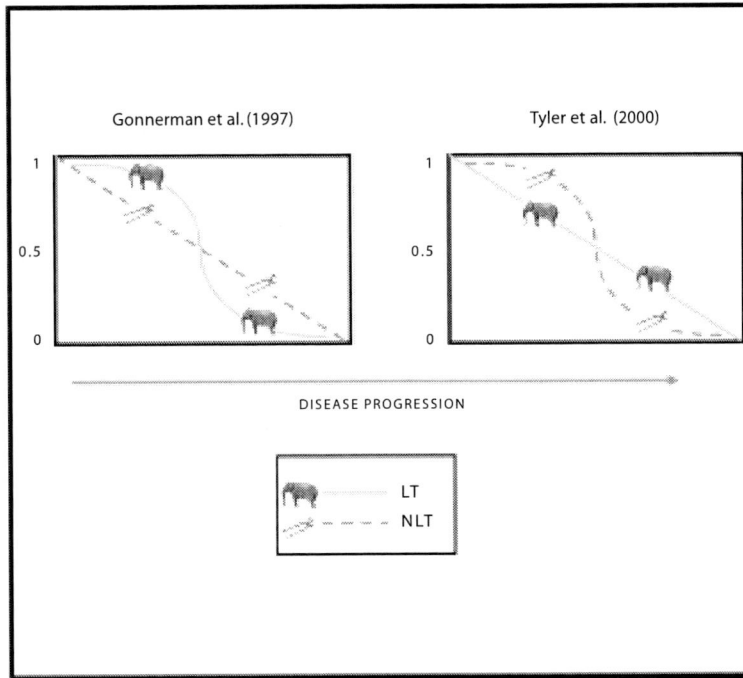

Figure 1. Progression of the disease and the naming of living thing (LT) and nonliving things (NLT), according to the proposal of connectionist models: Gonnerman et al. (1997) and Tyler et al. (2000).

If the interaction proposed by connectionist models is genuine, this effect should be detectable in longitudinal studies with AD patients. In general, most studies on category-specificity in AD have been cohort ones (but see Cuetos, Rosci, Laiacona, and Capitani, 2007; Garrard, Lambon Ralph, Watson, Powis, Patterson, and Hodges, 2001). Nevertheless, longitudinal studies are more appropriate to detect reliable changes across time, since they exclude individual differences as a confound. Although more difficult to carry out than cohort studies, longitudinal ones are especially useful to investigate diseases progressive and insidious, such as AD is (Braak and Braak, 1991). Our target was to investigate the relevant factors during the evolution of AD by carrying out a longitudinal study and carefully controlling the confounding effects of intrinsic variables.

METHOD

Participants

Two groups taken part in this study: a control group of 16 healthy elderly volunteers (8 women and 8 men) and an experimental group of 14 AD patients (9 women and 5 men) (table 1). The group of patients did not differ statistically from the control participants with regard to age $t(28) = -0.54$, n.s., or educational level $t(28) = .39$, n.s. The Mini Mental State Examination (MMSE: Folstein, Folstein, and McHugh, 1975) scores, after correcting for age and educational level in the Spanish population (Blesa et al., 2001), were of course significantly lower in the group of patients $t(28) = 7.18; p < .001$.

Table 1. Demographic characteristics of the groups

	Controls (n=16)	Patients (n=14)
Age mean (*SD*)	71.1 (7.7)	72.8 (9.0)
Education mean (*SD*)	8.8 (3.9)	8.1 (6.2)
MMSE mean (*SD*)	28.4 (2.1)	21.2 (3.3)

SD = Standard deviation.

The patients were diagnosed by senior neurologists at the Neurology Section of the Hospital "Divino Vallés" in Burgos, Spain. These patients underwent neurological examination, laboratory tests and brain imaging to rule out other possible causes of dementia. All the patients fulfilled the NINCDS-ADRDA criteria (McKhann, Drachman, Folstein, Katzman, Price, and Stadlan, 1984) and DSM-IV-TR for probable AD. No patient showed depression or any other medical or neurological condition which might have affected their cognitive performance.

The control group consisted of healthy elderly volunteers with no history of alcoholism, drug abuse, psychiatric or neurological disorders. An additional exclusion criterion was a score below 25 in the MMSE, since according to Blesa et al. (2001), a score under 25 could indicate cognitive impairment in Spanish speakers. All the participants, or their families, gave their informed consent to participate in the study. All participants were native Spanish speakers.

The patients were evaluated twice with a temporal interval of approximately a year. The first evaluation was carried out between January and April of 2004, the second one between February and April of 2005. The participants of the control group were evaluated once. All the patients were given the same list of photographs as well as the MMSE, in each evaluation.

Task

The participants had to individually name the items in the photograph naming task of the *Nombela* semantic battery (Moreno and Cañamón, 2005). This task is formed by 112 colour photographs of stimuli: 56 from the LT domain and 56 from the NLT domain (see Appendix 1 and 2). All the items were rated according to Spanish norms by asking 62 healthy elderly Spanish speakers to rate for the following intrinsic variables (Moreno-Martínez and Peraita, 2007): (a) age of acquisition, which reflects how early in life a word is acquired. Scores were obtained by asking participants to rate age of acquisition of each word on a scale (range: 0-13 years or more); (LT = 5.5, NLT = 6; t = -1.11, p = .3); (b) familiarity, which reflects how usual instances of a given concept are in one's realm of experience. Scores were obtained by asking participants to rate on a 5-point scale (5 = very familiar) how often they encounter instances of a given concept or think about it (LT = 2.9, NLT = 3.3; t = -1.54, p = .13); (c) name agreement, which reflects the percentage of times each name was given by the participants (LT = 84.6%, NLT = 91.5%; t = -2.36, p = .02); (d) manipulability, which reflects the degree the use of the human hand is necessary for this object performs its function. Scores were obtained by asking participants to rate on a 5-point scale (5 = very manipulable) how manipulable they found a thing (LT = 2.2, NLT = 3.7; t = -8.3, p = .0001); (e) visual complexity, which reflects the amount of detail or intricacy of lines in the photographs on a 5-point scale (5 = very complex); (LT = 2.6, NLT = 2.5; t = 0.3, p = .8).

The following intrinsic variables of the photographs were also considered: (a) prototypicality of the stimuli according to Soto, Sebastián, García, and del Amo (1994). In their study, 356 normal controls were given a limited amount of time to name as many items as possible belonging to a given category. The frequency of each item was recorded as a measure of its prototypicality (LT = 154.3, NLT = 176.4; t = -1.8, p = .14); (b) lexical frequency of the stimulus words in the Spanish lexicon (Sebastián, Martí, Carreiras, and Cuetos, 2000) after logarithmic transformation (LT = 3.4, NLT = 4.1; t = -2.38, p = .02).

The images were presented randomly one by one on a computer monitor, where they remained until the participant gave a response; this was followed by a three-second inter-stimulus interval before the next item. If no answer was forthcoming, there was a 10-second interval before moving on to the next item. When a patient was unable to name the photograph, she/he was encouraged to keep trying, but they were never provided with any cues. An answer was considered correct when the participant gave the name of the stimulus or other names considered (by the authors and an independent judge) to be synonymous with the target item name. For example, saying 'pot' for the stimulus 'pan' (in Spanish, *cazuela* for *cacerola*). Proportion of correct answers for each participant and group was calculated.

RESULTS

Table 2 shows the proportion of correct answer for the participants. A multiple regression analysis was conducted for each group and, in case of the AD patients, two regression analyses were conducted (Albanese, 2007; Perri, Carlesimo, Zannino, Mauri, Muolo, and Pettenati, 2003; Silveri, Cappa, Mariotti, and Puopolo, 2002; Zannino, Perri, Carlesimo, Pasqualetti, and Caltagirone, 2002). The dependent variable was the proportion of items correctly named. The independent variables or predictors of naming were the seven intrinsic variables mentioned above with domain coded as a dummy variable (1 = living, 0 = nonliving).

Table 3 shows the results obtained; in the group of patients, the variables age of acquisition, lexical frequency, manipulability and name agreement significantly predicted item naming. With regard to the controls, only name agreement predicted item naming. As a general rule, normal controls better named items with a greater name agreement; while AD patients better named items with a higher lexical frequency, manipulability and name agreement, and an earlier age of acquisition. Notably, domain was not a predictor in either of the group.

Table 2. Naming proportion of the normal controls and the patients at first (Patients-1) and second (Patients-2) evaluations

	Controls				Patients-1				Patients-2		
	LT	NLT	Total		LT	NLT	Total		LT	NLT	Total
C1	.84	.96	.90	P9-1	.64	.77	.71	P9-2	.54	.79	.67
C2	.93	.96	.95	P15-1	.61	.73	.67	P15-2	.61	.71	.66
C3	.84	.95	.90	P16-1	.73	.84	.79	P16-2	.64	.77	.71
C4	.70	.93	.82	P17-1	.82	.89	.86	P17-2	.73	.86	.80
C5	.95	.96	.96	P18-1	.38	.41	.40	P18-2	.30	.16	.23
C6	.80	.86†	.83	P21-1	.57	.93‡	.75	P21-2	.63	.88	.76
C7	.86	.93	.90	P23-1	.46	.68	.57	P23-2	.38	.52	.45†
C8	.80	.91	.86	P24-1	.59	.88	.74	P24-2	-	-	-
C9	.88	.98	.93	P25-1	.64	.68†	.66	P25-2	.57	.63	.60
C10	.95	.98	.97	P26-1	.46	.70	.58	P26-2	.43	.63	.53
C11	.86	.98	.92	P27-1	.70	.89	.80	P27-2	.73	.93	.83
C12	.93	.98	.96	P29-1	.71	.93	.82	P29-2	.68	.93	.81
C13	.95	.95	.95	P32-1	.71	.75	.73	P32-2	.57	.77	.67
C14	.95	.96	.96	P33-1	.75	.84	.80	P33-2	.82	.88	.85
C15	.86	.96	.91								
C16	.77	.98‡	.88								

- = not tested. † Better LT naming. ‡ Better NLT naming.

Table 3. Multiple correlation and semi-partial coefficient for controls and AD patients

	Controls		Patients-1		Patients -2	
R^2 Adjusted	.78		.69		.68	
$F_{(8.111)}(p)$	51.4 (.001)*		32.4 (.001)*		30.1 (.001)*	
Semi-partial correlation coefficient rs (p)						
Name agreement	.552	(.001)*	.342	(.001)*	.354	(.001)*
Visual complexity	.008	(.9)	-.048	(.36)	-.001	(.9)
Age of acquisition	-.016	(.71)	-.144	(.007)*	-.138	(.01)*
Familiarity	.034	(.45)	-.029	(.58)	-.003	(.96)
Lexical frequency	.087	(.05)	.167	(.002)*	.146	(.008)*
Manipulability	.053	(.23)	.077	(.15)	.117	(.03)*
Prototypicality	-.018	(.69)	-.009	(.86)	-.004	(.94)
Domain	-.044	(.32)	-.034	(.52)	-.013	(.8)

Analysis of the groups revealed no evidence of category-specific effects; however, some authors have proposed that because individual variability, category-specific effects may be masked in group analyses (Garrard, Patterson, Watson, and Hodges, 1998; Gonnerman et al., 1997; Moreno-Martínez et al., 2007). Hence, we conducted a logistic regression analysis to examine individual performance. The dependent variable was the individual naming performance (1 = correct, 0 = incorrect). Independent variables were the same used in the previous analysis (Perri et al., 2003; Zannino et al., 2002); table 4 shows the results of this new analysis.

Five cases with significant category-specific effects were found: two normal controls (2/16) and three AD patients (3/14). The pattern was similar in both groups: a participant of each group showed a better performance with living thing items and another one with nonliving thing items; notably, these five cases represented a small proportion of the total sample. Furthermore, only a case of category-specific effects (better performance with living thing items) was detected in patients at the second evaluation.

As with the group analysis, intrinsic variables were a determining influence in predicting naming of items: it was observed a significant influence of the variables age of acquisition, familiarity, lexical frequency, manipulability and name agreement. The better named items were those with a greater familiarity, lexical frequency, manipulability, name agreement, and an earlier age of acquisition.

Finally, to objectify patient's impairment, we compared MMSE scores and naming performance obtained in the first and the second evaluations; both comparisons were statistically significant (MMSE-1 mean = 21.2, MMSE-2 = 17; $t(13)$ = 2.81; $p < .001$. Naming-1 mean = .70, Naming-2 = .65; $t(13)$ = 2.96; $p < .01$).

Table 4. Predictor variables and significance for individual naming in AD patients (P) at the two evaluations and controls (C)

	Name agree.		Visual complexity		Age of acq.		Familiarity		Lexical frequency		Manipulability		Prototypicality		Domain	
	β	p	β	P	β	p	β	p	β	p	β	p	B	p	β	p
Patients-1																
P9-1	.0	.04*	-.5	.3	-.0	.9	.7	.1	1.2	.002*	.4	.4	-.0	.5	1.4	.2
P15-1	.1	.005*	-.1	.8	-.4	.04*	.0	.9	.2	.5	.0	.9	.0	.6	-.4	.6
P16-1	.1	.002*	.3	.5	-.3	.2	.3	.4	-.1	.6	.1	.7	-.0	.6	-.2	.8
P17-1	.0	.02*	-.9	.2	-.1	.6	-.7	.1	.5	.1	.3	.5	.0	.9	.5	.7
P18-1	.0	.4	-.1	.8	-.3	.1	.4	.2	.7	.02*	.0	.9	-.0	.3	.4	.6
P21-1	.0	.06	-1.3	.1	-.4	.1	-1.0	.04*	.7	.1	.1	.9	.0	.4	-3.2	.02*‡
P23-1	.0	.7	-.2	.6	-.6	.004*	.1	.7	.4	.1	.1	.8	-.0	.2	1.1	.2
P24-1	.0	.05*	-.3	.5	-.2	.2	-.7	.1	.3	.1	.1	.7	.0	.9	-1.4	.08
P25-1	.1	.001*	-.0	.9	.2	.4	.3	.4	.5	.1	.5	.2	.0	.3	2.4	.03*†
P26-1	.0	.1	.7	.2	-.8	.002*	-.3	.5	.3	.4	1	.02*	.0	.7	.1	.9
P27-1	.0	.3	.06	.9	-.1	.5	-.5	.2	.5	.1	1.2	.02*	.0	.2	.4	.6
P29-1	.1	.02*	-.6	.4	-.2	.4	-.2	.7	.8	.04*	.0	.3	-.0	.3	-1.8	.1
P32-1	.1	.004*	.0	.9	.2	.4	1.5	.002*	.4	.2	.2	.5	-.0	.6	1.8	.1
P33-1	.0	.1	-.8	.2	-.2	.2	-.4	.3	.5	.1	.4	.2	-.0	.4	.5	.6
Patients -2																
P9-2	.0	.09	.3	.6	-.2	.3	.0	.9	.5	.1	.9	.02*	.0	.8	.5	.5
P15-2	.1	.001*	-.2	.7	.1	.8	1.1	.008*	.3	.3	.1	.1	.0	.9	.7	.5
P16-2	.1	.001*	.1	.1	-.3	.1	.3	.4	-.2	.5	.3	.4	.0	.8	.0	.9
P17-2	.0	.01*	.5	.4	-.3	.1	-.8	.1	.1	.7	.6	.1	.0	.3	.0	.9
P18-2	.0	.07	1.5	.05*	-.6	.01*	.6	.2	.2	.6	.2	.6	-.0	.2	1.8	.07
P21-2	.0	.04*	-.4	.5	-.1	.5	-.2	.6	.4	.2	.2	.5	.0	.9	-1	.4

	Name agree.		Visual complexity		Age of acq.		Familiarity		Lexical frequency		Manipulability		Prototypicality		Domain	
	β	p	β	p	β	p	β	p	β	p	β	p	B	p	β	p
P23-2	-.0	.6	-.3	.9	-.8	.004*	.2	.6	1.2	.002*	1.7	.003*	-.0	.1	2.2	.05*†
P25-2	.1	.001*	-.2	.7	-.0	.9	.5	.9	.2	.5	.4	.2	.0	.9	1.3	.1
P26-2	.1	.007*	.3	.5	-.6	.005*	-.2	.6	.1	.8	.2	.6	.0	.9	-.1	.3
P27-2	.1	.008*	.2	.8	.0	.8	-.9	.1	.6	.1	.9	.1	.0	.1	.0	.9
P29-2	.1	.02*	-.7	.3	-.0	.9	-.1	.8	.9	.02*	-.4	.4	-.0	.1	-1.9	.1
P32-2	.1	.002*	-.0	.6	-.1	.5	-.2	.6	.5	.1	.3	.4	.0	.3	.0	.9
P33-2	.0	.5	-1.2	.1	-.0	.1	.6	.3	.6	.1	-.1	.9	-.0	.6	-.2	.9
Controls																
C1	.1	.01*	.9	.4	-.6	.1	2.3	.04*	-.5	.3	-.2	.7	-.0	.1	-3.1	.1
C2	.0	.3	-7.2	.1	-.7	.3	-1.8	.2	2.5	.1	.9	.5	.0	.5	-.3	.9
C3	.0	.1	1.2	.2	-.8	.7	.8	.3	1.6	.004*	1.1	.1	-.0	.2	2.4	.1
C4	.1	.02*	1.7	.1	-.3	.2	.1	.8	.9	.02*	.3	.6	-.0	.4	-.8	.5
C5	.0	.3	-2.1	.2	-.2	.6	-1.4	.2	.1	.8	1.1	.4	.0	.3	.6	.8
C6	.1	.009*	.6	.5	.2	.4	.3	.5	1.4	.04*	.5	.3	.0	.4	3.0	.03*†
C7	.1	.009*	.5	.5	.2	.5	1.2	.1	-.0	.9	-.0	.9	.0	.7	.2	.9
C8	.1	.01*	.7	.4	.5	.04*	.8	.1	.5	.2	.8	.1	-.0	.8	2.0	.09
C9	.1	.04*	.1	.9	-1.5	.05*	.7	.5	-.7	.3	-1.3	.2	-.0	.2	-5.8	.07
C10	.0	.9	-.9	.6	-.8	.1	.9	.5	-.1	.9	-.5	.5	.0	.6	-3.2	.2
C11	.1	.03*	.9	.6	-.2	.5	1.1	.5	-.2	.7	1.2	.5	.0	.1	-1.9	.4
C12	-.0	.5	-2.4	.1	.1	.8	-.2	.2	1.0	.2	3.0	.2	-.0	.2	.4	.9
C13	.1	.1	-.0	.9	.1	.7	1.7	.1	.7	.2	-1.0	.2	.0	.8	-.6	.8
C14	.1	.04*	-.3	.8	-.2	.5	-.2	.8	-.4	.3	-.8	.2	.0	.7	-1.2	.5
C15	.1	.1	-5.4	.1	1.3	.03*	4.1	.05*	2.2	.1	-.7	.4	-.0	.2	-1.2	.7
C16	.1	.02*	-.1	.9	-1.1	.007*	.4	.7	-.4	.5	-.8	.3	-.0	.6	-6.7	.02*‡

† Better living thing naming. ‡ Better nonliving thing naming..

DISCUSSION

This longitudinal study of AD patients aimed to clarify the theoretical debate with respect to the relationship of category effects to the progressive impairment in AD. Three important results were observed: first, that category-specific effects were sparse; second, intrinsic variables had a greater influence on naming than semantic domain; and finally, we found no evidence of a relationship between category effects and time or illness severity (as measured by MMSE) and hence, no support for the proposed connectionist models (see figures 2 and 3).

Turning first to the sparse number of category-specific effects found, our work gives empirical support to recent and methodologically well-controlled studies that did not find such effects in AD patients (Cuetos et al., 2005; Laws, Gale, Leeson, and Crawford, 2005; Moreno-Martinez et al., 2007; Perri et al., 2003; Tippett et al., 2007; Moreno-Martinez and Laws, 2007, in press). Remarkably, a similar conclusion was obtained in our recent meta-analysis (Laws et al. 2007) of 21 group-studies comparing over 500 AD patients and 500 control participants. Unexpectedly perhaps, this review reported similar levels of impairment in both the living and the nonliving domains in AD patients. Nevertheless, it is known that category-specific effects can be masked when a sample include patients with opposite impairments (Garrard et al., 1998; Gonnerman et al., 1997) or "double dissociations" (Shallice, 1988). Precisely this was observed in our study: a lack of category-specific effects in the group analysis, but a small number of significant cases after doing individual analyses. This result emphasizes the importance of analysing individual performance of the participants, since group analysis could mask the presence of category-specific effects. At same time, however, the fact that so few category-specific cases were observed, suggests that this phenomenon is still relatively uncommon. Furthermore, significant effects were also found in healthy participants (Moreno-Martínez et al., 2007). This all suggests that category effects may not reflect a qualitatively different phenomenon that emerges with neurological injury, but perhaps a quantitative exaggeration of *normal* effects (cf. Moreno-Martinez and Laws 2007; in press).

Our work confirms the importance of intrinsic variables as naming predictors and suggests an almost irrelevant role for semantic domain (Cuetos et al., 2005; Moreno-Martínez et al., 2007; Tippett et al., 2007). In particular, our study underlines the importance of lexical frequency and name agreement, whose (confounding) covariation with category has been well established (Funnell and Sheridan, 1992; Moreno-Martínez et al., 2007; Stewart et al., 1992; Tippett et al., 1996). Recent naming studies with AD patients have showed the importance of these variables (Albanese, 2007; Moreno-Martínez et al., 2007; Silveri, et al., 2002; Tippett et al., 2007). As yet, however, the reason for their importance is a matter of debate. It has been proposed that concepts more frequently used have been learnt earlier. As the subjects are learning new information, this knowledge would join to the previously acquired, as a result, oldest concepts would be richer and would have more interconnected networks that newest ones (Steyvers and Tenenbaum, 2005). It seems to be probable that aforementioned variables, and especially the age of acquisition of concepts, potentially provide a greater capacity for resistance to the disease process.

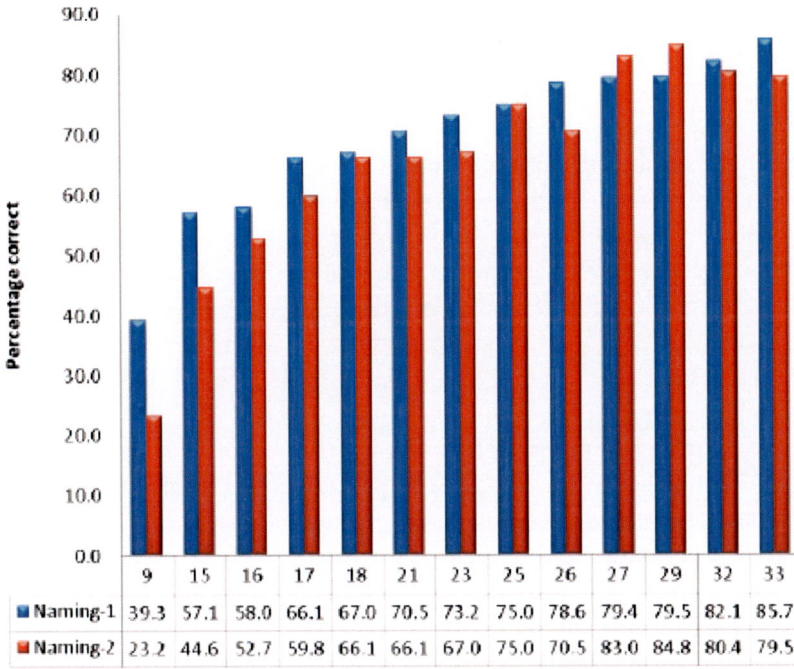

Note. Patients are organised according to naming at Time (patients are indicated by their patient number).

Figure 2. Percentage of total items named by AD patients at Time 1 and Time 2.

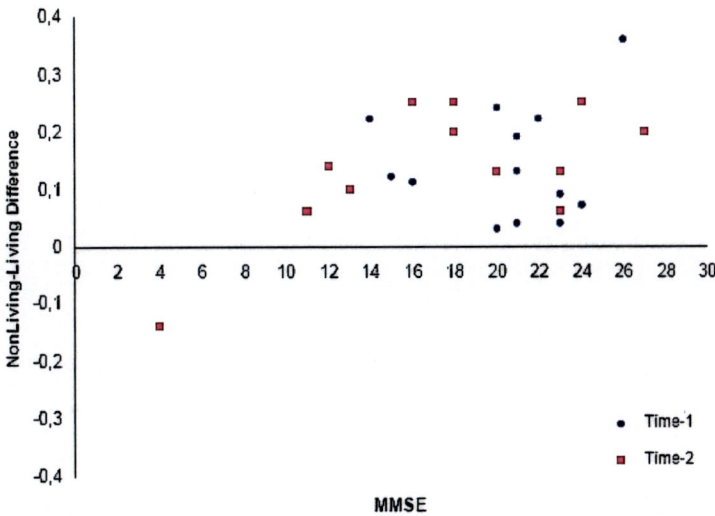

Figure 3. Scattergram showing lack of relationship between dementia severity (as measured by MMSE scores) and domain (nonliving minus living) performance in AD patients at Time 1 and 2.

Connectionist models have proposed an interaction between ability of patients to name items of the semantic domains and the level of brain damage (Durrant-Peatfield et al., 1997; Gonnerman et al., 1997). Increasing neuronal damage will cause either living or nonliving thing impairment. To the author's knowledge, the sole support for the Gonnerman model comes from the study of AD patients by Laura Gonnerman's group (Gonnerman et al., 1997) -although the results from a recent paper by Hernández, Costa, Juncadella, Sabastián-Gallés, and Reñe, 2008, fitted partially with Gonnermans' model-. On the other hand, although the pattern predicted by Tyler et al. (2000) -worse performance of patients with living thing items- is the more usual in the literature (see Capitani, Laiacona, Mahon, and Caramazza, 2003), no relationship emerged between level of impairment and semantic domain in our AD patients. Of course, it might be argued that our patients were not at a sufficiently severe stage of dementia for any category change to be observed or that the time gap analysed was too short to detect change. While we cannot eliminate these possibilities, over a one-year period, the patients as a group did show a significant drop in MMSE scores from 21.2 to 17. The latter represents a large and clinically significant decline, which although matched by a significant naming decline, still revealed no category shift one way or the other. Additionally, both connectionist models propose that a category effect is observable in the earlier stages (either living or nonliving); however, our data provide little evidence of category effects in any patient at any stage and certainly no greater proportion of significant category effects than we observed in healthy controls.

Although our naming data across the two domains provides no support for a change in the direction of any category effect with dementia severity, we should note that effects may be more notable in specific subcategories. According to Moss, Tyler and Devlin (2002), living and nonliving things are more faithfully represented by the subcategories of animals and tools, because animals have many shared correlated properties, whereas tools have little shared information and strong correlations among pairs of highly distinctive form and function properties. By contrast, they argue that fruits and vegetables will be the most vulnerable at all levels of damage because they are close to each other in semantic space and have very few poorly correlated distinctive properties, as well as fewer shared properties than other living things such as animals. Within the artefact domain, vehicles pattern more closely to living things than other artefacts such as tools, in that they have more shared correlated properties. Hence at severe levels of damage, it is tools that will most strongly show the nonliving disadvantage (because of their small number of shared properties). Again, however our results provide no support for these patterns and certainly no evidence of cross-over in any of these subcategories i.e. parallel decline occurs in all four subcategories (see figure 4).

As noted above, tables 2 and 4 document the small number of category-specific effects found and that these effects were found in *both* patient and control groups. The connectionist models mentioned here do not predict performance in the *normal* population; and this is true, in fact, for all models of category-specificity (Laws, Moreno-Martínez, and Goñi-Imízcoz, 2007). The second main finding was the evidence of opposing category effects in patients with a similar level of impairment (P21-1 and P25-1). Similarly, patients with both good (P17-1 and P29-1) and bad (P18-2 and P26-2) semantic performance did not show category-specific effects. Therefore, we would argue against any obvious interaction between the level of impairment and the semantic domain

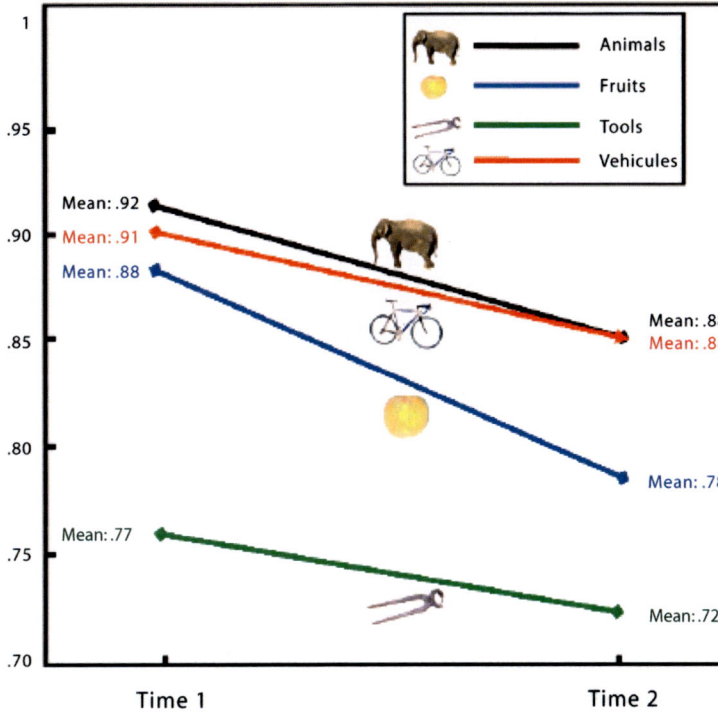

Figure 4. Performance (mean) of AD patients in both evaluations in the critical categories referenced by Moss Tyler and their collaborators: animals, fruits, tools and vehicles.

Summarising, this study has showed some important aspects related to the phenomenon of categorical effects in AD. The first is that intrinsic variables are important predictors of naming performance in both AD patients and neurologically intact participants. This highlights the importance of carefully controlling such variables in studies that focus on category-specificity. The second concerns the almost irrelevant role for semantic domain of the items; this is particularly notable respect to the active role played by intrinsic variables. Furthermore, it is important to stress that categorical effects can be found not only in patients, but also in healthy participants. Finally, our one-year longitudinal follow-up study failed to find support for either of the two principal connectionist models proposed to explain the phenomenon of categorical effects. In fact, our data failed to reveal any interaction between domains, as suggested by these models. Moreover, despite the fact that patients showed a significant deterioration in their cognitive abilities (as measured by MMSE and naming performance), our cross-sectional analysis also failed to find evidence of the proposed interaction. We would conclude therefore that category effects are rare in AD and seem largely to reflect the influence of intrinsic cognitive linguistic variables that covary across category rather than the impact of semantic category itself.

REFERENCES

Albanese, E. (2007). The "hidden" semantic category dissociation in mild-moderate Alzheimer's disease patients. *Neuropsychologia, 45*, 639-643.

Blesa R., Pujol M., Aguilar M., Santacruz P., Bertran-Serra I., Hernández G., et al. (2001). Clinical validity of the 'mini-mental state for Spanish speaking communities. *Neuropsychologia, 39*, 1150-57.

Bowles, N.L., Obler, L.K., and Albert, M.L. (1987). Naming errors in healthy aging and dementia of the Alzheimer type. *Cortex, 23*, 519-524.

Braak, H., and Braak, E. (1991). Neuropathological stageing of Alzheimer-related changes. *Acta Neuropathologica, 82*, 239-259.

Capitani, E., Laiacona, M., Mahon, B., and Caramazza, A. (2003). What are the facts of semantic category-specific deficits? A critical review of the clinical evidence. *Cognitive Neuropsychology, 20*, 213-261.

Chertkow, H., and Bub, D. (1990). Semantic memory loss in Alzheimer's-type dementia: What do various measures measure? *Brain, 113*, 397-417.

Cuetos F., Dobarro A., and Martínez C. (2005). Deterioro de la información conceptual en la enfermedad de Alzheimer. *Neurología, 20*, 58-64.

Cuetos F., Rosci, C., Laiacona, M., and Capitani, E. (in press). Differente variables predict anomia in different subjects: A lonfgitudinal study of two Alzheimer's patients. *Neuropsychologia,*

Daum, I., Riesch, G., Sartori, G., and Birbaumer, N. (1996). Semantic memory impairment in Alzheimer's disease. *Journal of Clinical and Experimental Neuropsychology, 18*, 648-665.

DSM-IV-TR Manual diagnóstico y estadístico de los trastornos mentales. (2002). Texto revisado. Barcelona: Masson, S.A.

Durrant-Peatfield, M.R., Tyler, L.K., Moss, H.E., and Levy, J.P. (1997). The distinctiveness of form and function in category structure: A connectionist model. I In: *Proceedings of the Nineteenth Annual Conference of the Cognitive Science Society* (pp. 193-198). Stanford University, Mahwah, NJ: Lawrence Erlbaum Associates Inc.

Folstein, M.F., Folstein, S.E., and McHugh, P.R. (1975) "Mini-Mental State": a practical method for grading the cognitive state of patients for the clinician. *Journal of Psychiatric Research, 12*, 189-198.

Fung, T.D., Chertkow, H., and Templeman, (2000). Pattern of semantic memory impairment in dementia of Alzheimer's type. *Brain and Cognition, 43*, 200-205.

Funnell, E., and Sheridan, J. (1992). Categories of knowledge: unfamiliar aspects of living and nonliving things. *Cognitive Neuropsychology, 9*, 135-153.

Gainotti, G., Daniele, A., Nocentini, U., and Silveri, M.C., (1989). The nature of lexical-semantic impairment in Alzheimer's disease. Journal of Neurolinguistics, 4, 449-460.

Garrard, P., Lambon Ralph, M.A., Watson, P.C., Powis, J., Patterson, K., and Hodges, J.R. (2001). Longitudinal profiles of semantic impairment for living and nonliving concepts in dementia of Alzheimer's type. *Journal of Cognitive Neuroscience, 13*, 892-909.

Garrard, P., Patterson, K., Watson, P.C., and Hodges, J.R. (1998). Category specific semantic loss in dementia of Alzheimer's type. Functional-anatomical correlations from cross-sectional analyses. *Brain, 121*, 633-646.

Gonnerman, L.M., Andersen, E.S., Devlin, J.T., Kempler, D., and Seidenberg, M.S. (1997). Double dissociation of semantic categories in Alzheimer's disease. *Brain and Language*, 57, 254-279.

Hernández, M., Costa, A., Juncadella, M., Sebastián-Gallés, and Reñe, R. (2008) Category-specific semantic deficits in Alzheimer's disease: A semantic priming study. *Neuropsychologia, 46*, 935-946.

Hodges, J., Patterson, K., Graham, N., and Dawson, K. (1996). Naming and Knowing in dementia of Alzheimer's type. *Brian and Language, 54*, 302-325.

Hodges, J., Salmon, D., and Butters, N. (1992). Semantic memory impairment in Alzheimer's disease: Failure of access or degraded knowledge? *Neuropsychologia, 30*, 301-314.

Laws, K.R., Adlington, R.L., Gale, T.M., Moreno-Martínez, F.J., and Sartori, G. (2007). A meta-analitic review of category naming in Alzheimer's disease. *Neuropsychologia, 45*, 2674-2682.

Laws, K.R., Gale, T.M., Leeson, V.C., and Crawford, J.R. (2005). When is category-specific in Alzheimer's disease. *Cortex, 41*, 452-463.

Laws, K.R., Crawford, J.R., Gnoato, F., and Sartori G, (2007) A predominance of category deficits for living things in Alzheimer's disease and Lewy Body dementia. *Journal of the International Neuropsychological Society, 13*, 401-409.

Laws, K.R., Moreno-Martínez, F.J., and Goñi-Imízcoz, M. (2007). Revisión teórica del deterioro categorial y los problemas metodológicos asociados a su estudio. *Revista de Neurología, 44*, 747-754.

Mauri, A., Daum, I., Sartori, G., Riesch, G., and Birbaumer, N. (1994). Category-specific semantic impair men in Alzheimer's disease and temporal lobe dysfunction: A comparative study. *Journal of Clinical and Experimental Neuropsychology, 16*, 689-701.

McKhann, G., Drachman, D., Folstein, M., Katzman, R., Price, D., and Stadlan, E. (1984). Clinical diagnosis of Alzheimer's disease: Report of the NINCDS-ADRDA Work Group under the auspices of the Department of Health and Human Services Task Force on Alzheimer's disease. *Neurology, 34*, 939-944.

Moreno F.J., and Cañamón S. (2005). Presentación y resultados preliminares de la Batería Nombela (I): Un nuevo instrumento para evaluar el deterioro semántico categorial. *Revista de Psicopatología y Psicología Clínica, 10*, 205-19.

Moreno-Martínez, F.J., and Laws, R.K. (2007). An attenuation of the 'normal' category effect in patients with Alzheimer's disease: A review and bootstrap analysis. *Brain and Cognition, 63*, 136-142.

Moreno-Martínez, F.J., and Laws, K.R. (in press). No category-specificity in Alzheimer's disease: a normal aging effect. *Neuropsychology*.

Moreno-Martínez, F.J., and Peraita, H. (2007). Un nuevo conjunto de ítems para la evaluación de la disociación ser vivo / ser no vivo con normas obtenidas de ancianos sanos españoles. *Psicológica, 28*, 1-20.

Moreno-Martínez, F.J., Tallón-Barranco, A., and Frank-García, A. (2007). Enfermedad de Alzheimer, deterioro categorial y variables relevantes en la denominación de objetos. *Revista de Neurología, 44*, 129-133.

Moss, H.E., Tyler, L.K., and Devlin, J.T. (2002). The emergence of category-specific deficits in a distributed semantic system. In E. M. E. Forde and Humphreys (Eds.), *Category-specificity in mind and brain* (pp.115-146). East Sussex, UK: Psychology Press.

Perri, R., Carlesimo, G.A., Zannino, G.D., Mauri, M., Muolo, B., Pettenati, C., and Caltagirone, C. (2003). Intentional and automatic measures of specific-category effect in the semantic impairment of patients with Alzheimer's disease. *Neuropsychologia, 41*, 1509-1522.

Sebastián N., Martí M.A., Carreiras M.F., and Cuetos, F. (2000). *LEXESP, Léxico informatizado del Español*. Barcelona: Ediciones de la Universitat de Barcelona.

Shallice, T. (1988). *From Neuropsychology to Mental Structure*. Cambridge: Cambridge University Press.

Silveri, M.C., Cappa, A., Mariotti, P., and Puopolo, M. (2002). Naming in patients with Alzheimer's disease: Influence of age of acquisition and categorical effects. *Journal of Clinical and Experimental Neuropsychology, 24*, 755-764.

Soto P, Sebastián M.V., García E., and del Amo T. (1994). *Las categorías y sus normas en castellano*. Madrid: Visor Distribuciones.

Stewart, F., Parkin, A.J., and Hunkin, N.M. (1992). Naming Impairments Following Recovery from Herpes Simplex Encephalitis: Category-specific? The Quarterly *Journal of Experimental Psychology, 11A*, 261-284.

Steyvers, M., and Tenenbaum, J.B. (2005). The large-scale structure of semantic networks: Statistical analyses and a model of semantic grown. *Cognitive Science, 29*, 41-78.

Tippett, L.J., Grossman, M., and Farah, M.J. (1996). The semantic memory impairment of Alzheimer's disease: Category-specific? *Cortex, 32*, 143-153.

Tippett, L.J., Meier, S.L., Blackwood, M.K., and Diaz-Asper, C. (2007). Category- specific deficits in Alzheimer's disease: fact or artefact? *Cortex, 43*, 907-920.

Tyler, L.K., Moss, H.E., Durrant-Peatfield, M.R., and Levy, P (2000). Conceptual structure and the struture of concepts: A distributed account of category-specific deficits. *Brain and Language, 75*, 195-231.

Zannino, G.D., Perri, R., Carlesimo, G.A., Pasqualetti, P., and Caltagirone, C. (2002). Category-specific impairment in patients with Alzheimer's disease as a function of disease severity: a cross-sectional investigation. *Neuropsychologia, 40*, 2268-2279.

ACKNOWLEDGEMENTS

The writing of this chapter was supported in part by a postdoctoral fellowship from the Spanish Ministry of Education and Science (*programa José Castillejo* -JC2007-00248-) to F.J.M.M. and by the foundation "*Burgos por la Investigación de la Salud*". The authors would like to thank Sara Cañamón for helping in several ways and to all the participants and their families for their generous contribution.

APPENDIX 1. CATEGORIES AND STIMULI USED IN THE STUDY

Living things			Nonliving things	
Animals	*Insects*		*Buildings*	*Tools*
Cat	Ant		Castle	Hammer
Cow	Bee		Cathedral	Monkeywrench
Dog	Butterfly		Chalet	Nail
Elephant	Cockroach		Church	Pincers
Hen	Fly		House	Pliers

Living things			Nonliving things	
Horse	Mosquito		Palace	Screwdriver
Lion	Spider		Shanty	Saw
Tiger	Wasp		Skyscraper	Shovel
Body parts	*Trees*		*Clothing*	*Vehicles*
Arm	Cypress		Coat	Airplane
Eye	Fir		Jacket	Bike
Finger	Oak		Shirt	Boat
Foot	Olive		Skirt	Bus
Hand	Palm tree		Sock	Car
Leg	Pine		Sweater	Motorbike
Mouth	Polar		Trousers	Train
Nose	Willow		Vest	Truck
Flowers	*Vegetables*		*Furniture*	
Bellflowers	Artichoke		Armchair	
Carnation	Cabbage		Bed	
Daisy	Cauliflower		Bedside table	
Geranium	Chard		Bookcase	
Orchid	Endive		Chair	
Poppy	Green bean		Lamp	
Rose	Lettuce		Table	
Tulip	Spinach		Wardrobe	
Fruits			*Kitchen utensils*	
Apple			Casserole	
Banana			Fork	
Melon			Fry pan	
Orange			Knife	
Pear			Pot	
Peach			Plate	
Strawberry			Saucepan	
Watermelon			Spoon	

APPENDIX 2. EXAMPLES OF STIMULI USED FROM THE NOMBELA BATTERY

ITEMS FROM LT DOMAIN

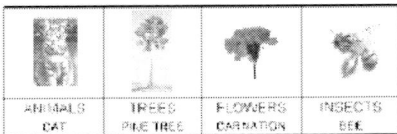

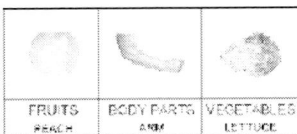

ANIMALS	TREES	FLOWERS	INSECTS
CAT	PINE TREE	CARNATION	BEE

FRUITS	BODY PARTS	VEGETABLES
PEACH	ARM	LETTUCE

ITEMS FROM NLT DOMAIN

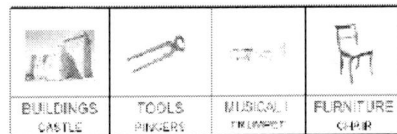

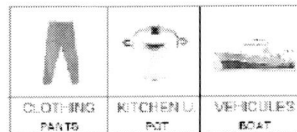

BUILDINGS	TOOLS	MUSICAL I	FURNITURE
CASTLE	PINCERS	TRUMPET	CHAIR

CLOTHING	KITCHEN U.	VEHICLES
PANTS	POT	BOAT

In: Alzheimer's Disease in the Middle-Aged
Editor: Hyun Sil Jeong, pp. 209-223

ISBN: 978-1-60456-480-8
© 2008 Nova Science Publishers, Inc.

Chapter 9

DIFFERENTIATING DEMENTIA SYNDROMES IN THE MIDDLE-AGED PATIENT

Cecile A. Marczinski[*1] *and Estee C. Grant*[2]
[1] University of Kentucky, Lexington, KY, US
[2] University of Calgary, Alberta, Canada

ABSTRACT

Distinguishing between the various degenerative dementias often poses a diagnostic dilemma for clinicians. This problem is a particular concern in the accurate assessment of the middle-aged patient. A growing body of research is establishing that nearly one quarter of degenerative dementias, particularly those with a presenile onset, can be caused by diseases variously termed Pick's disease, frontotemporal dementia, primary progressive aphasia, and semantic dementia. Thus, distinguishing these various syndromes from the more common causes of dementia, such as Alzheimer's disease, is critical for making appropriate treatment decisions and accurately communicating prognosis with patients and caregivers. Thus, this chapter reviews the literature on the various degenerative dementias that often present in middle age. This review highlights the obstacle of distinguishing these various dementias from one another using general cognitive screens and neuroimaging, particularly at the early stages of disease onset. Results from a study are then described which illustrate that category and letter fluency tasks may be more helpful in distinguishing various dementia syndromes from normal controls and from one another. These fluency tasks may outperform more general cognitive screens that are typically used to assess dementia. In summary, this chapter expands and improves upon the currently accepted methodology used in the diagnosis of dementia, particularly in the middle-aged patient.

---

[*] Cecile A. Marczinski, Ph.D.; Department of Psychology; 206 Kastle Hall; University of Kentucky; Lexington, KY 40506-0044; P. (859) 257-4977; F. (859) 323-1979; E. cecile.marczinski@uky.edu

OVERVIEW

Distinguishing between the different dementia syndromes is a common diagnostic dilemma facing the clinician assessing a patient presenting with symptoms of a dementia syndrome (Feldman and Kertesz, 2001; Pasquier, 1999). Alzheimer's disease (AD) is often foremost in mind as it is one of the most common causes of dementia. AD has memory impairment as one of its defining features, and memory impairment is often synonymous with dementia in the general public. Routinely forgetting where one parked his car or forgetting to turn off the stove may indicate dementia. Therefore, observed memory impairment is often what leads family members to request assessment of their relative. However, a growing body of research is establishing that nearly one quarter of degenerative dementias, particularly those with a presenile onset, can be caused by diseases variously termed Pick disease (Pick, 1892), frontotemporal dementia (Gustafson, 1987; Neary et al., 1986), primary progressive aphasia (Mesulam, 1987), and semantic dementia (Hodges et al., 1992). These syndromes do not have episodic memory impairment as a primary feature (although memory problems can be secondary), but do seem to have considerable overlap with each other (Kertesz, 2001). Since these syndromes often present in late middle age, there is often a misperception that the patient is still too young to be diagnosed with dementia. An additional challenge for diagnosis is that the characteristic features of behavioral changes and/or language difficulties are less likely to be considered as part of the dementia spectrum, resulting in delays in identification of a problem or misdiagnosis (e.g., as a psychiatric problem). Further difficulty in distinguishing these various dementias from one another and from AD is caused by the problem that general cognitive screens and neuroimaging are not particularly helpful in diagnosis at the early stages of disease onset (Heidler-Gary et al., 2007; Perry and Hodges, 2000). The overlap in clinical profiles of the degenerative dementias, particularly as dementia progresses, makes clinical differential diagnosis a challenge (Jobst et al., 1997). With so many problems with the traditional approaches at differential diagnosis, it has been suggested that a new and different approach is warranted (Blair et al., 2006; Wichlund et al., 2004).

EPIDEMIOLOGY OF EARLY ONSET DEMENTIA

Inconsistencies in terminology in the literature create some difficulty in establishing accurate prevalence estimates of dementia syndromes. For example, it has been suggested that Primary Progressive Aphasia is the left-hemisphere variant of Frontotemporal Dementia (Neary et al., 1993; Snowden and Neary, 1993), leading to some cases of Primary Progressive Aphasia in the literature being referred to as Frontotemporal Dementia, meaning a language disorder form of Frontotemporal Dementia and not the disinhibition disorder. However, despite confusion over terminology, it is clear that the group of dementia syndromes without episodic memory loss as the primary feature contribute to a large proportion of patients presenting with dementia. It has been reported that up to 20% of cases of degenerative dementias on autopsy are due to frontotemporal dementia alone (Heston and Mastri, 1982; Gustafson, 1993). Furthermore, the changing age structure of the U.S. population will markedly affect the future incidence and prevalence of all dementia syndromes. Prevalence estimates of Alzheimer's disease using 2000 census data indicated that there were 4.5 million persons with AD in the U.S. population. By 2050, this number is estimated to triple to 13.2 million (Hebert et al., 2003).

Thus far, there has been a paucity of research on the epidemiology of early onset dementia (onset at an age less than 65 years), so the rates of frontotemporal dementia, primary progressive aphasia, and semantic dementia in the U.S. and world population are unknown. However, one study reviewed medical records from 1,683 patients at a large Veteran's Affairs Medical Center Memory Disorders clinic over a 4-year period. The study was the largest to date on early onset dementia and the authors reported an unexpectedly large number of patients who were below the age of 65 and had with cognitive deficits (30% of all patients). Frontotemporal dementia was the leading cause of dementia not attributable to preventable causes, such as alcohol abuse. This contrasted with the causes of late-onset dementia where Alzheimer's disease prevailed (McMurtray et al., 2006). A similar study from Japan also concluded that early-onset dementia is not rare and that the clinical characteristics and causes of early onset dementia differed from late onset dementia. In a sample of 668 demented patients, 28% were early onset cases, with frontotemporal dementia as a leading cause of dementia in this group (Shinagawa et al., 2007). While the exact rates of the other dementia syndromes, besides Alzheimer's disease, in the general population are not known, it is becoming increasingly clear that approximately 1/3 of dementia cases present before the age of 65 and in most cases the predominant cause of the dementia in all age groups is something other than Alzheimer's disease.

DEGENERATIVE DEMENTIAS WITH PRESENILE ONSET

Arnold Pick was the first to report of a patient with progressive aphasia (loss of the ability to produce and/or comprehend language) and this report was the basis of the concept of Pick's disease (Pick, 1892). In his report, he described the aphasia as being caused by a single circumscribed atrophic process in the brain and established the concept of focal atrophy causing a specific behavioral syndrome. Today, Pick's disease is often reserved for the pathological description of frontotemporal atrophy with silver staining, globular inclusions (Pick bodies), swollen neurons (Pick cells), superficial cortical spongiosis, neuronal loss and gliosis (Kertesz, 2001). However, these diagnostic criteria present some difficulties. First, the pathologic findings are only known at autopsy, which is clearly not helpful to the clinician faced with a symptomatic patient. Second, only 25% of cases have the typical inclusions. To address these challenges, patients with focal atrophy are better described by their clinical presentation. Furthermore, it is now understood that although some cases have Pick bodies, the majority do not, and the clinical syndrome is not affected by the pathological variant. There are several clinical presentations that are widely described. A patient with a primarily apathy - disinhibition dementia is said to have Frontotemporal Dementia (FTD) or Frontotemporal Dementia – frontal variant (FTD-fv), since the focal atrophy is largely in the frontal lobes. A patient with a progressive aphasia is said to have Primary Progressive Aphasia (PPA) or Frontotemporal Dementia – temporal variant, since the focal atrophy is in the temporal lobes. A patient with loss of meaning and words is said to have Semantic Dementia (SD) and the atrophy is often initially in the left temporal lobe. There is considerable overlap in all three conditions and over time, patients acquire the symptomatology of another condition as atrophy spreads. Thus, a patient that starts with FTD may eventually develop the aphasia of PPA or a patient that initially presents with PPA may develop the disinhibition characteristic of FTD (Blair et al., 2007; Kertesz, 2001; Marczinski et al., 2004).

Age of onset for FTD, PPA, and SD is most commonly between 45 and 65 years (Neary and Snowden, 1996). In general, a family history of a similar disorder in a first-degree relative occurs in approximately half of cases (Neary and Snowden, 1996) and familial cases tend to have an earlier onset (Kertesz and Munoz, 2002). There are case reports of very young onset in patients who were age 25 (Coleman et al., 2002) and 27 (Jacob et al., 1999) when diagnosed with FTD. Unfortunately, optimal treatment for FTD, PPA and SD has been difficult to establish. Failures to recognize the widespread existence of these conditions have potentially contributed to the slow emergence of effective treatments.

Diagnosis of these early onset dementias is challenging. Often, the characteristic clinical findings often lead individuals to be inappropriately treated as depressed or psychotic before considering referral to a neurologist. However, there are some indications that specific cognitive tasks, such as category and letter fluency tasks, and specific behavioral assessments, such as the Frontal Behavioral Inventory, may be more helpful in distinguishing various early onset dementia syndromes from normal controls and from one another (Diehl et al., 2005; Marczinski et al., 2004; Marczinski and Kertesz, 2006). This rest of this chapter will describe these lesser-known dementia syndromes in greater detail, and will then present new ways to distinguish these various syndromes from one another.

FRONTOTEMPORAL DEMENTIA (FTD)

The core symptoms of Frontotemporal Dementia (FTD) are personality change, apathy, blunting of emotions, lack of insight, and disinhibition (Brun et al., 1994). Other symptoms include loss of personal hygiene, loss of social awareness, hypersexuality, hyperorality, perseverative behavior, utilization behavior (i.e., excessive touching), and distractibility. Affective symptoms include indifference, remoteness, inertia and aspontaneity (Kertesz et al., 1997). Early diagnosis of FTD can be extremely difficult because cognitive functioning may be initially well preserved in these patients. Any poor performance on psychometric tests is often due to the patient being uncooperative or easily distracted when given task instructions. Psychiatric symptoms may predate the onset of FTD by many years (Neary and Snowden, 1996). The hallmark feature of disinhibition can range from childish rude behavior to kleptomania. Patients can come in contact with the law when they steal, grope strangers or expose themselves. The social inappropriateness frequently makes family members uncomfortable and embarrassed. Hypersexuality may only be verbal or gestural in the middle-aged patient. Hyperorality often manifests as overeating or development food fads, particularly for things like sweets. As atrophy is occurring in the frontal lobes, some executive dysfunction is evident in psychometric testing. However, for the most part, cooperative patients, despite their grossly abnormal behavior, can perform well on most psychometric tests (Kertesz and Munoz, 2002).

PRIMARY PROGRESSIVE APHASIA (PPA)

Primary Progressive Aphasia (PPA) is characterized by an isolated and gradual dissolution of language function. PPA symptoms start with anomia (word finding difficulty), progress to a loss of fluency, and are ultimately followed by mutism (Kertesz et al., 2003; Mesulam, 1987). Anomia is also a feature of Alzheimer's Disease. Therefore, the operational definition of PPA includes a period of two years of progressive aphasia with relative preservation of other functions and activities of daily living (Weintraub et al., 1990). Even in fully mute patients, relatively well-preserved memory and visuospatial orientation is often evident and PPA patients may function surprisingly well in the community if they do not start developing the disinhibition of FTD when atrophy spreads from the temporal lobes into the frontal lobes (Kertesz and Munoz, 2002).

SEMANTIC DEMENTIA (SD)

Semantic Dementia (SD) is characterized by a pattern of profound deterioration of semantic memory that disrupts the meaning, recognition, and comprehension of objects (Hodges et al., 1992; Snowden et al., 1989). For example, a patient may no longer know what a 'steak', a 'tool' or a 'vehicle' is (Kertesz et al., 1998). This lexicosemantic language impairment is in striking contrast to the relatively preserved phonological and syntactic process of language and cognition in general (Hodges et al., 1994). In other words, patients can speak fluently and coherently, yet they have lost the meaning of some words. The lexical and semantic aspects of the representation progressively deteriorate in a frequency dependent manner, with the loss of lower frequency words first (e.g., the word 'antelope' is lost before the word 'dog'). However, with disease progression, higher frequency words become increasingly lost (Bird et al., 2000). The neuropsychological profile of patients with SD contrasts greatly with other dementias (such as AD), as the patients have well-preserved episodic memory and visuospatial skills (Graham and Hodges, 1997).

ALZHEIMER'S DISEASE (AD)

In contrast to FTD, PPA and SD described above, the core features of AD include episodic memory deficits and visual-spatial deficits (Hodges et al., 1999; Storey et al., 2002). While episodic memory deficits are often severe in AD, more subtle impairments in semantic memory and visuospatial skills are often observed (Hodges et al., 1999). The other dementias are difficult to distinguish from AD clinically because AD exists in several variants. A patient can present with a predominant impairment of executive, visuospatial, or language skills (Storey et al., 2002). Word finding difficulties in AD are often present, at times quite early on in the disease process (Appell et al., 1982). Impaired verbal and semantic fluency have been documented in AD patients compared to controls (Chertkow and Bub, 1990; Diaz et al., 2004; Duff Canning et al., 2004; Martin and Fedio, 1983; Nebes, 1989). Structural imaging in AD generally shows global cortical atrophy, including hippocampal atrophy (Black, 1996), compared to the focal frontal and temporal atrophy seen in patients with FTD, PPA and SD (Kertesz et al., 1997).

GENERAL COGNITIVE TESTING

In the assessment of various degenerative dementias, the examination of cognition is often carried out with brief psychometric tests. The Mini-Mental Status Examination (MMSE) has been shown to be a useful and highly popular instrument (Folstein, Folstein and McHugh, 1975). Since this short test includes questions that query orientation (what is the date today) and visuospatial skills (draw a clock), results from the MMSE often identify quickly when AD is a possibility. However, this test is often insensitive to the earliest changes in individuals with dementia, particularly in high-functioning and/or highly educated individuals. Furthermore, the MMSE and even longer mental status exams, such as the Mattis Dementia Rating Scale (MDRS) (Mattis, 1988), have been shown to fail to distinguish between various degenerative dementias, such as AD, FTD, PPA and SD (Kertesz et al., 2003). As such, clinicians have sought better diagnostic neuropsychological assessments that still incorporate brevity as a key feature necessary for administration in a clinical setting.

DIAGNOSTIC UTILITY OF FLUENCY MEASURES

Verbal fluency tasks consist of generating words from a semantic category (e.g., animals) or words beginning with a given letter (e.g. letter 'S') with a specified time limit, such as 60 seconds. While both category and letter fluency task performance is impaired by degenerative dementias, there are some differences in performance between these two tasks, suggesting that letter and category fluency tasks rely on both some common and some distinct cognitive processes (Pompeia et al., 2002; Rende et al., 2002). It has been suggested that the category tasks may rely more heavily on access to lexical representations of semantic concepts, whereas the letter task may rely more heavily on the central executive component of working memory (Baddeley, 1992; Baddeley et al., 1975), and this distinction appears to have anatomical correlates (Gold and Buckner, 2002).

The first study to suggest the utility of category and letter fluency tasks in distinguishing dementia syndromes from controls and from one another was published by Duff Canning et al. (2004). The authors compared patients with AD to patients with vascular dementia (VaD) and normal controls. The one-minute category task involved naming as many animals as possible. The one-minute letter fluency task involved naming as many words that began with the letter 'F' as possible. The authors reported that both patient groups generated fewer animal names compared to normal elderly controls. Furthermore, letter fluency scores differentiated AD from VaD, with patients with AD able to generate more 'F' words compared to patients with VaD.

The success of this approach led to the suggestion that the fluency test might be a powerful test to aid in diagnostic decisions, and could be deemed the one-minute mental status examination (Cummings, 2004). The appeal of the fluency task as a one-minute mental status exam is, at least in part, that it is extremely brief to administer and while yielding a tremendous richness in the data. For instance, patients' responses can provide several pieces of information such as: (1) the raw number of words generated with the one minute trial, (2) the actual word frequencies of the words generated, based on published norms of the English language, and (3) the numbers of errors made of repeating a word within the one minute trial. Duff Canning et al. (2004) only reported the raw number of words produced by the patients in the trial. However, it has been hypothesized that this potential rich data may be useful in distinguishing the various degenerative dementias, particularly those with an early onset, that pose diagnostic dilemmas for clinicians (Marczinski and Kertesz, 2006). For instance, the number of errors of repetition (where there is at least one intervening item) could indicate deficits of working memory. Imagine two patients who both score 7 on the animal task. The first patient has a response list of 'giraffe, cow, dog, cat, lion, beaver, snake' while the second patient has a response list of 'dog, cow, horse, dog, sheep, snake, dog'. Clearly, the two lists are not equal. The second patient demonstrates a deficit in working memory in that the patient 'forgets' that he has already produced a particular exemplar from a category. By only scoring raw numbers of words produced, this important memory error is not captured. Furthermore, word frequencies indicate access to lexical representations with impairment indicated by failures to generate lower frequency exemplars. For example, a generated three word animal list of zebra, squirrel, and frog, includes lower frequency exemplars from the English language in comparison to a generated three words animal list of horse, dog, and bear. Again, while matched in the number of words generated, the two lists are qualitatively difference in access to lexical representations.

With this new approach, performance on category and letter fluency tasks was compared in patients with SD, PPA and AD (Marczinski and Kertesz, 2006). While it could easily be predicted that all these dementia patients would perform more poorly on both types of fluency tasks compared to normal elderly controls, more specific predictions about differences in performance between the groups could be made. Since profound deterioration of semantic memory is the key feature in SD, SD patients would be expected to produce the fewest number of words in a category task and produce more words in a letter task that relies more on the central executive component of working memory. Furthermore, the words generated in the category task should be higher in word frequency, since the lower word frequency words have been lost due to the disease process. Finally, errors of repeating a word within a list would be expected to occur very infrequently in patients with SD, as they characteristically have well-preserved working memory and would be less likely then AD patients to forget that they had just generated a particular exemplar from a category within a one minute trial.

Since verbal fluency is significantly impaired in PPA, it could be predicted that patients with PPA would produce the fewest number of words in both the category and letter fluency tasks. In particular, letter fluency might be dramatically impaired as patients with PPA have a deficit in accessing phonemes (the sound-based representation of speech) (Mendez et al., 2003). The mean word frequencies produced should be lower in PPA compared to SD patients, as the disease process of PPA impairs speech production more than access to lexical representations (e.g., a patient with PPA is more likely to produce a low frequency exemplar like antelope than a patient with SD). Furthermore, errors or repeating words within a list would be unlikely, as episodic and working memory remains relatively intact in patients with PPA.

As the core features of AD include episodic memory deficits and visual-spatial deficits, performance on fluency tasks should contrast greatly to the performance of patients with PPA and SD. Impaired verbal and semantic fluency has been documented in AD patients compared to controls (Chertkow and Bub, 1990; Diaz et al., 2004; Duff Canning et al., 2004; Martin and Fedio, 1983; Nebes, 1989). Low letter fluency scores discriminate AD patients from controls and are a reliable predictor of subsequent dementia status in elderly patients (Hodges and Patterson, 1994). However, results from previous studies would suggest that AD patients would generate more words in category and letter tasks compared to PPA patients (Kertesz et al., 2003; Mendez et al., 2003). Mean word frequencies should be lower in AD compared to SD, as semantic retrieval deficits are primary in SD and secondary in AD (Hodges et al., 1999). Finally, errors of repeating words within a list should be most impaired in AD as the disease process results in impairments in episodic memory.

RESEARCH STRATEGY

The aim of the following study was therefore to demonstrate that the category and letter fluency tasks distinguish patients with SD, PPA, and AD from controls and from one another (see Marczinski and Kertesz, 2006). Three fluency tasks (two category fluency tasks of animals and groceries and one letter fluency of words that start with the letter S) were administered. For animal category fluency, participants were asked to name as many different animals as they could within 60 seconds. For grocery category fluency, participants were instructed to name as many different items that they might purchase in the grocery store as they could within 60 seconds. Instructions emphasized that they should name individual items and not just a category label such as meat. For 'S' words letter fluency, participants were asked to name as many different words that start with the letter 'S' as they could within 60 seconds. Instructions emphasized that words generated should not include proper names such as Sally. Responses were tape-recorded and each word was generated was then assigned its appropriate word frequency based on the Kucera-Francis word frequency norms (Kucera and Francis, 1967). An error was recorded if the individual repeated a word within a list. From these verbatim responses, there were three dependent measures of interest: (1) the number of words generated, (2) the mean word frequency of the words generated, and (3) the number of errors of repetition divided by the total number of words generated. Thus, the current methodology used in fluency tasks was expanded upon for this study. By recording word frequencies, one might have more information about the status of lexical representations of semantic concepts. By recording the number of errors made, one might have more information about the status of episodic memory.

STUDY PARTICIPANTS

Twenty clinically diagnosed AD patients, 8 clinically diagnosed SD patients, 12 clinically diagnosed PPA patients, and 20 normal elderly controls participated in this study. The demographic characteristics of these groups are presented in table 1. The clinical diagnosis was made according to the criteria suggested for AD by the National Institute of Neurological Communicative Disorders and Stroke-Alzheimer's disease and Related Disorders Association (NINCDS-ADRDA) (McKhann et al., 1984), SD by Neary et al.

(1988), and PPA by Mesulam (1987). Diagnostic decisions were made independent of fluency scores. Spouses and caregivers were recruited as normal control participants if they were healthy individuals older than 65 years of age without any history of psychiatric or neurological disease.

Table 1.Means (M) and standard deviations (SD) of various demographic characteristics of patients and controls

	Controls		Alzheimer's disease (AD)		Semantic Dementia (SD)		Primary Progressive Aphasia (PPA)		
	M	*SD*	*M*	*SD*	*M*	*SD*	*M*	*SD*	*Sign.*
Sample size (N)	20		20		8		12		
Gender (M:F)	10:10		10:10		4:4		6:6		.99
Age at test (yrs)	73.8	5.9	74.7	7.6	65.9	9.3	63.1	7.1	<.001
Age of onset (yrs)	n/a		71.5	7.0	61.9	9.7	59.4	7.5	<.001
Duration ill (yrs)	n/a		3.2	2.3	4.0	2.1	3.5	1.6	.63
Education (yrs)	13.5	2.8	9.9	3.0	14.0	3.4	14.1	2.7	<.001
MMSE	28.8	1.1	21.3	4.0	22.6	8.6	15.3	6.5	<.001
MDRS	137.7	4.3	111.9	11.7	102.4	27.9	74.6	32.8	<.001

Note: MMSE = Mini Mental Status Exam; MDRS = Mattis Dementia Rating Scale.

RESULTS

Fluency task performance differed as predicted (see Marczinski and Kertesz, 2006). As shown in figure 1, controls generated the most exemplars in all three fluency tasks, followed by AD, SD and PPA patients. Interestingly, SD and PPA patients did not differ statistically for the two category fluency tasks. By contrast, AD and SD did not differ from one another on the letter fluency task.

Significant differences in the patient groups were obtained for the mean word frequency of the words generated in the animal and grocery category tasks. Figure 2 illustrates that the controls generated the lowest frequency exemplars in the animal task, followed by AD, PPA and SD patients. For the grocery task, a slightly different pattern emerged as AD patients generated words with higher mean word frequencies compared to all other groups. There were no significant differences between the groups for the mean word frequency from the S letter task.

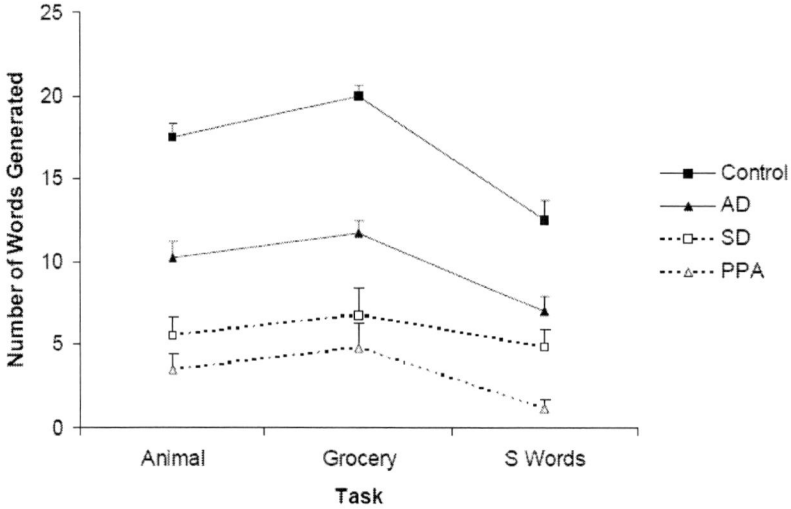

Figure 1. Mean number of words generated in the animal, grocery and 'S' words fluency tasks for controls, patients with Alzheimer's disease, patients with Semantic Dementia, and patients with Primary Progressive Aphasia. Error bars reflect standard errors of the mean.

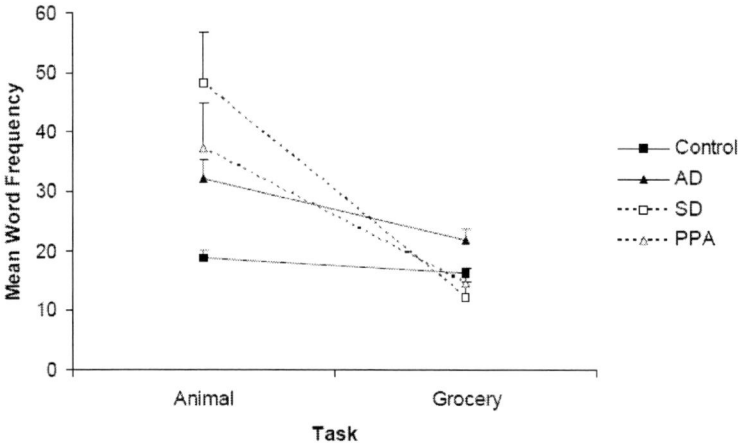

Figure 2. Mean word frequencies of words generated in the animal and grocery fluency tasks for controls, patients with Alzheimer's disease, patients with Semantic Dementia, and patients with Primary Progressive Aphasia. Error bars reflect standard errors of the mean.

The proportion of repetition errors generated in the animal category task revealed a significant difference between groups. Figure 3 illustrates that AD patients generated more errors compared to the other three groups. PPA and SD patients made no repetition errors on any of the three tasks. There were no significant differences found in the proportion of errors generated in the grocery category or the S letter task.

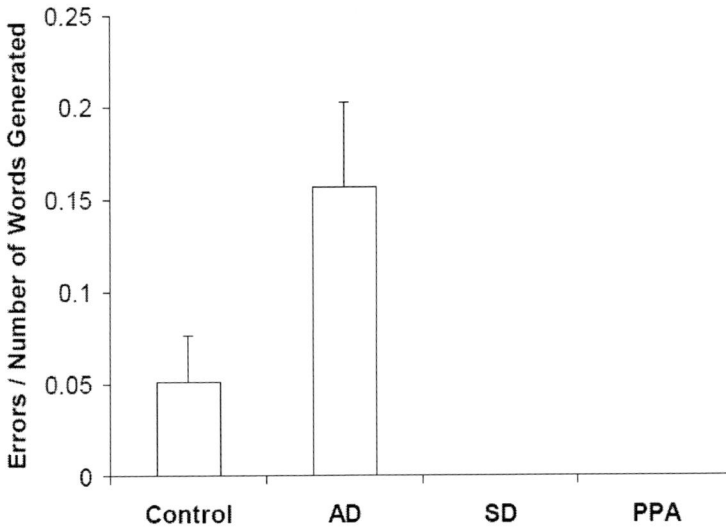

Figure 3. Mean number of perseveration errors divided by the total number of words generated in the animal fluency task for controls, patients with Alzheimer's disease, patients with Semantic Dementia, and patients with Primary Progressive Aphasia. None of the patients with Semantic Dementia or Primary Progressive Aphasia made any errors in this task. Error bars reflect standard errors of the mean.

DISCUSSION OF RESULTS

The results provide support for the hypothesis that category and letter fluency tasks can be used to distinguish various dementia syndromes from normal controls and from one another. All patient groups generated fewer words in all three tasks (animals, groceries, 'S' words) compared to normal controls. In all three tasks, AD patients generated the most exemplars, followed by the SD and PPA patients, consistent with hypotheses regarding the extent of language involvement in these three conditions. The category tasks did not differentiate the SD and PPA patients. However, the SD patients generated more exemplars in the letter task compared to the PPA patients, which further supports the phonological impairment in PPA in contrast to the semantic deficit in SD. When the mean word frequencies of the words generated were compared for the animal task, controls generated lower frequency exemplars, followed by AD, PPA and then SD patients generating the higher frequency exemplars, as predicted. Surprisingly, this pattern was not replicated in the grocery task where the higher frequency exemplars were generated by the AD patients. Finally, errors of repeating a word within a list in the animal category task were significantly higher for the AD patients compared to all other groups, as hypothesized based on deficits in short term working memory.

CONCLUSION

Distinguishing between the various degenerative dementias has long posed significant diagnostic challenges to the clinician. As the population ages and numbers of patients with new onset of dementia symptoms rise, clinicians will increasingly require efficient and effective methods for distinguishing between these dementia syndromes to provide accurate and timely diagnosis and treatment. Through a better understanding of the clinical and pathological distinctions between these syndromes, it has been possible to develop and test a novel method for using previously established category and letter fluency tasks to generate new data that can be used to help clinicians faced with this problem. Through not only recording the number of words generated, but also recording word frequencies and repetition errors, not only can patients with all forms of dementia be more easily differentiated from those with usual symptoms of normal aging, but patients with Alzheimer's Disease can now be differentiated from those with Semantic Dementia and Primary Progressive Aphasia. The ability to make such distinctions despite modest sample sizes and the use of only three fluency tasks provides great encouragement for the possible future benefit of this new methodology. Within the time constraints of a screening assessment in a memory clinic, the category and letter fluency tasks may therefore provide the clinician key information to allow quick and accurate diagnosis, and ultimately better access to appropriate treatment for this difficult group of diseases.

REFERENCES

Appell, J., Kertesz, A., and Fisman, M. (1982). A study of language functioning in Alzheimer patients. *Brain and Language, 17*, 73-91.

Baddeley, A. (1992). Working memory. *Science, 255*, 556-559.

Baddeley, A.D., Thomson, N., and Buchanan, M. (1975). Word length and the structure of short-term memory. *Journal of Verbal Learning and Verbal Behaviour, 14*, 575-589.

Bird, H., Lambon Ralph, M.A., Patterson, K., and Hodges, J.R. (2000). The rise and fall of frequency and imageability: Noun and verb production in semantic dementia. *Brain and Language, 73*, 17-49.

Black, S.E. (1996). Focal cortical atrophy syndromes. *Brain and Cognition, 31*, 188-229.

Blair, M., Kertesz, A., McMonagle, P., Davidson, W., and Bodi, N. (2006). Quantitative and qualitative analyses of clock drawing in frontotemporal dementia and Alzheimer's disease. *Journal of the International Neuropsychological Society, 12*, 159-165.

Blair, M., Marczinski, C.A., Davis-Faroque, N., and Kertesz, A. (2007). A longitudinal study of language decline in Alzheimer's disease and frontotemporal dementia. *Journal of the International Neuropsychological Society, 13*, 237-245.

Brun, A., Englund, B., Gustafson, L. et al. (1994). Clinical and neuropathological criteria for frontotemporal dementia. *Journal of Neurology Neurosurgery and Psychiatry, 57*, 416-418.

Chertkow, H., and Bub, D. (1990). Semantic memory loss in dementia of Alzheimer's type. What do various measures measure? *Brain, 113*, 397-417.

Coleman, L.W., Digre, K.B., Stephenson, G.M., and Townsend, J.J. (2002). Autopsy-proven, sporadic pick disease with onset at age 25 years. *Archives of Neurology, 59*, 856-859.

Cummings, J.L. (2004). The one-minute mental status examination. *Neurology, 62*, 534-535.

Diaz, M., Sailor, K., Cheung, D., and Kuslansky, G. (2004). Category size effects in semantic and letter fluency in Alzheimer's patients. *Brain and Language, 89*, 108-114.

Diehl, J., Monsch, A.U., Aebi, C., Wagenpfeil, S., Krapp, S., Grimmer, T., Seeley, W., Forstl, H., and Kurz, A. (2005). Frontotemporal dementia, semantic dementia, and Alzheimer's disease: the contribution of standard neuropsychological tests to differential diagnosis. *Journal of Geriatric Psychiatry and Neurology, 18*, 39-44.

Duff Canning, S.J., Leach, L., Stuss, D., Ngo, L., and Black, S.E. (2004). Diagnostic utility of abbreviated fluency measures in Alzheimer disease and vascular dementia. *Neurology, 62*, 556-562.

Feldman, H., and Kertesz, A. (2001). Diagnosis, classification and natural history of degenerative dementias. *Canadian Journal of Neurological Sciences, 28 Supplement 1*, S17-S27.

Folstein, M.F., Folstein, S.E., and McHugh, P.R. (1975). 'Mini-Mental State': A practical method for grading the cognitive state of patients for the clinician. *Journal of Psychiatric Research, 12*, 189-198.

Graham, K.S., and Hodges, J.R. (1997). Differentiating the roles of the hippocampal complex and the neocortex in long-term memory storage: Evidence from the study of semantic dementia and Alzheimer's disease. *Neuropsychology, 11*, 77-89.

Gustafson, L. (1987). Frontal lobe degeneration of non-Alzheimer type, II: clinical picture and differential diagnosis. *Archives of Gerontology and Geriatrics, 6*, 209-223.

Gustafson, L. (1993). Clinical picture of frontal lobe degenerescence of non-Alzheimer type. *Dementia, 4*, 143-148.

Hebert, L.E., Scherr, P.A., Bienias, J.L., Bennett, D.A., Evans, D.A. (2003). Alzheimer disease in the US population. *Archives of Neurology, 60*, 1119-1122.

Heidler-Gary, J., Gottesman, R., Newhart, M., Chang, S., Ken, L., and Hillis, A.E. (2007). Utility of behavioral versus cognitive measures in differentiating between subtypes of frontotemporal lobar degeneration and Alzheimer's disease. *Dementia Geriatric and Cognitive Disorders, 23*, 184-193.

Heston, L.L., and Mastri, A.R. (1982). Age at onset of Pick's disease and Alzheimer's dementia: implications for diagnosis and research. *Journal of Gerontology, 37*, 422-424.

Hodges, J.R., and Patterson, K. (1994). Is semantic memory consistently impaired early in the course of Alzheimer's disease? Neuroanatomical and diagnostic implications. *Neuropsychologia, 4*, 441-459.

Hodges, J.R., Patterson, K., Oxbury, S., and Funnell, E. (1992). Semantic dementia. Progressive fluent aphasia with temporal lobe atrophy. *Brain, 115*, 1783-1806.

Hodges, J.R., Patterson, K., and Tyler, L.K. (1994). Loss of semantic memory: Implications for the modularity of mind. *Cognitive Neuropsychology, 11*, 505-542.

Hodges, J.R., Patterson, K., Ward, R., Garrard, P., Bak, T., Perry, R., and Gregory, C. (1999). The differentiation of semantic dementia and frontal lobe dementia (temporal and frontal variants of frontotemporal dementia) from early Alzheimer's disease: a comparative neuropsychological study. *Neuropsychology, 13*, 31-40.

Jacob, J., Revesz, T., Thom, M., and Rossor, M.N. (1999). A case of sporadic Pick disease with onset at 27 years. *Archives of Neurology, 56*, 1289-1291.

Jobst, K.A., Barnetson, L.P., and Shepstone, B.J. (1997). Accurate prediction of histologically confirmed Alzheimer's disease and the differential diagnosis of dementia: the use of NINCDS-ADRDA and DSM-III-R criteria, SPECT, X-ray CT, and APO E4 medial temporal lobe dementias. The Oxford Project to Investigate Memory and Aging. *International Psychogeriatrics, 9 Supplement 1*, 191-222.

Kertesz, A. (2001). Pick's disease. *The Canadian Journal of Continuing Medical Education, September*, 141-155.

Kertesz, A., Davidson, W., and Fox, H. (1997). Frontal behavioral inventory: Diagnostic criteria for frontal lobe dementia. *Canadian Journal of Neurological Sciences, 24*, 29-36.

Kertesz, A., Davidson, W., and McCabe, P. (1998). Primary progressive semantic aphasia: A case study. *Journal of the International Neuropsychological Society, 4*, 388-398.

Kertesz, A., Davidson, W., McCabe, P., Takagi, K., and Munoz, D. (2003). Primary progressive aphasia: Diagnosis, varieties, evolution. *Journal of the International Neuropsychological Society, 9*, 710-719.

Kertesz, A., and Munoz, D.G. (2002). Frontotemporal dementia. *Medical Clinics of North America, 86*, 501-518.

Kucera, H., and Francis, W.N. (1967). *Computational Analysis of Present-day American English.* Providence, RI: Brown University Press.

Marczinski, C.A., Davidson, W., and Kertesz, A. (2004). A longitudinal study of behavior in frontotemporal dementia and primary progressive aphasia. *Cognitive and Behavioral Neurology, 17*, 185-190.

Marczinski, C.A., and Kertesz, A. (2006). Category and letter fluency in semantic dementia, primary progressive aphasia, and Alzheimer's disease. *Brain and Language, 97*, 258-265.

Martin, A., and Fedio, P. (1983). Word production and comprehension in Alzheimer's disease: The breakdown of semantic knowledge. *Brain and Language, 19*, 124-141.

Mattis, S. (1988). *Dementia rating scale.* Odessa, FL: Psychological Assessment Resources Professional manual.

McMurtray, A., Clark, D.G., Christine, D., and Mendez, M.F. (2006). Early-onset dementia: frequency and causes compared to late-onset dementia. *Dementia Geriatric and Cognitive Disorders, 21*, 59-64.

Mendez, M.F., Clark, D.G., Shapira, J.S., and Cummings, J.L. (2003). Speech and language in progressive nonfluent aphasia compared with early Alzheimer's disease. *Neurology, 61*, 1108-1113.

Mesulam, M.M. (1987). Primary progressive aphasia – differentiation from Alzheimer's disease. *Annals of Neurology, 22*, 533-534.

Neary, D., and Snowden, J. (1996). Fronto-temporal dementia: Nosology, neuropsychology, and neuropathology. *Brain and Cognition, 31*, 176-187.

Neary, D., Snowden, J.S., Bowen, J.S. et al. (1986). Neuropsychological syndromes in presenile dementia due to cerebral atrophy. *Journal of Neurology Neurosurgery and Psychiatry, 49*, 163-174.

Neary, D., Snowden, J.S., and Mann, D.M.A. (1993). The clinical pathological correlates of lobar atrophy. *Dementia, 4*, 154-159.

Nebes, R.D. (1989). Semantic memory in Alzheimer's disease. *Psychology Bulletin, 106*, 377-394.

Pasquier, F. (1999). Early diagnosis of dementia: neuropsychology. *Journal of Neurology, 246*, 6-15.

Perry, R.J., and Hodges, J.R. (2000). Differentiating frontal and temporal variant frontotemporal dementia from Alzheimer's disease. *Neurology, 54*, 2277-2284.

Pick, A. (1892). Uber die beziehungen der senilen hirnatrophie zur aphasie. *Prag Med Wochenschr, 17*, 165-167.

Pompeia, S., Rusted, J.M., and Curran, H.V. (2002). Verbal fluency facilitated by the cholinergic blocker, scopolamine. *Human psychopharmacology, 17*, 51-59.

Rende, B., Ramsberger, G., and Miyake, A. (2002). Commonalities and differences in the working memory components underlying letter and category fluency tasks: A dual-task investigation. *Neuropsychology, 16*, 309-321.

Shinagawa, S., Ikeda, M., Toyota, Y., Matsumoto, T., Matsumoto, N., Mori, T., Ishikawa, T., Fukuhara, R., Komori, K., Hokoishi, K., and Tanabe, H. (2007). Frequency and clinical characteristics of early-onset dementia in consecutive patients in a memory clinic. *Dementia Geriatric and Cognitive Disorders, 24*, 42-47.

Snowden, J.S., Goulding, P.J., and Neary, D. (1989). Semantic dementia: A form of circumscribed cerebral atrophy. *Behavioral Neurology, 2*, 167-182.

Snowden, J.S., and Neary, D. (1993). Progressive language dysfunction and lobar atrophy. *Dementia, 4*, 226-231.

Storey, E., Slavin, M.J., and Kinsella, G.J. (2002). Patterns of cognitive impairment in Alzheimer's disease: assessment and differential diagnosis. *Frontiers in Bioscience, 7*, e155-e184.

Weintraub, S., Rubin, N.P., and Mesulam, M.M. (1990). Primary progressive aphasia: Longitudinal course, neuropsychological profile, and language features. *Archives of Neurology, 47*, 1329-1335.

Wichlund, A.H., Johnson, N., and Weintraub, S. (2004). Preservation of reasoning in primary progressive aphasia: further differentiation from Alzheimer's disease and the behavioral presentation of frontotemporal dementia. *Journal of Clinical and Experimental Neuropsychology, 26*, 347-

In: Alzheimer's Disease in the Middle-Aged
Editor: Hyun Sil Jeong, pp. 225-253

ISBN: 978-1-60456-480-8
© 2008 Nova Science Publishers, Inc.

Chapter 10

MID-LIFE TRANSITIONS: SPOUSAL EXPERIENCES OF COPING WITH DEMENTIA OF THE ALZHEIMER TYPE

*Colleen MacQuarrie**

Psychology Department; University of Prince Edward Island;
550 University Ave. Charlottetown, PEI, C1A 4P3

ABSTRACT

A diagnosis of possible or probable Alzheimer's Disease has repercussions at any age, however, coping with this diagnosis at mid-life can be particularly challenging. This chapter explores the coping experiences of a middle-aged couple over a period of six months. A phenomenological hermeneutic approach to analyzing the interviews reveals the individual as well as the shared impact of the disease in their lives. Experiences with Alzheimer Disease are typically portrayed either from the caregiver's perspective or the care-recipient's perspective. This chapter focuses on the longitudinal impact of living with a diagnosis of AD from a couple's perspective. The analysis reveals the impact of the diagnostic process from both a caregiver and a care-receiver's perspective and the longer term impacts on self image, adaptation, resilience, and coping to questions about relationships with spouse and others, to care, the meaning of the disease, and existential meaning. This chapter can provide insight for couples in middle-age who are learning how to cope when one of them is diagnosed with dementia of the Alzheimer Type.

INTRODUCTION

Historically, Alzheimer's Disease (AD) has been identified for close to a century (Alzheimer, 1907). However it has only been in the latter part of the twentieth century that the symptoms of AD have been distinguished from other types of dementia. The American Psychiatric Association (1994) defined it as a degenerative disorder of insidious onset, which is characterised by loss of intellectual abilities, changes in personality, and behavioural disturbances. Although the clinical definition of AD is clear, the practice of diagnosis is open

---

* phone: (902)566-0617;fax: (902)628-4359;Email: cmacquarrie@upei.ca

to interpretation. Currently a medical doctor makes a clinical diagnosis after ruling out competing explanations, taking an in-depth personal history, and conducting a series of cognitive and other tests as required (Gauthier and Panisset, 1998). Even with a battery of testing, clinicians qualify their diagnosis as possible or probable AD, reserving definitive diagnosis until autopsied brain tissue can be examined for the characteristic plaques and tangles of AD.

A diagnosis of possible or probable Alzheimer's disease (AD) has repercussions at any age, however, coping with this diagnosis at mid-life can be particularly challenging. In middle age as opposed to older age onset of dementia the challenges can be fraught with the simultaneous balancing of mid life tasks such as raising a family, managing career and work pressures, and shifts in the trajectory of the spousal relationship (Duvall, 1977).

This chapter presents a case study which has been extracted from a larger research project examining transitions in early stage AD for community dwelling couples[1]. In this chapter, I explore the coping experiences of a middle-aged couple over a period of six months. Their interviews reveal the individual as well as the shared impact of the disease in their lives. Experiences with AD are typically portrayed either from the caregiver's perspective or, less often, the care-recipient's perspective. This case study focuses on the longitudinal impact of living with a diagnosis of AD from a couple's perspective. The analysis deepens our understanding of the coping process from the experience of diagnosis to the way that awareness, vigilance, and monitoring operate to both facilitate and hinder self esteem and relationships. In particular, the narratives show how couples and individuals come to terms with the changes associated with AD at midlife and at this stage in their family life cycle. This chapter can provide insight for couples in middle-age who are learning how to cope when one of them is diagnosed with early stage dementia of the Alzheimer Type.

Pseudonyms are used for people and places to protect anonymity. Diagnosis was through an accredited research university with an Alzheimer's Clinic in a large Canadian city. Ethical approval for this study was granted by a university research ethics board at a teaching hospital in Canada. Partial funding was through a Provincial Alzheimer's society.

MEASURES

The primary source for the case study information came from two semi-structured interviews that served as a conversational guide. These interviews, Transition Interview for Persons with DAT (TIPD; MacQuarie, 2005) and the Transition Interview for Spousal Care-givers (TISC) were developed specifically for the larger research project. These were designed to explore a series of questions ranging from queries about self image, adaptation, resilience, and coping to questions about relationships with spouse and others, to care, the meaning of the disease, and existential meaning.

The interviews were augmented with established quantitative measures from the larger project. Some of the quantitative measures are reported to enable readers to draw parallels to existing literatures but form a mere backdrop for the qualitative analysis and provide a methods based form of triangulation (Willig, 2004). Briefly, a subset of the measures

[1] Analyses of the experiences of AD participants have been published in MacQuarrie (2005).

included the following: A one item Perceived Health Likert-type scale ranging from 1 to 7 with higher scores indicating better health. A Geriatric Depression Scale, (GDS) (Yesavage, et al., 1983) with 30 yes/no items designed to tap the domain of depressive symptoms. The number of depressive responses were tallied, and the score of 0-30 indicated the level of depression (0-10 = normal; 11-20 = mild depression; 21-30 = moderate or major depression). A Quality of Relationships Inventory (QRI) (Pierce, Sarason, Sarason, Solky, and Nagle, 1993) with a 25 item Likert-type scale designed to measure interpersonal relationships. The QRI's three subscales assessed relationship-specific social support, conflict, and depth. The Screen for Caregiver Burden (SCB) (Vitaliano, Russo, Young, Becker, and Maiuro, 1991) with 25-items measured objective and subjective burden specifically for spousal care-givers of AD persons.

INITIATING AND SETTING THE CONVERSATIONS

My first contact with the couple was through a letter that I sent inviting their participation in my PhD research project on the experiences of living with AD. The Clinic had given me permission to contact potential participants after their family conference was completed. Two weeks after I sent the letter to the couple, I phoned and asked to speak to the caregiver spouse, Mary. I explained the purpose of the research, answered any questions, and asked if there was interest in participation. Mary and Dan had talked about participating and they were both interested. Mary invited me to their home the following week to discuss the project and to proceed with interviews if they were both in agreement. I phoned the morning before I went to their home to re-confirm that it was still convenient for them to have me come that day.

When I arrived at their home, we spent approximately 15 minutes together at their kitchen table, establishing rapport, talking in general terms about the project, and getting settled. I discussed the informed consent process with the couple together. After the informed consent process, Mary took her packet of questionnaires to fill out independently while Dan and I had our conversation in private. All conversations took place in the couple's home in a quiet spacious area in a comfortable family room in the basement. A door at the top of the stairs was closed so there would be no interruptions. Dan and I started with the interview and concluded with the questionnaires over the course of about two hours with a break. When we were finished, Dan went upstairs and Mary and I started our conversation. We started with any questions she had about the measures, discussed them, and then proceeded for approximately an hour and a half with the interview. I arranged to follow up with some questions they had about community resources and to return in six months to repeat the interview process. Six months later I returned, repeated the informed consent process and again had approximately a two hour conversation with Dan and about an hour and a half with Mary.

DATA ANALYSIS

All conversations were tape recorded and transcribed using a double iteration approach. The first transcription was verbatim; the second iteration added timed pauses and some conversational context such as overlapping conversation, voice inflections, and laughter. A guide to transcription marks is included at the end of this chapter to aid the reader's understanding of the quotations. All quotations are marked with either a (T1) or a (T2) to indicate whether the quote came from the first or second interview. Excerpts presented as data are verbatim from the transcribed narratives.

The cornerstones for this inductive project are based in methodological hermeneutics (Gergen, 1989, Heidegger, 1927/62, Packer and Addison, 1989, Rennie, 2000), an interpretive approach that seeks overarching themes, and phenomenological methodologies (Gadamer, 1975, Mills, 2001, Willig, 2004) which guide analyses first within individuals and then across participants. I approached the interpretation by first creating an analysis of each participant's narrative over time and secondly looking across the individual narratives for the couple's similarities and differences in their experiences. Using this hermeneutic approach to the dyadic coping, the case study centers around how the couple understands their situation from their unique individual standpoints.

CASE STUDY OVERVIEW

Dan and Mary, a middle aged Caucasian couple, have been married for 26 years. Their two daughters, in their early twenties, lived at home. The oldest daughter worked full time after having graduated from university and the youngest was in her second year of university. They have lived in a bungalow in their upper middle class neighbourhood for well over a decade and they were in close proximity to a large metropolitan city in Canada. Neither spouse had parents alive. They did not live in close proximity to their siblings, the nearest being several hours by car away and the furthest a full day's international flight. They both mentioned they were not particularly close to their siblings, preferring to keep to themselves.

Mary, age 52, had been a full time homemaker until her youngest child entered high school. She reentered the paid work force as a bank teller just months prior to Dan's difficulties becoming noticeable. Her position at the bank was part time and precarious. She hoped to hold her job so their family would have some income and medical benefits.

Dan, age 64, was forced to retire early from his career as a stock broker. The company was downsizing and he was let go approximately four years ago. At least five years ago, Dan suspected something was not quite right with his memory. He wondered if his high pressure job was affecting him. At first he put it down to exhaustion, or some other excuses. He started to prepare to leave his job as the rumours at work of layoffs circulated. In our conversations, Mary speculated that Dan's concern with his ability to do his job well lead him to go for early retirement when he did not seek out another stock brokerage house: "but I think perhaps he just didn't feel even then able to cope …but it was only a matter of a few months after (his layoff) that he was diagnosed." In our conversations, Dan spoke about giving things up so as to 'cause no harm.' At home, Mary noticed changes in him. Unbeknownst to her, he had already approached his doctor and friend of over 15 years and confided his fears to him. Dan received a preliminary diagnosis from a neurologist of early onset dementia but was then referred to a special clinic for a more thorough set of tests that spanned two days.

After extensive testing at an Alzheimer and related dementias clinic, Dan's diagnosis of probable dementia of the Alzheimer's Type was confirmed 6 months prior to entering my project. I invited him to participate because his files at the clinic contained measures indicative of a very highly functioning person. For example, his Mini Mental State Exam (Folstein, Folstein, and McHugh, 1975) at the time of diagnosis was 25. In consultation with the team at the clinic, they affirmed that he would be a good candidate for a talk-based research project. I was aware he had decided to participate in clinical drug trials associated with the clinic and wondered if he and Mary might already be burdened with research participation and less inclined to take part in my project which involved considerable time commitments from both of them. I mailed an invitation to the couple and both he and Mary agreed to participate in my research project on understanding the experiences of couples living in the community where one spouse had the diagnosis of dementia of the Alzheimer type.

Dan's conversational ability was very high, spending approximately two hours with me in an engaged discussion for both of our meetings. His narrative showed a great deal of pride in holding others' trust and confidence. These were important aspects that were highlighted when he talked about his career and his volunteerism with his service club. It seemed that had dementia not entered the picture he would have been still going strong in his career and he would not have altered his leadership and considerable responsibility with his volunteerism.

Mary too was thoroughly engaged in our conversations using them as an opportunity to reflect on her experiences. Her narrative showed her resolve to make the best of what they have and she struggled against feeling overwhelmed.

While our conversations were central to my research project, I did use some established measures to add another layer of triangulation to the project. Dan and I completed the measures together discussing some of the items more than others and using it as an opportunity to elaborate on issues. Thus it was more like an extension of our conversation than a standardized test. Dan indicated his health was quite good. In our conversations he did not present as depressed and our discussion of the items on the Geriatric Depression Scale showed he was in the normal range for both interviews (scoring 5 and 6 respectively). Mary reported excellent health as well. Her GDS scores were in the normal range for the first (6) and second (4) interviews, yet she spoke at length about a depression she had been treated for a few years earlier. She described using a medicinal herb to assist with her feelings of depression. Throughout our conversations she did not appear to be depressed.

In looking across Dan's and Mary's experiences that they shared with me throughout their interviews, 5 major themes emerged from their narratives. These five themes are about 1) diagnosis, 2) awareness (with a sub-theme on dyadic coping), 3) relationships, 4) stage of life, and 5) work. In the remainder of this chapter I will explore what these themes entailed.

1. The Journey to Diagnosis and beyond

As a couple, diagnosis was experienced very differently for Dan and Mary. In the beginning, approximately 5 years ago, diagnosis was pursued independently by Dan. Mary only came into the picture later. In both our conversations I invited Dan to describe his experience of the diagnostic process. Dan described an initial diagnosis "when I went through this cylinder thing, then when they x-rayed everything" (T1). Of note was his description of "the doctor comes in, and has a bunch of tricks that he plays on you" (T2). His understanding of how "it's simple as can be" but "I still can't do it" (T2) was also balanced by his statement that there were others with Alzheimer's who would do more poorly than he, "It's probably better than some of them (laughs through words)" (T2). Thus he was coping with the diagnosis by simultaneously acknowledging it and resisting it; that he was not as bad off as some people.

Mary described her experience of the diagnostic process as peripheral where Dan "of his own volition, unknown to us, he went to the doctor um to ask him about his failing memory and his family doctor sent him for, referred him to a neurologist I guess it was, who did tests and ahhm he diagnosed him" (T1). Mary explained how "when Henry (family doctor) got the results from the (tsk) neurosurgeon, he asked us both to go into the office to get the results." There was no medication offered at the time and Mary's experience was one where "they just sort of say, well this is what you have, go home, tough and that and that's it. You're not offered anything. There's nothing you can (raises voice) do, take" (T1). She confides, "there was denial in the beginning but ahh that's not denial, it's just (5 sec) coping I guess." (T1). I asked her to explain:

> (T1) Mary: Well yes, after his diagnosis, nothing ahh nothing
> was done I didn't, we didn't see anybody about it, didn't go back
> to the doctor, didn't do anything and I think that was denial and I
> think too in a way, that was wrong. I, I, looking back, he, he
> obviously needed some support then and I think it would have
> been helpful if ahh, (tsk) we'd looked for some. I wish the doctor
> had said something about that, thinking about it now. It would
> have been kinder than just abandoning him (3 sec) to it. (10 sec)
> But nothing, nothing was done til ahh (4 sec) I had my
> depression.

Mary's depression was diagnosed approximately a year later and treated for approximately a year and a half at which time a counselor spoke with Dan as well. Dan's initial diagnosis of possible or probable AD was followed up with referrals and more extensive testing at the Alzheimer Clinic. Dan's the last diagnosis occurred about 6 months prior to entering my project. Dan described his reaction to the diagnosis at the clinic:

> (T1) Dan: (3 sec) I, I, I just think, thought that well I'm gonna
> have to go with it and but do everything in my power to ahh
> (inhales) to work to get something done about it. I, you know I
> was ah ah (4 sec) gung ho to help and that's how it is because I
> have volunteered myself to these particular things (referencing
> research participation) that may run out on me but it may help
> somebody else someday.

I asked Dan about his perspective on whether people with dementia should be told about their diagnosis, "I think the doctor should, yes." He was glad to be told, "because I'd be wondering what's going on" and "Now I know how to (inhales) attack it on my own way. (T1)"

Dan preferred to keep his diagnosis within his immediate family, "But I don't think the people should go, go around spouting, "I've got Alzheimer's disease," I don't think the patient should be doing that" (T1). Dan did not discuss it with his daughters even though they know:

(T1) Interviewer: At some point do you think you'll want to talk to them more about what's going on for you or that's/

Dan: (inhales) I, I've, I've, I think that maybe their mother would probably put it in nicer words than that I would. I would put it down bluntly.

Interviewer: What would you say to them?

Dan: Just ahh (4 sec) I'm not what I used to be (laughs through words). No I, that's it, I I've I don't think I'd really say too much. (3 sec) No, I wouldn't say too much (sniffs somewhat teary).

He was very private about his life, "Nobody knows that I have this problem" (T1). Not even his brothers know. And as far as he is concerned, no one in his service club knows as he covers up his mistakes, explaining to me: "because I'm trying to hedge you know so they don't know (lowers voice) what's going on" (T1). I wondered why:

(T1) Interviewer: What, what do you think umm why, why is it that you don't want to talk to or let other people know that Alzheimer's disease is/

Dan: I don't think it's any

Interviewer: happening to you?

Dan: I don't think it's their business.

Interviewer: It's your personal

Dan: It's pers, yeah, and I've gotta, yeah, (inhales) or they ahh, I don't, I don't (3 sec), maybe they want to challenge you or something. I know my limitations ahh what I can do.

Dan knew that he was putting on an act pretending to fit in with people:

(T2) Dan: (lowers voice) Oh no, it's not easy. No. This is a false face. A lot of it is false. Here this laughing or anything like that, a lot of it is false.(5 sec) And you just go along with the crowd. Don't get lost from it. Don't get separated. Or you can laugh just the same as the other people can laugh, (lowers voice) but you don't know what you're laughing for.

Unfortunately the act came at a cost to his self esteem. In his service club he described how "At one time I had my own division as they say with the souvenirs" (T1). But he had relinquished responsibilities because "And ahh that's my main concern that I won't hurt anybody and ahh that I won't have any money because I, (3 sec) if I reached in my pocket, I wouldn't know how much of it was mine" (T1). Rather than tell his service club brethren about his dementia he maintained silence and modified his contributions to loading the truck:

(T1) Dan: But they don't, they don't know, they (inhales), I just play, play dumb (laughs through words) which I am (laughs) down there. No, I've got a job to do (loading the truck) and know when I can be, who I'll be working with and no, no problems.

Interviewer: You laughed when you said play dumb cause you're not dumb

Dan: Oh, no (lowers voice). I just ahh yeah I, you know it's something to, that you can brush it off with.

2. Awareness Lead to Sets of Strategies

Both Dan and Mary were paying attention to lapses and shifts in Dan's abilities. Dan noted the changes he's observed, "But with my condition, it's hard. A lot of things are hard. Everyday living here is hard. Ahh harder than what I was used to say 5 years ago" (T1). In our first conversation, Mary described the changes she has seen since the first signs of dementia:

(T1) Mary: Well (raises voice) the memory gets worse, and more forgetful and less able to do things he used to be able to do, more anxious, more fearful, less (raises voice) connected. (3 sec) Not the guy he was, that's for sure (somewhat teary)!

Dan described and illustrated how he watched himself. During our interview he explained, "I just don't know how, their names, that's all, that's why I stumbled" (T1). And in talking about his abilities he says he does not think he talks well anymore, and that he is vigilant about what he does: "See that's the only thing that bothers me is getting mixed up in something that I don't know my way out" (T1). He reported on the frequency of his experiences, "It doesn't happen very often" (T1). Dan's awareness was from a metacognitive perspective in which he had insight into his lapses:

(T1) Dan: if I sssstumble on something, that maybe it would be a connection but nobody outside the house like family, would have any indication. But in, at home, here ahh sometimes I have to stop and think of (3 sec) of a person's name and have to ask, probably have to ask again and

Interviewer: Do you notice when you're asking the same question more than once?

Dan: Yes. (4 sec) Yeah. I don't notice as often as Mary would.

He openly acknowledged his limitations with his family:

(T1) Dan: (inhales) (7 sec) I I don't know the time, but I know that I could ask the question and then remember the answer, but now it's it's getting ah getting a little harder to ahh, the timing is coming closer that I would forget. You know, they, I'd ask,

they'd ask me or Mary or somebody would ask me to do
something and sure I'd go over and do it and ahh have it
completed. They'd ask me something now, by the time I get
there, I've forgotten what it, (lowers voice) what it was.

Interviewer: So then what do you do?

Dan: Ask them what it was.

His awareness also extended into an understanding of situations where he was
compromised in terms of his abilities to think:

(T1) Dan: Gettin around in the (7 sec) I get uptight when I get
challenged.

Interviewer: Challenged in terms of?

Dan: Talking ahh names, ahh dates, ahh or just (3 sec) if Mary
says, "Oh we're gonna go somewhere," then I'll go away and do
something else and I'll have to come back and go, "Where were
we going?" (4 sec) And I would say, (5 sec) especially it's, it's
hard especially when there's pressure coming from it. From the,
say Mary or one of the kids or ahh you know. They want the
answer right now and they can't understand why I can't give it to
them, a simple question. It's because I can't think fast enough.
Not as fast as I used to be able to at work. (3 sec) Ahh I'm
noticing that (3 sec) quite often now. (inhales) And but if, if I'm
re relaxed and I'm not ahh interrupted or anything like that, I can
usually remember something. But it's when the pressure is on it,
the pressure has just got to be slight. It, it will turn my thinking
off and completely, completely off the object that we're
discussing.

Furthermore, his awareness lead him to use strategies to prevent problems for himself:

(T1) Dan: I'm in the ahh Lodge and quite active in the Lodge and
ahh they will give me dates and things like that and if I don't
write them right down, I've lost it. If it's a strange mall, I get
concerned. Say I forgot.

Interviewer: Concerned about what?

Dan: Yeah, well, where put the, where the car is. Not, I, I've I've,
although I can drive, I refuse to drive.

Interviewer: Because?

Dan: In case I hurt somebody. No (lowers voice) I don't want to
ahh be responsible for driving.

Interviewer: Are you concerned that you might forget a certain
rule or

Dan: That's right! Or ah yeah, or not, not thinking fast enough or you know, it may be somebody else's fault but ahh it would be still an accident and I don't want to be driving and it be my fault. Ahh (lowers voice) I wouldn't feel very happy about it at all. And no, I don't, I don't do any driving, although I can. My license hasn't been taken away. It might be one of these days, but I haven't, I haven't driven I guess for about 6 months or.

Interviewer: So it was your decision to stop driving?

Dan: (inhales) I, I think so. Yeah, I think so. Yeah. Yeah.

Mary's experience of this transition was different:

(T1) Interviewer: How was the driving issue handled?

Mary: (11 sec) (exhales) Well it was mine because I, he was ahh (3 sec) I thought getting to be not quite safe in that (5 sec) he was getting more and more hesitant and ahh less confident. I can't say he really actually made any mistakes but he was getting, he's always been a very defensive driver and ahh I could see the potential there where he would be getting ready to make a mistake and I just didn't feel (tsk) (3 sec) that it was really safe for him to be driving. (5 sec) (raises voice) And he always drove when we were together and he always, always drove and one day I just said, "Shall I drive?" (lowers voice) and he said, "Ok." I've driven ever since. He did (clears throat) after I started to do that, occasionally he would still drive up to the subway to meet one of the kids. If it was daylight, if the weather was good, if it wasn't rush hour, he would drive up to the station and ahh meet them. But he hasn't done that for (4 sec) months. (3 sec) He doesn't, he doesn't suggest it, driving. (8 sec)

Interviewer: So the decision happened almost by consensus.

Mary: Yeah, he's never, he's never said, "I think I should," or "I wish I could" or

Interviewer: Is his driver's license coming up for renewal.

Mary: (3 sec) I don't, I don't think so. Umm I think it hadn't long been renewed when he stopped driving. (6 sec) If it comes up, (lowers voice) I think I'll probably let him renew it cause he doesn't drive. So I think I'll let him have that (lowers voice). Just let him have the license. I don't think I would say he can't have it. You can't just take him away from having it. (6 sec) Like carrying a cheque book when you've got no money, you still got the cheques and it makes you feel better (shared laughter).

Interviewer: (shared laughter) What a great analogy.

Mary: Well you, you know. You've got to give them what they've got left.

In addition to relinquishing driving, Dan was also relinquishing other cherished activities like traveling with his service club. "I'll miss going up there, (inhales) but" (T1) he gave it up because, "Yeah, I'm not comfortable. At one time I was right into it, no problems, but (inhales) now I'm not comfortable with it" (T1). He feels torn, "Although they, all the guys, want me to come," he feels, "I could, I could handle it going with the crew to, to these ceremonials but ahh (4 sec) if, if I had to go into a large mall or something, I'd get all twisted around" (T1). Mary was aware of the importance of this activity for her husband and noted the significance of this change for Dan, "And he doesn't do much else. So he likes to do that, but this year for the first time, he isn't going out of town" (T1).

Dan indicated that his awareness of what he needed and his personal coping strategies sometimes created problems. For example, Dan's primary coping strategy was to walk:

> (T2) Dan: I've had a good long life and (raises voice) it's still
> good! And, and I can enjoy it and do it (lowers voice) the best
> way I can. And as I say I, just as long as I, (raises voice) I've got
> to walk! (3 sec) (lowers voice) I've got to walk and I've got to
> walk hard. (4 sec) When I walk I try to tire myself out. So and
> the thing is if I have a good walk, I have a good sleep at night. I
> have a good appetite.

Yet, because awareness for Mary meant that she had to monitor his well being, this was a source of conflict between them:

> (T2) Dan: Ahh, oh yeah. She, she may think, she may think that I
> do too much walking but I've got to! ...And if that's taken away
> from me, I've had it! (lowers voice) Really had it! I've got to do
> it, yeah!

His strategy for not getting lost also seemed to create conflicts with others. For example, he described finding his way through the mall, "I know then I can work around the perimeter to, to find myself. There's little things that you have to ahh, to give yourself lots of time and to ahh that's if you get turned around. (T1)" He described the implications of that strategy:

> (T1) Dan: And the thing is, (5 sec) it's a lot slower. If
> somebody's waiting for you, they want to know why it took 20
> minutes to get here when it should only taken 10. It's because,
>
> Interviewer: So what do you say to that?
>
> Dan: I say well I just got a little turned around. But as I say, it's,
> it's more than a little turned around it's, (raises voice) it's pretty
> serious.

Six months later, Mary described how "He's had one hallucination, that's all. That was the biggest change." (T2) She reported no, "changes in his behaviour. I do think he is getting worse slowly. He has ahh a little trouble with his speech now. In, in finding the right word and a bit of st stuttering and ahh sometimes he'll use the wrong word and not be aware that he has. That's a little bit more frequent than it used to be. (3 sec) But, not really any other new symptoms" (T2). In our second interview, Dan seemed to be using more minimization of his symptoms which could be a precursor to a loss of insight into his limitations:

> (T2) Dan: No, actually, there's (laughs) really been not, no changes. Ahh maybe forgetting a little bit more, but, possibly and I'm, (3 sec) I think it's ahh, other people forget more than I do. But no I don't ahh I, I forget and ahh (4 sec) call myself a fool because it's so minute and ahh but I, it's not very often. Ahh the only time that I (raises voice) really forget or anything is if I'm challenged or ahh something like that. Everything will disappear out of my mind, and erase everything.

Clearly problems and conflicts could arise as Dan loses his ability to judge his limitations. He still maintained his responsible stance with regard to driving but he entertained the notion that he could use the car in an emergency. In our conversation he reconsidered his idea about driving and reminded himself why he gave it up:

> (T2) Dan: No. I gave that up as soon as I knew (lowers voice) what my problem was. (inhales) I, (raises voice) I stopped right then because and that's (3 sec) three or four years ago ah. No! I ahh (3 sec) I (raises voice) could do it up to (mall) or something. Just in my own area. (inhales) And, ahh, in an emergency or something. If one of the kids were hurt or they were sick or something, I could drive down to the hospital. But I, but I don't think I'd even think of it. I'd just take a cab. (3 sec) See that's when I'm phasing everything out that could hurt anybody on my behalf.

There was little doubt that Dan's insight into his abilities and his attitude of caution combined to make Mary's experience easier. And any changes were balanced by Mary's assessment that Dan seemed to be holding up rather well:

> (T1) Interviewer: (9 sec) Is there something that's been surprising for you in this? Five years ago it started. You had ideas about what was going to happen.
>
> Mary: (inhales) Well, he progressed so slowly. At the beginning, he seemed to be on a plateau for a long, long time. It didn't seem to get much worse. I guess I'd expected it to just, him to deteriorate more quickly but then in the last (inhales) (3 sec) 6 months or so, he has deteriorated more. (3 sec) So I wonder, you know, how long? Course they can't tell you. At one of these meetings I was at, they say ahh 6 years from diagnosis to stage 7, well obviously I don't feel that's (inhales) going to happen. So I, I really think they can't put slots on this and say it takes X number of years to go from stage this to stage that. I think ahh some people can have it for 30 years and still die of something else. (4 sec) (tsk) So you just wait and see.

Interviewer: So that's a big surprise for you?

Mary: (5 sec) Not a surprise it's just umm maybe I'd expected, 5 years ago, I guess I'd expected him to be worse by now.

Another strategy that they used was to enter a clinical drug trial to have access to medication and that seemed to have an impact:

(T2) Mary: We've finished the 6 month where it was the double blind. Personally I think he was not on it. But now he is on the medication for sure and has been since well, when, when did we start? We started it last December, so he'd been almost 6 months now on the medication. And perhaps we weren't, perhaps he wasn't on it when you were here. December, Jan. So it would have been June, July when we went on, on, on it for sure. (inhales) Anyway, at the very beginning, I thought I saw an immediate ahm improvement in his mood. He seemed to me to be more cheerful when he first went on it.

Awareness for Mary meant she had to find ways to cope with what she was witnessing in her husband because, "Well it can get a bit depressing I guess" (T1). Some of her strategies were familiar ways of dealing with stress, finding joy in, "My garden (laughs), (5 sec) the kids when they have their successes and see them getting on and developing and growing, that's always nice to watch, (3 sec) just little things now, good weather, holidays" (T1). Mary's Screen for Caregiver Burden scores indicated her objective burden decreased slightly from 10/25 to 8/25 over 6 months. Similarly she indicated a decrease in her feelings of subjective burden from 20/100 to 12/100 at the 6 month follow-up. Her narrative showed that she seemed to have adapted to her circumstances. She reflected back on her adaptation:

(T2) Mary: I'm (inhales), I'm feeling better than I, than I have done depression wise, I'm fine right now. So I'm glad about that.

Interviewer: How did you get out of your depression?

Mary: The original one? I, I took Prozack and then ahh I felt after 6 months, it was my suggestion that I discontinued it ahh the doctor was a little bit leery about it, but um I've been ok and there were, sometimes it's difficult but now I take St. John's Wart and it's ahh I think it's helping. Whether it's psychological or psychosomatic, or whatever, I don't know, but I do feel (inhales) better, so it's harmless, so I take that now. It's supposed to have the same effects on the ahh Serotonin is it in the brain that Prozac does so.

Her narrative showed how she used her sense of humour to cope and a long standing coping identity she shared with her mother:

(T2) Interviewer: What are some of the things that give you strength?

> Mary: St. John's Wart. (lowers voice) I don't know, I think I've
> always been a, a coper, really. My mother was like that you
> know. Whether it's the genes or just the attitude that ahh this is it,
> deal with it. But so far, that's, that's all I'm doing really. (8 sec)
> So far, so good.

Her dominant coping pattern was more clearly understood when I specifically focused on a significant shift in Dan's reality testing:

> (T2) Interviewer: How did you cope with that shift, with the
> hallucination? How did you, you said it was difficult how did
> you get through that?
>
> Mary: (lowers voice) Oh well, I didn't do anything, you just,
> there it is. It's not over yet so you get used to the idea.

She was searching for other ways to cope:

> (T1) Mary: (inhales) Well they say you're not sent anymore than
> you can cope with, that guy up there that's got it all planned
> (shared laughter) somebody once said that so maybe they know
> something (7 sec) and maybe not. (31 sec) I'm thinking of
> looking in, in the fall when they bring the parks and recreation
> brochures out to find one on the power of positive thinking, I
> think that might be something to focus on.

She found comfort in comparisons of her spouse's abilities relative to other's, "But ahh he helps lost people on the street though, so I guess it's not his turn yet (smiles) (T2). She also found comfort in comparison with others' predicaments:

> (T2) Mary: Yeah, it's such a shame for these people who don't
> have anyone and ahh you think, how, how is it that they're out
> there alone in the streets when they don't know where they live.
> But maybe there's somebody at home, I don't know.

Dyadic Coping Forms Part of the Set of Strategies

This couple managed a simultaneous open acknowledgement of AD with a reluctance to have it take on too much significance. There was a tenuous balance between open discussion and avoidance of focus on distressing events or their implications. None-the-less, this couple demonstrated dyadic coping. Dan described how he relied on Mary:

> (T1) Interviewer: Are you, do you find that you rely on her
> more?
>
> Dan: (raises voice) [Oh yeah! Yes, yes, yes, yeah..]
>
> Interviewer: [than you used to?]
>
> Dan: I've got to! (lowers voice) I've got to.

He gave the example of being out in public:

(T1) Dan: the only thing is if she disappears in a crowd of
people, and I don't know where she is, then, then I start to panic,
because I panic if she's in a crowd of people, and I may not have
seen her go in or where she'd go I just stop right there and let her
go through and eventually realize that I'm not there she'll come
looking for me (3 sec). I just stay still!

Mary was trying hard to help Dan cope with his symptoms, describing how she helped
him to deal with the lingering worry of a hallucination:

(T2) Mary: So I said that if he, that not to keep it to himself and
worry for days. That if anything worried him about it, then I
begged him to tell me so that we can talk about it and if it's true,
well let's talk about it anyway and if it's not, then you can sort it
out....But it's (inhales) silly for him to, to keep it in and worry
about it. Anyway, he hasn't mentioned it since, so as far as I
know, that's the only, the only one. It was sort of surprising
because I wasn't ready for that yet. I know that they do that. This,
this happens but I thought it much later. I was really surprised
that it had happened.

She understood and was compassionate about his emotional world:

(T2) Mary: He just gets a bit frustrated when he can't remember
things. He doesn't seem depressed or, or particularly anxious.
Just you know, he, when he knows he should remember things
and he can't. Or he thinks he should be some place and he doesn't
know, then he gets anxious. (4 sec) But other than that, his
behaviour isn't really any, (lowers voice) any different. (8 sec)
But as I say, it is frustrating and of course you're anxious when
you don't ahh you're not sure what you've forgotten or whether
you've forgotten.

She was Dan's confidante when he had problems but the discussion of his challenges was
fraught with tension for her. The surface content of their discussion was not typically open to
a deeper discussion of the implications of such challenges. For example, Dan had confided his
disorientation while traveling with his service club, but he framed it as the fault of a poorly
laid out hotel. Mary knew the disorientation was a symptom of his failing cognition but she
did not engage Dan in a discussion of this, nor did she pursue the implications. Rather, it was
Dan who made the decision to stop traveling:

(T1) Mary: But last year, I guess he had a lot of difficulty being,
(inhales) because of course they're in a strange place and I guess
he couldn't find his motel room and he had difficulty
remembering where he had to be at such and such a time, so I

guess he found it difficult. Anyway, he just said he wasn't going
to go this year.

Interviewer: How did you find out about his difficulties?

Mary: Well he told me. Yeah. Of course he blamed it on the
hotel, having a very confusing layout and things weren't marked
as they should be (tsk), (lowers voice) "Ok."

Mary helped to maintain his sense of pride, "I let him do as much as he can." (T1). Mary
elaborated how Dan had always been responsible for paying the bills and that she wanted to
facilitate his maintenance of that task:

(T1) Mary: I let him write the cheques that he can. I always
supply him with the date and help him make it out and make sure
that he writes it down in his record keeper but I like him to do as
much as he can for as long as he can. They tell you not to ahh
make him totally dependent before his time, so I try not to.

Mary worked hard to keep up the facade for Dan of his independence. For example, she
explained how the social worker needed to make contact with both of them:

(T2) Mary: Yeah, as long as, as long as she, but. Call him by all
means, but then let me know too. Because you know if he, if he.
Like I don't know he talked to you and people give him messages
thinking I'll get them. Well I don't. So she must realize you must
talk to me if she wants him to know (inhales) about it. Then I'll
have to know as well so that I can reinforce it.

However, as a couple the façade could become more stressful and involve more effort
than it was worth. Part of dyadic coping may be to hold on to some activities while
relinquishing others. Mary described how on their walks "now and then, he, he'll say
something funny or pertinent, (T1) and "We go for walks, not as often lately because I have
had so much stuff to do, but we go out for dinner" (T2). Dan and Mary have both noticed
changes in his ability to be with others in social settings. Dan explains that he is fine, "as long
as there's (raises voice) no people around" (T1). And this has not gone unnoticed by Mary:

(T1) Mary: He's not umm (inhales) very comfortable in social
situations so I don't ahh pursue that as much. We don't have
people over for dinner very often anymore.

Interviewer: So that's something as a result of the memory loss?

Mary: I suppose it is. I have less energy for that kind of thing so,
that's partly why, and then he doesn't, he would never object so
he says, "Don't do it." But you know he doesn't keep up with the
conversations very well. (lowers voice) So you don't get the
same pleasure out of it. So you think, "Why do all that work?"

3. A Disrupted Relationship

For this middle age couple, early onset dementia of the Alzheimer's type represented a considerable disruption in the expected trajectory of their relationship. The experience of this shift will be ongoing and on multiple levels as they are faced with changes in the meaning of reciprocity, companionship, independence, protectiveness, care, and in the balance of power in the relationship. Overall Dan's narrative showed little insight into how his dementia was impacting on their relationship. In contrast, Mary's narrative revolved around the loss of their relationship as she had known and expected it to be.

In addition to their narratives I examined their Quality of Relationships Inventory to compare their responses. I calculated dyadic differences between their relationship ratings at both interviews. Time 1 differences indicated Dan perceived more social support, conflict and depth in their relationship than did Mary. Six months later the dyadic differences showed the same pattern. It would be difficult to know if these differences were endemic to their relationship across the last 26 years or if they were new changes introduced in the last few years of transitions; Dan's retirement, Mary's reengagement with work outside the family; Dan's diagnosis. For Dan these transitions may have created a shift so that his wife became a more central person in his world and for Mary they may have had an opposite influence where she may have been anticipating less in their relationship across time. Perhaps, and most likely, all of these factors were operating simultaneously.

Each spouse needed to come to terms with what the marriage held in the face of dementia. For example, Dan's experience of their relationship, "I think we're closer together" (T1) does not match with Mary's:

> (T2)Mary: (3 sec) I don't confide in him a great deal. Like when you've told him three times, you know, (4 sec) you tend to, to not do that because if you're looking for support you're not going to get any.
>
> Interviewer: So, from what your relationship was where you were able to talk about things to where it is now, how is that for you?
>
> Mary: (exhales) (7 sec) Well you, you miss that, you know. You don't have the conversations that we used to. Or he doesn't get the jokes you know. It's cause he's not ahh, (inhales) he doesn't remember things. So when I'll say something and the kids will immediately ahhm relate it to something and laugh. Say it to him and it has no meaning for him. He doesn't have that memory of things or relating (3 sec) back so you, you miss that. So you still do the mundane talking or the day to day stuff but um (lowers voice) you miss that. But I've accepted it. It's, you've got to haven't you?

They needed to renegotiate, personally, what the marriage held in terms of each partner's roles and expectations. Mary described her new protective vigilance and monitoring role:

(T1) Mary: But I haven't made a point of going ahh around and informing everybody about this, no. (5 sec) (inhales) I mean what's the point? I don't. I'm afraid of the way that they might relate to him. You know treat him differently. (3 sec) And if he doesn't ahh tell, he's told no one as far as I know, then I don't like to do it.

Interviewer: So you try to protect him from being maligned.

Mary: Ohh sure.(inhales) Well I don't go out of my way to cover it up. I mean it must be apparent to people who've known him for some time. Obviously it is. Ahh well I just remind him of things that he forgets and supply names to the faces that he doesn't ahh remember. But I mean I don't try and cover it up. They must know. I guess they're reluctant to say anything (laughs through words) unless I do. (raises voice) But then I think, what's the point? So you tell everybody, so it doesn't change anything.

She monitored his functioning in terms of his behaviour and activities:

(T1) Interviewer: You said some days are better than others for his functioning.

Mary: (exhales) Maybe a little, a little bit, yeah, yeah. Situations you know if the, the more ahh depending on where he's been and what he's been doing. Like he, he goes still to, he's a Shriner and he goes still to the meetings. And if he's been (raises voice) out to something like that, when he comes in he's more confused and a little bit more forgetful because he seems with all this (raises voice) stimulation coming at him, then he seems to be a bit worse after that whereas if he's been just out for a walk and been quiet then he seems to to cope better. And from what I hear, this is quite common. They can't ahh take a lot of stimulation, it's too confusing.

For a while, both partners can be part of the renegotiation of roles and decision making. For example, Dan explained how he still felt like he had a say in "Decisions or, I can still make those." And that "I get to put it out on the table to them. Aah if it's you know a decision to be made, I'll have my chance to, what I think of it, of adopting something" (T1).

Not only will the renegotiation of roles and responsibilities be ongoing, it will also take place in the context of shifting cognitive abilities for one spouse. At some point, the partner who does not have dementia will have to face the responsibility of making decisions that may be against what their partner wants. The challenge will be how to continually readjust responsibilities in the face of cognitive decline, balancing between respect for the partner with dementia and monitoring for significant shifts in memory and judgment abilities that could be potentially harmful. Finding the balance between respect for one's spouse and peace of mind will be a struggle. Clearly the relationship that existed prior to the onset of dementia will have a direct bearing on how the couple adjusts to cope with the challenges of early stage dementia. Throughout both spouse's narratives, it was clear that they both held deep regard for one another as Dan described, "I think one respects the other" (T1).

Indicators of stresses and strains in the relationship emerged where the struggles of balancing between care and over-protectiveness were revealed. In speaking about how she allowed him to do as much as he can, she showed that she was in the 'overseeing' role. Mary illustrated a couple identity when she described their coping but her language shifted throughout our conversations from 'we' to 'he' to 'them' as she described her experiences. These shifts in language illustrated the struggles she faced between a reciprocal relationship to one where she must assume authority over her spouse. For example:

> (T2) Mary: ...so far we're managing. (9 sec) He seems to be progressing very slowly (3 sec) some of them do, you know. Some of them are quick.

This signaled a shift in the balance of power in the relationship, "but I try to let him do whatever he can, umm I recently got Power of Attorney but I haven't used it" (T1). Mary has to live with this unequal balance of power and with the dread of her spouse's blame should she be forced to make a decision against his will:

> (T2) Interviewer: What's your worst fear?
>
> Mary: That he's gonna get a lot worse. (5 sec) (lowers voice) And that I, that it, that I wouldn't be able to cope. That he'll be so much worse that he, I can't you know go to work and leave him here, that I won't be able to get (inhales) good help (4 sec) for him here and that he'll deteriorate to the point where he'll have to go in one of these (exhales) homes and I, I dread that! The worst, I think that he will be aware that he'll hate it there and that he'll blame me that he's there. That I think is the wor, the thing that I dread the most.

Relationships are the place where the past and the future co-mingle in the present. With a relationship there is an expectation for sustained interaction and commitment but dementia disrupts that trajectory by foreshortening the future. When the future shifted for the relationship, it also robbed Mary of some of the pleasure in her present experiences:

> (T1) Mary:.. one friend that I, I told she um (inhales), we visited her and I said he'd just been for a check up and his cholesterol was really low and everything was just fine. He had wonderful blood pressure. And I said, "What kind of a comfort is that? What's the good of being 93 and having a really healthy ahh body if you've lost your marbles?" So really I don't take as much comfort in these wonderful check ups as I normally would have done. Cause it's not like you can look forward (3 sec) to a, an old age with the same anticipation as you would have done otherwise.

Preparing for a dreaded future takes an emotional toll on the caregiver spouse. Finding a long term care facility was part of the preparation for the future that Mary resisted, "but I've never been able to force myself to do that yet" (T1). This was a major challenge because on the one hand Mary was getting advice, "They tell me I should be touring these places to find out," (T1) And yet:

> (T1) Mary: They don't (sniffs) I understand they don't let you put your name down until you're ready. It's not like I could go and look at this place in Bingham and say, "Yes," that "this is what I want for him. Put his name down and when he's ready I'll let you know." You have to be ready before they put you on a waiting list. But then the long, the list is lengthy. So he's ready now. What happens? Well, I don't know.

> (T2) Mary: Sort of vaguely aware that things are out there, but I haven't pursued because I don't feel that there's anything for him yet (3 sec) and I, I think there then I think well, I should get going on this because they did tell me that ahh it takes ages to get into the system and you can't just say well I'd like to enroll him in this day care two mornings a week. You have to go through a, a dozen hoops first; be assessed and do this, that and the other before you're allowed to maybe participate in not daycare, there were, they used to call it adult day care, they've got a better name for it now.

Counselors generally would encourage and advise a couple to talk about these issues early but this couple found that did not work well for them:

> (T2) Mary: People seem to think that we should be discussing this between us. People seem to be surprised and, and to think that ahh it would be beneficial, but ahh anytime I bring it up, he doesn't, he just sort of shrugs. He doesn't seem to want to talk about it to me. So I don't pursue it. (6 sec) When ahh I was seeing a therapist for a year and a half, I'd go and she'd ahh try to have him talk and he wouldn't talk to her about it. He didn't seem to want to. (8 sec) So I don't, I don't see how you can make people (voice rises) talk about it, if (lowers voice) if he doesn't want to. I mean it would be nice if he could just open up and some people can. But I'm not comfortable with it and neither is he, so I don't see that happening. (14 sec)

> Interviewer: Yeah. It's a life long pattern

> Mary: Yeah, you can't change your behaviours.

> Interviewer: All you can do is create opportunities

> Mary: Umhm

> Interviewer: (12 sec) You did talk about the hallucination.

Mary: Yes, I was just going to say that, that perhaps, when he feels a need then he will do but just as for a conversation piece, then it it's not beneficial (inhales) to him to keep umm (3 sec) talking about it, you know. He refers to it all the time when he can't find anything. Or you know, he refers to it. It's not that he can't say the word (Alzheimer's) (lowers voice) We just sort of say ahh, we joke about it or just say something about it you know, but he doesn't ahh he doesn't seem to want to just to keep discussing it. What's to say?

Interviewer: But he likes to be able to acknowledge that/

Mary: Oh yeah.

Interviewer: this happened. And these are things that he's experiencing. And that's talking about it.

Mary: Oh yeah, oh yeah, we do that all the time. Lots of opportunities for that! (laughs through words) (raises voice) Or I'll, I'll, ahh not lose something, but can't think of a word or something, but can't think of a word or something, I'll say, "You know this thing's catching don't you?" And stuff like that, you know. The kids'll say, "Oh God, both of you! Now what are we gonna do?" (6 sec)

Interviewer: It sounds a lot to me that you are discussing it

Mary: Yeah, acknowledging it. Yes, right. You can't be in tears all the time either. (inhales) Some people, as you say, you do what's right for you and if, if talking about it is right for some people (raises voice) then great, (lowers voice) but I don't think that's for us. Not yet anyway, not ahh (9 sec). It doesn't seem to be. (18 sec) But then maybe, you know there's some, (3 sec) go to one of these ahh support groups and maybe he can talk to people in there more easily. (lowers voice) If that would help him, that would be great.

Despite the fact that counseling seemed to fall short of what Mary and Dan needed, Mary's advice to another spouse facing her situation would be to "suggest that they got counseling because some people are helped a great deal by that and if they do need to do some talking, a good therapist could really get that going," (T1). She also recommended support groups even though she did not personally find them helpful.

While it is likely in the early stages of dementia where a couple could most benefit from counseling to help them negotiate this transitional period, it must be sensitive to the context of the need. When Mary struggled with the implications for her and went to counseling for feelings of depression, Dan had been included in sessions with the counselor but this did not seem to be helpful from Mary's perspective. At the time of our conversations, Dan was searching for support but felt reluctant to move forward on this, stating he was not at that stage yet. A specialized kind of couple counseling would be required to meet the unique needs of this stage of a relationship in the context of the transition in the early stages of dementia. The right kind of support and counseling is important in this transitional period:

> (T1) Mary: (lowers voice) …No good being, being miserable
> before you have to be. (3 sec) This is, I think, why (inhales) (3
> sec) I don't really get much yet out of these umm support and
> this talking because then it's a constant thing, it's there all the
> time, whereas not, ignoring it but (4 sec) having a life. I mean it's
> there. It's not gonna go away. It's only gonna get worse, but why
> anticipate it? Why be (raises voice) really miserable now, before
> you have to be?

> (T2) Mary: (inhales) Very, early on in the diagnosis one of the
> doctors said well ahh, it was at the Alzheimer Clinic, he said ah
> there's a support group but you're not ready for that yet and that
> was really all that's been (raises voice) offered if that's the word.
> Offered for that (inhales) but I am aware that there is one but I
> haven't ahh I haven't found the need for it, but I didn't realize that
> ahh there was an ongoing one for Dan. I'd like him to try that if
> it's possible.

4. Not what You Expected at this Stage of Life

Both Dan and Mary talk about the fact that they are younger than most people who are dealing with dementia of the Alzheimer's type, "it's a bit young for this, isn't it?" (Mary T1). Dan is quite aware that there are other men who seem to have memory problems in his service club but "they're older than I am." Mary feels off time in her experience of dealing with dementia too:

> (T1) Interviewer: You're quite a young woman.

> Mary: Yes, younger than most at this stage. I think. (4 sec) I
> don't know if that's good or bad. (4 sec) I know ummm (inhales)
> some women are in their 80s when this happens. Of course that's
> got to be very difficult for them. (8 sec)

When they have children, part of a middle age couple's stage of life is often centered around launching their adult children into independent lives. In Mary's case, she had decided to make her children and their family life a central part of her world. Negotiating what early onset dementia means to this stage of a family life cycle is also an area where families can have considerable challenge:

> (T1) Mary: Well they're in their twenties, you know, you can't
> keep them at home for forever, although I'd like to. (inhales)
> Ashley (Oldest daughter) graduated from university and she has
> a full time job now, so I don't know how long we can keep her.
> Linda's (Youngest daughter) still, she's just in second year, so
> I've got her here for a bit. (3 sec) But it's unrealistic to expect

them to live here all their lives. (4 sec)... Maybe it won't be as bad as I think it will be when they leave, but .. you miss them. (8 sec) I've told them I'm like an American Express Card and they can't leave home without me, but they insist that someday they will (laughs)! (8 sec)

Interviewer: Are you close with your daughters?

Mary: (smiling) Yeah, yeah, we get along pretty well. (8 sec) Yeah, they're nice people. (9 sec)

Interviewer: Do you think they'll help with their dad as he progresses?

Mary: (inhales) I don't know. (3 sec) I think Linda might, maybe. I don't know about Ashley, she seems to be more comfortable distancing herself from all of this. (3 sec) They don't, they don't spend any time with him now. Really you know, they don't (tsk) (3 sec) (raises voice) seek out to spend time with him while they still can.

Interviewer: Do you try to create moments when they can?

Mary: (lowers voice) Oh I have, they just laugh at me because I'm always trying to get this family time and ahh what's this other expression they have where they laugh at me for ahh, (inhales) not quality time, but they have this expression whenever I suggest doing, "Oh God, no. Mum's on one of her quality time kicks again (laughs)!" (3 sec) So they just laugh. "I'm not 8 years old anymore, you know! I don't want to spend time with my parents!"(shared laughter) (6 sec) And they're so busy you know, the jobs and school and whatever. (4 sec) Well that's just an excuse. They always have time to do what they want to do. (7 sec) Maybe they will. You don't know what people will do when it comes to (inhales) a crunch.

The dynamic between the daughters and their mother with regard to their father's dementia is one where the youngest daughter encourages her mother to not worry about covering up for Dan, "well it's obvious to people" (T2) and "the girls have told their close friends" (T2). So far their involvement is peripheral as Mary says, "I don't ahh ask them for any help. (8 sec) (lowers voice) What could they do? And we don't talk about it. I don't, I don't find it helpful to talk about it really" (T2). The youngest daughter "went to the library and got books out, but Ashley (oldest daughter) hasn't, as far as I know hasn't done any research on it. She, she's less likely to talk about it than, than Linda. (9 sec) But perhaps they find it easier to talk to their friends about it than to talk to me. I don't know. I haven't asked them" (T2).

5. The Changing Significance of Work

This theme served different purposes for Dan and Mary. Dan's work role was in the past, "I just loved every minute of it and every person that I worked with" (T1). Talking about work in our conversation served the purpose of pride "when I'm referring to me, it's not, it's the company and I'm responsible" (T1). He used it as an illustration of his competence and as a source of self esteem. For example, in this passage, he described his job as a broker, clearly illustrating its centrality to his identity:

(T1) Dan: Ahh, I ah I didn't have any ah (tsk) problem, I, you know over 15, 20 years you get into a little bit of a jam but I, I had a good clientele, knew everyone of them umm down to San Diego, up through here ah and I enjoyed my work. I was up at 4 o'clock in the morning and I was getting home here at about 6 o'clock at night for dinner. I but I did my ahh I was what they call a technical analyst. Ahh they ahh the technical is um you follow a particular stock and ahh the stock that's trading, ahh I plo, I plotted what it closed each day. And ahh it's just like writing a book. When you have it on a chart and any stock that's in it's possibly gonna that's gonna break the, the, the (raises voice) ssscale, you can tell how far it's gonna go down, but it also gives you a chance to get out, but that's only if you're a broker that's ahh charting because people see it on a screen that's trading here to here to here, now they don't know the number that, their take down (inhales), there's different ways of doing it. There's, closes that you chart, on the closing of the stock or there's also another stock or another method of doing it is the high lows. A lot of the ahh so called sophisticated people that are playing it big, go high (inhales) high low ahh trading (inhales) and that would (inhales) mean that they're not too cautious. They're just playing it, that ahh now I enjoyed every minute of it.

Interviewer: So how long have you stopped?

Dan: Ahh.. I guess it would be about 3 years now. I may be out a year but it's about 3 years.

Interviewer: Did you stop because you were having memory problems or you just decided to stop.

Dan: No, I, no, the doctor, no, the doctors ahh spotted it, and the ahh company told me it was better just to get out.

Interviewer: So do you miss it?

Dan: Oh yes! Ohhh (laughs), yeah, yeah, much..

Interviewer: So what do you do//

Dan: I don't, I don't think ahh, I don't think I could handle it down there, now after being off for say two to three years, I couldn't handle it, I'd ahh I'd I I'd (inhales) another thing, as I say, I charted the stocks and they never lied and that's what I miss. Is just

Interviewer: the fun of that?

Dan: Yeah, yeah, yeah, yeah, of just knowing what's going to happen with the stock.

Interviewer: Do you still do that?

Dan: No, no, no.

Interviewer: By reading in the papers?

Dan: Oh I read the papers, (laughs through words) oohh yes, everyday, but (exhales) I don't think my wife would like it if I started drawing charts.

Interviewer: Oh really?

Dan: No.

Interviewer: Cause she, what does she say?

Dan: She (inhales), no, she just ended. You're finished, it's finished and that's it. So I contemplated for a few minutes and I said well I guess that's it! Psssh. I just.

Interviewer: That must have been hard

Dan: Ohhh! (exhales) That was the hardest thing in my life (teary)! Yeah. (4 sec) The hardest thing. But, it's all over, in the past now and (4 sec) mind you I had many many good days though.

Dan's current involvement in his service club and his familial role of facilitating mornings serve his current esteem needs. For example,

(T1) Dan: I do the housework.

Interviewer: And that's probably a change for you too.

Dan: Oh yeah, yeah.

Interviewer: Tell me about those changes.

Dan: In the, (inhales) well no, I just ahh I'm an early waker from my brokerage days. I used to get up at 4 o'clock, and ahh but no, today I can sleep in til about 6:30, 7.

Interviewer: That's sleeping in?

Dan: yeah, yeah

Interviewer: I guess for you it is. For me that's getting up early (laughs)!

> Dan: Yeah, and I, I, I enjoy that time of day and I get things
> ready for the two girls and Mary and the mornings, whatever I
> can, sometimes they don't want to eat.

In contrast, Mary's work had not been her life's career, having chosen to reenter the paid work force within the last 5 years after her youngest child entered high school:

> (T1) Mary: Yeah, (7 sec) but fortunately, I had just gone back to
> work, so that helped. I stayed home for 15 years to raise the kids
> (clears throat) and when Linda, the younger one, went to high
> school, I ahh I think I started doing 8 hours a week, just you
> know a bit of interest. And then just before he was diagnosed, I
> found this position that was ahh the 20 hours a week. So, I'd just
> taken that and it had benefits which hadn't been an issue but
> thank goodness it did because it just came (inhales) at the right
> time. So I'm still doing it, for how long, I don't know but it's been
> helpful.

Her narrative showed her identity was not connected to her work. Mary's description of her work life changed over the project. Initially she was quite worried about her future work prospects and the threat of losing her job was just one more source of concern as she was describing her fears for the future, "A lesser fear is losing my job" (T1). In fact she had already started confiding this stressor to me in our off tape conversation:

> (T1) Interviewer: And on top of all that, you've got what's going
> on at work (Threatened job loss due to downsizing - earlier
> discussed off the tape and referred to as a very stressful
> business.)
>
> Mary: Oh yeah. Yeah. (exhales) (9 sec) I guess when ahh shit
> happens, it really happens eh?

Work was something she did to assist the family income, not something that defined her:

> (T1) Mary: I'd like to keep my job, but then I wonder what we'll
> do if I lose that. (4 sec) It's not easy to ah get another job at my
> age. That would make things difficult, financially.

When the stressor of being laid off was removed, this improved her outlook. So while work may not have been an identity factor, it was central to her feelings of being overwhelmed by stress:

> (T2) Mary: Yeah, it looks a little more secure now, or let me say
> I'm no more insecure of my job than anybody else in the branch
> now. There's no security at the bank anymore, but I'm no, I don't
> think I'm any more at risk than the others now. It seems to have
> leveled off a bit.

Interviewer: So has your stress level come down as a result of that?

Mary: (3 sec) I, I guess it must have. You know wondering all the time if your job's there or not, is ahh (lowers voice) is ahh stressful.

Work, or rather the threat of not having it, set limitations for what they could do as a couple at this stage in their life. At a time when many in their upper middle class cohort might be looking at increased leisure they were not planning a vacation because, "Umm no, not now, I might lose my job" (T1). Work also represented limitations in terms of what she could do to support her husband. For example, she was excited about taking him to a support group meeting but it had a set time in the middle of her workday, "See, I work, (lowers voice) how would he get there?" (T2)

By the time of our second interview, work and her relationship with a coworker as a confidante, had become coping resources for her. For example, "when I'm, you know you always get down now and then and I said to my, my girlfriend, Donna, at work," (T2). When I asked about her future and how far she planned ahead, work figured prominently in her feelings of stability:

Mary: (inhales) Two weeks (laughs). No I don't ahh (5 sec) oh well we, we plan ahead. We're going away in January, we've planned that. But ahh (inhales) I don't do anything about the far future. I don't know what I could do. (6 sec) Sometimes I worry about that too, that I should be doing something, but I don't know what I think I ought to be doing. Well how can you plan when you don't know (4 sec) how much worse he's gonna be or when or what? What can you do about it? When it happens, it happens. I don't know about planning. (5 sec) What can you do for it? Yet sometimes I feel I should be doing something about it. (3 sec) (lowers voice) I don't know what. (19 sec) I hope I keep my job. Keep working. That's about the only concrete thing I think I can do as far as helping the future (laughs through words). (T2)

CONCLUSION

This case study represents one particular couple's experience in dealing with the diagnosis of dementia in an open awareness context. The themes that were salient here are likely to be relevant touchstones for other couples who are facing the implications of dementia in mid-life. Their narratives portray a dyadic perspective on the diagnostic journey and the differing tensions created by awareness of symptoms and their implications for caregivers as well as for their spouses with AD. Lives interrupted in their career and relationship trajectories are likely to be common themes for any couple grappling with the meaning of dementia in the mid-life time period. Coping with dementia in middle age will look different depending upon a confluence of factors such as the gender of the person, their marital relationship status, the quality of their relationship with their spouse, children, and extended family members, the kind and nature of formal and informal social supports that they have to draw from in their community, their socio-economic status, their interpersonal skills, their financial resources, existing and developing co-morbidities, and the kind of dementia they are dealing with to name a few of the more obvious factors. Lessons learned from this case study may be more or less applicable to others' situations. It is hoped that the challenges they faced can be instructive to others seeking to understand how a middle age couple navigates the terrain following diagnosis of dementia.

Guide to Transcription Marks for Chapter Quotations

(T1):	First interview
(T2):	Second interview
.... :	Ommited words for the quotation
(x seconds):	Length of pause in the conversation
/:	Interrupted sentence
[overlapping words]:	Spoken at the same time
(voice changes; laughter, conversational accoutrements):	enriched context for the words

ACKNOWLEDGMENTS

Thank you to the couple who participated in this case study for their time and candour in making this research possible. This project would also not have been possible without the extensive cooperation of a Canadian university based Alzheimer clinic. I also want to express gratitude for the generous funding from a provincial Alzheimer Society.

REFERENCES

Alzheimer, A (1907). A unique illness involving the cerebral cortex. In C.N. Hochberg and F.H. Hochberg (Eds.), Neurologic classics in modern translation (pp. 41-43). New York: *Hafner Press.*

American Psychiatric Association (1994). Diagnostic and statistical manual of mental disorders (4th ed). Washington, D.C.: *Author.*

Duvall, E.M. (1977). Marriage and family development (5th ed.). Philadelphia*: Lippincott.*

Gadamer, H. (1975). Truth and method (D.E. Linge, Trans.). Berkeley: University of *California Press.*

Gauthier, S. and Panisset, M. (1998). Current diagnostic methods and outcome variables for clinical investigation of Alzheimer disease. *Journal of Neural Transmission Supplement*, 53, 251-254.

Gergen, K. (1989). The possibility of psychological knowledge: A hermeneutic inquiry. In P. Martin and R. Addison (Eds.), Entering the circle: Hermeneutic investigation in psychology. (pp. 241-260). *New York: State University of New York Press.*

Heidegger, M. (1927/62). Being and time. (Translated by Macquarrie, *J. and Robinson*, E.) San Francisco: Harper-Collins.

Folstein, M.F., Folstein, S.E.,and McHugh, P.R. (1975). Mini-Mental State: A practical method of grading the cognitive state of patients for the clinician. *Journal of Psychiatric Residents,* 12, 189.

MacQuarrie, C. (2005). Experiences in early stage Alzheimer's Disease: Understanding the paradox of acceptance and denial. *Aging and Mental Health: An International Journal, 9(05),* 1-12.

Mills, J. (2001). Self-construction through conversation and narrative in interviews. *Educational Review*, 53(3), p. 285 - 301.

Packer, M., and Addison, R. (1989). Entering the circle: Hermeneutic investigation in psychology. *New York: State University of New York Press.*

Pierce, G.R., Sarason, I.R., Sarason, B.R., Solky, J.A., Nagle, L.C. (1993, unpublished). Assessing the quality of personal relationships: *The Quality of Relationships Inventory.*

Rennie, D. (2000). Grounded Theory Methodology as Methodical Hermeneutics: Reconciling realism and relativism. *Theory and Psychology, 10(4),* 481-502.

Vitaliano, P., Russo, J., Young, H.M., Becker, J., and Maiuro, R. (1991). The Screen for Caregiver Burden. *The Gerontologist*, 31(1), 76-83.

Willig, C. (2004). Introducing Qualitative Research in Psychology: Adventures in Theory and Method. Open *University Press*, pages 50 - 68.

Yesavage, J., Brink, T., Rose, T., Lum, O., Huang, V., Adey, M., and Leirer, V.O. (1983). Development and validation of a geriatric depression screen scale: A preliminary report. *Journal of Psychiatric Research*, 17, 37-49.

In: Alzheimer's Disease in the Middle-Aged
Editor: Hyun Sil Jeong, pp. 255-260

ISBN: 978-1-60456-480-8
© 2008 Nova Science Publishers, Inc.

Chapter 11

DEMENTIA IN THE MIDDLE AGED IN CHINA

Li Qi[1], Zhang Lihong[2,3], E. L. Forster[2] and D. T. Yew[21]

[1.] Stanley Ho Centre for Emerging Infections Diseases, School of Public Health,
The Chinese University of Hong Kong, Shatin, NT, HK
[2.] Brain Research Centre, The Department of Anatomy,
The Chinese University of Hong Kong, Shatin, NT, HK
[3] Department of Neurology, The First Hospital of Hebei Medical University,
Shijiazhuang, Hebei, China.

ABSTRACT

The prevalence of dementia in China, manifest as Alzheimer's disease (AD) and/or vascular dementia (VaD), is comparable to that of Western countries. Overall, AD has become the most common subtype of dementia in China, yet it is interesting to note that the diagnosis of AD is significantly lower than that of VaD, specifically in middle-aged (younger than 65) men. In this paper, we aim to highlight the potential causes of early onset dementia in order to emphasize the importance of improving diagnosis, treatment, and prevention of these forms of brain disease.

Epidemiological studies show the prevalence of cardiovascular diseases in middle-aged Chinese populations, especially males, has increased significantly in the past 30 years. Evidence suggests that various forms of cardiovascular disease, such as hypertension, diabetes, and cerebrovascular disease, may contribute to the development of dementia, yet there is a risk of underdiagnosis of AD in middle-aged men. Clinical physicians tend to pay much more attention to elderly, rather than middle-aged persons suffering from dementia. Also, there is greater access to computed tomography or magnetic resonance imaging for VaD (50.9%) compared to AD (6.8%). These imaging methods are sensitive to early detection of all forms of dementia. While apolipoprotein E (ApoE) remains the best-established risk factor for detecting late-onset AD, studies are progressing on finding genetic evidence for detecting early onset AD. The possibility of suffering from dementia in midlife may be increased by the vascular risk factors of dementia. It is essential that more efforts be employed to identify the genetic,

---

[1] Address for Correspondence:Department of Anatomy, The Chinese University of Hong Kong, Shatin, New Territories,Hong Kong S.A.R.,China.Tel:(852)2609-6899,Fax:(852) 2603-5031 Email: david-yew@cuhk.edu.hk

biochemical, neuroimaging and clinical markers for early detection and treatment of dementia in clinical practice.

INTRODUCTION

Dementia is defined as a clinical syndrome characterized by progressive deterioration in multiple cognitive domains. Developed countries have a higher reported prevalence of dementia than developing areas, yet the global majority of people with dementia are found in developing countries. With an enormous progressive increase in the proportion of old persons, China and its Western Pacific neighbors now have the highest actual population with dementia (6 million) [1]. Some researchers predict that by 2040, these areas of eastern Asia will have three times more people with dementia than Western Europe [1].

There is a similar pattern of dementia subtypes across the globe. Alzheimer's disease (AD) is the most common dementia disorder, followed by vascular dementia (VaD), with these two most common forms accounting for 50-70% and 15-25% of all dementia disorders respectively. The incidence of dementia has been reported as 3% in individuals aged 55 years in urban and rural areas of Shanghai, China, with Alzheimer's disease more frequently reported than VaD [2,3]. Using extensive case ascertainment procedures, Zhang et al. reported that the overall prevalence of AD and VaD in four regions of China was comparable to that in Western countries [3]. However, it is interesting to note in their study that the prevalence of AD in the middle aged (< 65 years old), especially in men, was significantly lower than that of VaD. Here we aim to highlight the potential causes of this situation from epidemiology studies, vascular risk factors, genetic studies and neuroimaging studies of dementia in order to improve the diagnosis, treatment, and prevention of dementia.

EPIDEMIOLOGY STUDIES OF THE PREVALENCE OF AD AND VaD IN THE MIDDLE AGED IN CHINA

Guo et al reported the prevalence of dementia in China from 1986 to 1996 by using Meta analysis [4]. Similar to most Western studies, the age-specific AD prevalence roughly doubled at 5-year intervals. The age-specific VaD prevalence was half that, with a 50% increase at 5-year intervals. Obviously, age was a major risk factor for dementia in this study (figure 1). However, the prevalence rate (%) for AD in the middle-aged males from 60 to 64 years old was much lower than that of VaD in the same age group (figure 2). In 1997, Zhang et al. also demonstrated that AD predominated in China [3], with samples from rural and urbanized communities of Beijing, Xian, Shanghai, and Chengdu. The target population included those of 55 years or older. In comparing these studies, we found that the rate of diagnosis of VaD in middle-aged males from 55 to 64 years old was much higher than that of AD (figure 3).

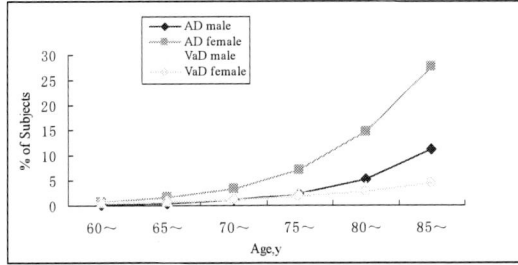

Figure 1. Age- and sex-specific prevalence of Alzheimer disease and vascular dementia in China (from 1986 to 1996). Estimation of Bayesian Meta analysis models by using WinBUGS implementation of MCMC simulation.

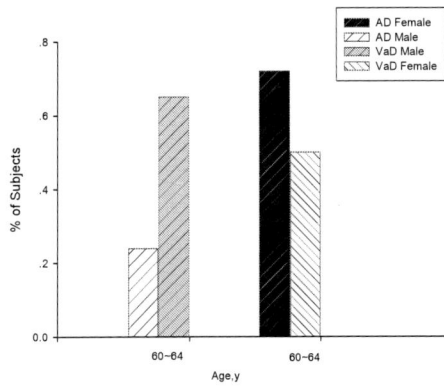

Figure 2. The prevalence rate (%) for Alzheimer disease and vascular dementia in China in the middle aged from 60 to 64 years old (from 1986 to 1996).

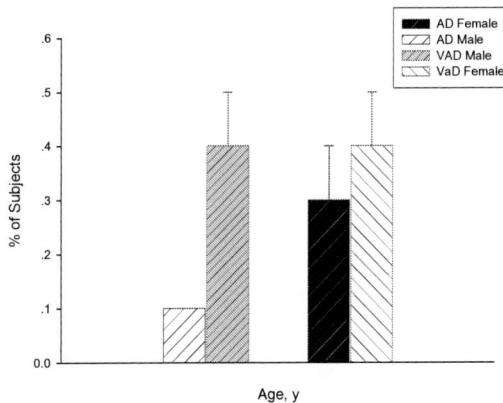

Figure 3. The prevalence rate (%) for Alzheimer disease and vascular dementia in China in the middle aged from 55 to 64 years old (1997).

VASCULAR RISK FACTORS OF DEMENTIA

Experimental and clinical evidence have suggested that vascular risk factors and vascular disorders might both be important for Alzheimer's disease and VaD [5,6]. Experimental data suggest that in AD, as in VaD, there is perturbation of cerebral blood flow and its regulation. Clinical studies suggest that AD and VaD share common cerebrovascular risk factors, such as high blood pressure, obesity, diabetes mellitus, heart disease, hypercholesterolemia, and hyperhomocystinemia [6-10]. These findings suggest that these deleterious vascular effects may play a role in both AD and VaD. Consequently, risk factor modification may be a valuable strategy for prevention of AD, as in VaD. This is particularly important for the middle-aged at risk for early onset dementia in China. According to epidemiology studies, the incidence of cardiovascular disease in the middle aged Chinese population, especially in men, has increased significantly in the past 30 years [11] .

GENETICS OF DEMENTIA

Much research attention continues to be focused on identifying the genetic factors underlying dementia. In particular, AD is believed largely to stem from predisposing genes. Thus far, the major susceptibility gene identified is the Apolipoprotein Epsilon gene (ApoE, or APOE) [12]. ApoE protein is involved in the transport of cholesterol during neuronal growth, after injury, and in the deposition of Amyloid Beta protein (Aβ), one of the hallmarks of AD. The ApoE gene has three alleles: ε2, ε3, and ε4. Those who inherit ApoEε4 allele have a greater risk for developing AD, as well as VaD. ApoEε4 allele is also a significant risk factor for AD as well as for VaD in the Chinese population [13].

NEUROIMAGING STUDIES OF DEMENTIA

Neuroimaging has become an important tool in the early detection and monitoring of AD and VaD. Various neuroimaging techniques can provide direct information of brain structure and function in AD and VaD, showing development and decline due to the disease processes. Magnetic resonance imaging (MRI) has the potential to detect focal signal abnormalities which may assist the clinical differentiation between AD and VaD [14]. MRI methods that are sensitive to the microstructural changes of white matter, called Diffusion Tensor Imaging (DT-MRI or DTI), may be helpful in correlating clinical manifestations of white matter abnormalities. Single-photon emission CT (SPECT) and positron emission tomography (PET) can directly or indirectly record regional cerebral blood flow (CBF) patterns [15]. Because regional cerebral hypoperfusion is one of the earliest, if not *the* earliest, markers of AD symptoms, these neuroimaging techniques enable detection of AD with only mild cognitive impairment. Even so, the risks of underdiagnosis of AD cannot be ignored. For example, there was greater access to Computed Axial Tomography (CAT) or MRI for VaD (50.9%), but much less access for AD (6.8%) patients in China.

CONCLUSION

In summary, the epidemiologic, basic, and clinical features of VaD and AD appear to represent the actual patterns of dementia in the middle-aged in China. Dementia represents a major challenge to public health in China due to the rapid growth of the elderly population. Vascular risk factors in the middle-aged significantly contribute to the development and progression of dementia, whereas extensive social networks and active engagement in social, physical, and mental activities may delay its onset in China. Therefore, more basic and clinical research on the vascular and metabolic features of dementia, more funding for these investigations, and more tolerance to new research ideas are urgently needed. Furthermore, extensive efforts are imperative to identify the genetic, biochemical, neuroimaging, and clinical markers that can be used for early detection of dementia in medical practice.

REFERENCES

[1]   Ferri CP, Prince M, Brayne C, Brodaty H, Fratiglioni L, Ganguli M, et al. Global prevalence of dementia: a Delphi consensus study. *Lancet* 2005 Dec 17, 366, 2112-7.

[2]   Fratiglioni L, Winblad B, von SE. Prevention of Alzheimer's disease and dementia. Major findings from the Kungsholmen Project. *Physiol Behav.* 2007 Sep 10, 92, 98-104.

[3]   Zhang ZX, Zahner GE, Roman GC, Liu J, Hong Z, Qu QM, et al. Dementia subtypes in China: prevalence in Beijing, Xian, Shanghai, and Chengdu. *Arch. Neurol.* 2005 Mar, 62, 447-53.

[4]   Guo X, Liu L, Xu YY. A Meta analysis of the prevalence of dementia and related risk factor in China: A Bayesian approach. *J. Fourth Mil. Med. Univ.* 2001, 22, 1185-6.

[5]   De la Torre, JC. Is Alzheimer's disease a neurodegenerative or a vascular disorder? Data, dogma, and dialectics. *Lancet Neurol.* 2004 Mar, 3, 184-90.

[6]   Qiu C, Winblad B, Fratiglioni L. The age-dependent relation of blood pressure to cognitive function and dementia. *Lancet Neurol.* 2005 Aug, 4, 487-99.

[7]   Newman AB, Fitzpatrick AL, Lopez O, Jackson S, Lyketsos C, Jagust W, et al. Dementia and Alzheimer's disease incidence in relationship to cardiovascular disease in the Cardiovascular Health Study cohort. *J. Am Geriatr. Soc.* 2005 Jul, 53, 1101-7.

[8]   Akomolafe A, Beiser A, Meigs JB, Au R, Green RC, Farrer LA, et al. Diabetes mellitus and risk of developing Alzheimer disease: results from the Framingham Study. *Arch. Neurol.* 2006 Nov, 63, 1551-5.

[9]   Gustafson D. Adiposity indices and dementia. *Lancet Neurol.* 2006 Aug, 5, 713-20.

[10]   Pappolla MA, Bryant-Thomas TK, Herbert D, Pacheco J, Fabra GM, Manjon M, et al. Mild hypercholesterolemia is an early risk factor for the development of Alzheimer amyloid pathology. *Neurology* 2003 Jul 22, 61, 199-205.

[11]   Liu L. Cardiovascular diseases in China. *Biochem. Cell Biol.* 2007 Apr, 85, 157-63.

[12]   Bertram L, McQueen MB, Mullin K, Blacker D, Tanzi RE. Systematic meta-analyses of Alzheimer disease genetic association studies: the AlzGene database. *Nat. Genet.* 2007 Jan, 39, 17-23.

[13] Lam LC, Tang NL, Ma SL, Lui VW, Chan AS, Leung PY, et al. Apolipoprotein epsilon-4 allele and the two-year progression of cognitive function in Chinese subjects with late-onset Alzheimer's disease. *Am. J. Alzheimers Dis. Other Demen.* 2006 Mar, 21, 92-9.

[14] Pantano P, Caramia F, Pierallini A. The role of MRI in dementia. *Ital. J. Neurol. Sci.* 1999, 20, S250-S253.

[15] Gualdi GF, Colaiacomo MC, Bertini L, Melone A, Rojas M, Di BC. [Neuroimaging of Alzheimer disease: current role and future potential]. *Clin. Ter.* 2004 Oct, 155, 429-38.

In: Alzheimer's Disease in the Middle-Aged
Editor: Hyun Sil Jeong, pp. 261-314

ISBN: 978-1-60456-480-8
© 2008 Nova Science Publishers, Inc.

Chapter 12

BIOMARKERS IN ALZHEIMER'S DISEASE

Amanda McRae[1], Gershwin K. Davis[2], Nelleen Baboolal[3] and John A. Morren[4]

[1] Department of Preclinical Sciences,
[2] Department of Paraclinical Sciences,
[3] Department of Clinical Medical Sciences,
Faculty of Medical Sciences, The University of the West Indies,
St. Augustine, Trinidad and Tobago.
[4] County St. George Central, Trinidad

ABSTRACT

Dementia and Alzheimer's disease in particular is fast becoming a major health issue in many countries where life expectancy is increasing and chronic non-communicable diseases have replaced infectious disease as the major cause of morbidity and mortality. To date a cure for Alzheimer's disease is yet to be found and the best that can be hoped for is to slow down the progression of the disease and improve the quality of life of the individual. These temporizing measures would postpone the onset of the final and debilitating stages of the disease. Interventions may be simple but profound. For example, encouraging results have been seen in pre-morbid and affected individuals in whom an active an cognitively-stimulating lifestyle has been facilitated. With this background it is easy to appreciate the need for early detection and intervention, justifying the spirited search for biomarkers. Predicting Alzheimer's disease is problematic due to the very nature of the disorder as clinical features only become apparent following a period of insiduous but substantial cell loss. Thus there is a need for biomarkers to flag early cell death as this may allow for treatment interventions which could arrest the neuropathological processes.

There are different types of biomarkers currently under investigation: ones that can predict susceptibility for dementia, those that can be used for a diagnosis, those that can help in the follow up of the patient i.e. monitor the progression of the disease, and finally those that can be useful in prognosis. Though the vast research effort has been directed towards finding a reliable diagnostic biomarker, no candidate investigated has satisfied all the recommended criteria thus far. To this end the object of this chapter   is to review prospective biomarkers for Alzheimer's Disease. The chapter will focus on, cerebrospinal fluid (CSF) and serum biomarkers, genetic indicators and imaging techniques. At the conclusion of the chapter the reader will appreciate the great challenges investigators are faced with in designing a biomarker for this complex neurodegenerative disorder. At the same time it will become apparent that even though some of the candidate biomarkers are not ideal, they may have some utility in distinguishing pathologies associated with Alzheimer's disease from those of other dementias. Finally, as suggested by this review and others- combinations of biomarkers may increase antecedent, diagnostic and prognostic capacity.

IMMUNE RESPONSE BIOMARKERS IN ALZHEIMER'S DISEASE

Introduction

Immune System

The immune system is amazingly well organized with soldiers to protect us against bacteria and other infectious agents. Actually there are two immune systems, a simple one and a complex one. The simple one or rather the innate immune system is our first line of defense. The complex one or the adaptive immune system is the second line of defense and offers protection against re-exposure to the same pathogen. Each of the systems rely on different cellular components to exert their protective functions. The Russian immunologist Elie Mechnikov discovered the innate immune system in 1883 (1). He performed his landmark discoveries by poking a starfish with thorns, which caused cells to mobilize and engulf the introduced bacteria. He described the process as phagocytosis ("cell eating") and was awarded a Nobel Prize for his cell- based theory of immunity. Thus the main player in the innate immune system is the phagocyte, This system is nonspecific in that it is directed against any pathogen, which enters the body.

Though now viewed as important the innate system has played a back burner role to the more sophisticated adaptive immune system or acquired immunity, which relies on B cells, T cells, lymphocytes and the production of antibodies. Equipped with immunologic memory the adaptive immune system mounts a stronger immune response against an antigen and through this process provides the body with a stronger defense for re-exposure to the same pathogen. The two systems do not function in isolation as there is interplay between them as well mutual influence.

For the reasons described above the adaptive immune system has been considered as the heart of immunology. Tables are turning and the innate immune system is now being perceived as one of great significance. The recent change in focus is due to understanding how innate immune system components such as macrophages, complement proteins, cytokines and toll receptors not only contribute to disease processes, defense mechanisms but are attractive therapeutic targets.

Inflammation can either be acute or chronic. An acute response is the initial response and is usually completed within a short period of time. During the response to an intruder there is an increased mobilization of plasma and leukocytes into the injured area. A cascade of biochemical events propagates and matures the inflammatory response, involving the local vascular system, the immune system, and various cells within the injured tissue. Chronic inflammation, leads to the recruitment of different types of cells, which, are present at the site of inflammation, and is characterized by simultaneous destruction and healing of the tissue from the inflammatory process. One of the hallmark features of chronic inflammation is the presence of macrophages in the injured tissue. These powerful defense agents of the body become toxic to the host tissue through the release of substances such as cytokines, oxygen free radicals and complement. Consequently, chronic inflammation is almost always accompanied by tissue destruction.

Macrophages are dispersed throughout body tissues in a variety of shapes or forms. Specialized macrophages include alveolar macrophages in the lungs, mesangial phagocytes in the kidneys, and Kupffer cells in the liver. What about the brain's specialized macrophages? They do exist under the name of microglia. It has taken approximately a century (1899-1999) to establish their role as the immune cell of the brain and their implications in neurodegenerative disorders in particular Alzheimer's disease (AD) pathology. Detailed investigations about the interactions of microglia and AD have been the impetus for employing components of immune responses as potential biomarkers for this disorder. To fully appreciate the concept of immune responses markers it is first important to trace the historical journey of microglia as they progressed from scavenger cell to the brain immune cell (see 2 for the above definitions and descriptions).

MICROGLIA

One of the earliest documented views of the immune function of microglia was that of Franz Nissl in 1899 (3) who used the term *stabchenzellen* or rod cells to describe microglia. He emphasized that rod cells appeared to be reactive glia cells and that their major attributes were that of migration, phagocytosis and proliferation. Nissl stated,

"It is highly likely that glia cells in addition to producing an intercellular substance have a second task which is approximately the same as the one leukocytes have in other tissues"

Interestingly microglia has been a cardinal feature of the hallmark lesions of AD pathology ever since its initial descriptions by Alois Alzheimer in 1906 (4). The formation of a microglia coffin around cortical pyramidal neurons was probably one of the first observations (5). Though about eighty years too early it was Oskar Fischer (6,7) who noted that plaque formation was an extra-cellular event, which provoked inflammation followed by regeneration. Morphological tools at the time did not allow him to observe an immune response around the plaques and he was also unable to observe complement.

Thus from the very beginning of the description of AD pathology microglia as well as astrocytes have been considered to participate in hallmark lesions in particular plaque formation (5, 8-10). It was even hypothesized that the formation of primitive plaques began around a central microglia cell (11).

While microglia was morphologically recognized in association with plaques, one of the longest running debates in the history of neuroscience was ongoing about the origin of the ramified microglia or the form, which resides in the brain. Based on beliefs four schools of thought were formed concerning the derivation of microglia: i) invasion of mesodermal pial elements, ii) neuroectodermal matrix cells together with the macroglia, iii) from pericytes and

iv) invasion of monocytes in early development. (for review see 12) How did this debate actually begin?

Rio Hortega (13) was the first to demonstrate ramified microglia. He was persuaded that these cells originated from the invasion of mesodermal pial elements. He postulated that pial elements invade the brain tissue to become the globose (rounded and amoeboid microgliocytes (young microglia) and subsequently develop into ramified microglia. He described the migratory and phagocytic properties of microglia (14). His method to reveal microglia, a sliver stain almost abolished the concept of a ramified microglia. However Mori and Leblond (15) adapted a weaker staining procedure, which allowed an electron microscopic analysis of ramified microglia in the brain. The accepted concept about the origin of ramified microglia that being from monocytes was proposed by Santha and Jiba (16). They noted that the arrival of ramified microglia coincided with the vascularization of the brain and considered that ramified microglia was derived from the circulating monocytes. Elegant studies conducted by Ling and his co-workers (17,18) established that ramified microglia are true entities of the brain.

It is be noted that amoeboid microglia in early postnatal development are reactive macrophages phagocytosing degenerating cells and processes (for review see 12). With the closure of the blood brain barrier these cells gradually take on a ramified shape or enter into a resting mode. In response to neuronal damage these cells change their morphology, immunophenotype and proliferate to become activated microglia or full-blown brain macrophages

The injection of carbon particles into the periphery in 5- day old postnatal rats revealed that amoeboid microglia were derived from circulating monocytes (17,18). During early postnatal development these amoeboid microglia are active or proliferate. In this respect one would expect that the number of amoeboid microglia would increase in the brain. However surprisingly there is a constant decrease in these cells and eventually by postnatal day 15 they disappeared. About thirty percent of amoeboid microglia transform into ramified microglia (17). The carbon labeling studies identified that both amoeboid microglia and ramified ones were laden with carbon. Thus this added significant support for a monocyte origin for ramified microglia (17, 18). The transformation of amoeboid microglial cells into ramified microglia results from a regressive phenomenon (19).

With the origin of the ramified microglia fairly well-established the next stages in the history of microglia saw it evolve from a scavenger cell to the immune cell. With the advent of immunocytochemistry and antibodies it was possible to reveal the immunophenotype of microglia (20-24). Even more important was the ability to associate antigen expression with morphological change. As the result of an injury immediate microglia morphological changes occur (20-24). In the first instant slender microglia processes begin to retract and look swollen. About a week later microglia begin to withdraw their process and take on a more rounded or activated form. By the time they are full blown macrophages the cells are rounded with no processes. Each of different stage of morphological changes is denoted by the expression of different antigens. In first proliferating stages microglia express complement- 3 (CR3) receptors in the next stages there is enhanced expression of major histocompatibilty complex (MHC) antigens with MHC I expressed by activated microglia and MHC II by the full blown macrophages (20-24). The expression of these antigens conferred antigen-presenting capacity to microglia. Thus by the late 1980s microglia had moved up the ranks as the accepted immune cell of the brain (20).

The long journey, which witnessed the progression of microglia from a scavenger cell to that of the immune cell of the brain was completed. Microglia was now to embark on another journey, which would place them as early participants in a cascade of events leading to the pathogenesis of AD. Interesting features in this cascade are the combination of innate immune responses and chronic inflammation.

The sections below will provide overviews of the participation of microglia in different phases of AD pathology

Microglia and Neurodegenerative Disorders

With today's wealth of knowledge concerning chronic inflammation in Alzheimer's disease (AD) (25-29) it may difficult to conceive that about 20 years ago there was scarcely any association between the immune system and neurodegenerative disorders. One reason for the delay in acceptance of inflammation in the brain is due to its historical definition and cardinal signs: rubor, calor, dolor and tumor (2). However we should be quickly reminded that the brain has no pain fibers so there can not be dolor nor can there be tumor since the blood brain barrier prevents swelling. Furthermore there is no lymphatic drainage in the brain but this is performed by cerebrospinal fluid (28). The reigning dogma of an immunological privileged central nervous system (CNS) hindered this connection. However evidence, such as the demonstration that activated lymphocytes cross the blood brain barrier (30) gnawed at the strength of this dogma. Even more immunocytochemical approaches began to quickly unmask immune related antigens in the human CNS (31). In a short time span an arsenal of immunocompetent cells were localized in AD brains (32, 33). These initial reports were followed by a series of reports that microglia cluster around senile plaques one of the hallmark lesions of AD but their mechanism in plaque formation is an ongoing debate (34-39). Consideration has been given that microglia may be the source of the beta amyloid (39,). One of the cardinal features in AD is the progression of the beign diffuse plaques to full blown neuritic plaques (40). During the transformation of diffuse plaques to neuritic plaques non-fibrillary amyloid beta becomes fibrillary. The core of amyloid is surrounded by dystrophic neuronal processes with neurofibrillary degeneration. Increasing numbers of neuritic plaques are associated with cognitive decline (40). Studies which quantified microglia in association with these different types of plaques demonstrated that microglia have a specific role in the formation of the neuritic plaques from the diffuse plaque (41). More recent results indicate that amyloid beta releases the monocyte chemotactic protein-1 (MCP-1) from microglia; MCP-1 is a major chemotactic protein that serves as a signaling mechanism for migrating microglia. Apparently this is the suggested pathway that microglia respond to the build up of amyloid beta (42). Thus the early build up of amyloid beta could be viewed as the intruder and this signals to microglia to mount a defense to clear up the intruder as it is the case with a standard innate immune response. However as amyloid beta deposits continue to build up and form a solid mass microglia become frustrated in front of the enemy and begin to release toxins to assist with the removal of the intruder. Thus microglia are not only present in the AD brains but they are also driving forces in the pathological processes. It is significant that the ramified or resting microglia, which provide no apparent function for the healthy CNS, can become activated and set out on a destructive pathway and contributes to chronic inflammation. The recognition that activated microglia participate in the cascade of events leading to the pathology of AD has provided new perspectives for the disease process, therapeutics and diagnostic tools. Taken together the data accentuate the importance of establishing biomarkers to predict ongoing immune processes during the course of the disorder or more significantly before the onset of clinical symptoms. The first use of peripheral markers as indicators of immune responses in dementia dates about 40 years ago. The innovative use of immunological indices as peripheral markers for AD and cognitive dysfunction provided interesting, but inconsistent findings (43-50). Inspite of the data the concept that inflammation plays a role in dementia has been considered for a lengthy period of time. These early pioneers need to be recognized as they were not impeded by dogmas and definitions of inflammation in proposing that inflammation is a player in dementia. As it will be demonstrated in the next sections with today's knowledge together with the acceptance that inflammation plays an integral role in AD pathology using components of immune responses such as complement proteins, cytokines, acute phase proteins and antibrain antibodies as peripheral markers for AD has gained momentum.

The sections below describe current immune response markers for AD. To appreciate why they are being scrutinized their participation in AD pathology is briefly described.

COMPLEMENT

Complement proteins play a major role in the destruction of invaders and to assist in phagocytosis. The adaptive immune system employs complement through antibodies that coordinate the humoral responses. The complement system is equipped with components which carry out fours major functions: recognition opsonization, inflammatory stimulation through anaphylatoxins and direct killing though the membrane attack complex. Complement activation is accomplished by a set of proteins, which are activated in a sequence when exposed to an intruder. Activation of the classical pathway commences by the attachment of C1q to as target. Once fully activated complement proteins finalize their mission by forming the membrane attack complex (MAC (for review and definitions of complement see 51) Complement is produced by neurons in particular cortical pyramidal neurons, which are quite vulnerable in AD (52). In response to an injury microglia express complement receptors (20-24, 51)

Further strong evidence that inflammation is involved in AD was the immuno-cytochemical localization of activated classical complement pathway proteins associated with hallmark lesions in AD (52-58). In AD brains dystrophic neurites are immunostained for MAC supporting the role of an autolytic attack (58, 59). Thus it seems likely that neurites are under complement self attack especially since there is no upregulation of self-defense proteins associated with complement inhibition. (60). Properdin and fraction Bb of factor B, two proteins that bind to tissue when the alternative complement pathway is activated, are not presence in AD brains (27-29)

AD was the first disorder described where complement activation leads to host tissue damage in the absence of antibodies (28, 50). In this respect McGeer describes AD as an autotoxic disorder (29). Rogers et al unraveled important mechanisms concerning complement activation in AD by demonstrating that the amyloid protein can initiate the complement cascade (61). Other substances which are also enhanced in AD brains such as pentraxins, amyloid P and C-reactive protein can perform similar feats (62,63). Immunocytochemical investigations carried out on AD brains reveal that a chronic inflammation is key factor in the pathology of this disorder (for review see 27). This is based on the presence of fundamental components in inflammation such as microglia, complement chemokines, cytokines and pentraxins and the local production of immune mediators (27). Quite interestingly neither the adaptive immune system nor the peripheral immune system is involved in AD inflammation. The work of McGeer and Rogers and others highly support that inflammation in AD is driven by the innate immune system and that amyloid drives the classical complement pathway (27-29, 51, 61). McGeer has recognized for a number of years that complement targeted drugs need to be developed and predict that they would be able to restrict the autotoxicity in AD (28, 29, 64). In view of this it is encouraging to note that the first complement specific drug has recently received FDA approval (65).

Complement Proteins as Biomarkers

The presence of complement proteins in AD brains suggested that measuring their levels in cerebrospinal fluid and serum may be a potential marker for ongoing immune responses. Use of complement proteins as markers in AD have not been very successful. Despite the fact that serum amyloid P (SAP) and complement C1 q are highly localized to hallmark lesions in AD brains no significant differences could be established between cerebrospinal fluid levels of SAP and C1q in healthy elders and those with AD. From this study it was then concluded that these factors should no longer be pursued as markers for AD (66). Another study has suggested that isoforms of complement proteins may provide some means to distinguish patients with neurodegenerative disorders (67). However it is the general consensus that complement proteins are not promising as markers for AD (68)

ACUTE-PHASE PROTEINS

Acute-phase proteins include C-reactive protein (CRP), serum amyloid A (SAA), amyloid P (AP), fibrinogen, and alpha 1-acid glycoprotein. AP is strongly associated with all forms of amyloid. CRP and AP are both produced by brain neurons, and are enhanced in AD (62). The amyloid deposits and extra-cellular tangles of AD are intensely immunostained by AP. CRP has less of an association with the extracellular lesions of AD. CRP is more recognized for its association with such inflammatory lesions as infarcted heart (69) and atherosclerotic plaques (63). Both AP and CRP are strong activators of complement (62). It may be, then, that the pentraxins act as key molecules in innate immune defense by identifying and binding to pathological tissue and then activating the complement system to mount a directed attack on the target. Plasma concentration of these proteins increases (or decreases) by 25% or more during certain inflammatory disorders. Though there are reports of measuring their levels, the data is quite variable and efforts to establish acute-phase proteins as markers in AD are not a high priority.

CYTOKINES

These are proteins that are secreted by various types of immune cells such as microglia and serve as signaling chemicals. The central role of cytokines is to control the direction, amplitude, and duration of the inflammatory response. There are two main groups of cytokines: pro-inflammatory and anti-inflammatory. Pro-inflammatory cytokines are produced predominantly by activated immune cells such as microglia and are involved in the amplification of inflammatory reactions.

The most potent of these are interleukin-1 (IL-1), IL-1α, IL-1β, IL-6 and tumor necrosis factor alpha (TNF-α). The first stage of the inflammatory response is recognition of the pathogen and activation of tissue macrophages that on stimulation produce among other cytokines. On the other hand anti-inflammatory cytokines mediators such as IL-10, IL-13, and IL-4, transforming growth factor beta (TGF-β) are summoned to decrease the immune response. Anti-inflammatory cytokines are involved in the reduction of inflammatory reactions. Thus in the brain as in the periphery there are balances between pro and anti inflammatory cytokines which together respond to intruders and then monitor the intensity and duration of the immune response. As one ages the balance tilts towards an increased expression of pro-inflammatory cytokines as opposed to anti-inflammatory cytokines.

Cytokines entered the AD pathology arena with reports that IL-1, IL-6, TGF-β and TNF-α are upregulated in AD brain and are mainly associated with lesions (27, 70-76). These cytokines are produced and their sustained release by activated microglia and astrocytes contributes to chronic inflammation (77, 78). Griffin et al first demonstrated that microglia and astrocytes over express IL-1 in AD brains (70). They further proposed that excessive amounts of IL-1 trigger a cascade of events leading to neurodegeneration. These landmark observations placed microglia as a pivotal cell in the neurodegenerative process of AD as they suggested that IL-1 positive microglia actual drive the evolution of plaque formation (71-73). Furthermore, the finding that IL-1 is overexpressed decades before the appearance of Alzheimer neuropathological changes in Down's syndrome (70) suggested that over expression of this cytokine in the brain may be associated with generation and progression of disease. IL-6 has a strong association senile plaques and it is speculated that amyloid plaques are derived from a IL-1/IL-6 mediated acute phase reaction (74-76). The degree of clinical dementia correlates with the immunocytochemical intensity of the expression of this cytokine (76). No expression is noted in plaques of non-demented individuals (76).

In regards to AD pathology the anti-inflammatory IL-10 has been shown in human and mouse microglia cell lines to suppress amyloid beta induced expression of inflammatory proteins such as IL-1α, IL-1β, TNF-α, IL-6 and the chemokine MCP-1 (79) These anti-inflammatory cytokines are present in the AD pathology and may attempt to offer protection against ongoing immune responses.

TNF-α is a pleiotropic cytokine produced by a variety of cells and has been recognized as playing an important role in neurodegenerative diseases and is present in AD brains (80). As other cytokines it is produced by microglia in response to injury. An acute release of TNF-α may offer neuroprotection whereas its chronic release contributes to inflammation.

Another significant multifunctional cytokine is transforming growth factor beta. This cytokine is considered to be neuroprotective and is localized in AD brains (81, 82). TGF-β has been suggested to promote amyloid deposition in transgenic mice and thus may play a similar role in AD (83). Recent investigations have disclosed that a defect in the signaling pathway for TGF-β in AD patients may cause it to loose its protective effects in this neurodegenerative disorder (84).

The extensive reports demonstrating the presence and role for various cytokines in AD have initiated a search for their use as markers for immune responses. It is still unclear whether these cytokines participate in late or early or through the entire disease process. While some investigators consider that cytokines have an early role in the pathogenesis of AD (70) others propose that they intervene in the later stages (85). The presence of cytokines suggested that measuring circulating cytokines could be a means to follow the progression of the disease as well as to identify ongoing immune responses.

Cytokines As Markers For Dementia

Due to the relationship of cytokines and AD pathology volumes of information have been generated about levels of circulating cytokines in AD and other dementias For the most part the use of circulating cytokines has been inclusive with scattered data. There are reports of elevated levels, decreased levels and no change at all. This has been interpreted as a reflection of the disease, methodologies and probably to great extent subsets of dementia. (73, 86, 87). Findings of differential roles of cytokines in relationship to AD pathology in the later stages of the disorder further support these inconsistencies (85)

Another factor that may be responsible for reported discrepancies is the population under investigation. Three European studies on the elderly have reported three different outcomes. In a study from Amsterdam the authors reported that serum inflammatory protein alpha1-antichymotrypsin is associated with cognitive decline in older persons, whereas IL-6 , CRP, and albumin are not." (88)

Investigations conducted in the elderly in Rotterdam and Leiden concluded "that systemic markers of inflammation are only moderately associated with cognitive function and decline and tend to be stronger in carriers of the APOE epsilon4 allele. Systemic markers of inflammation are not suitable for risk stratification" (89).

Finally in Edinburgh investigators reported that "systemic markers of inflammation and hemostasis are associated with a progressive decline in general and specific cognitive abilities in older people, independent of major vascular co-morbidity". (90)While measuring the levels of circulating cytokines may have produced inconclusive results about the current state of the pathogenesis of AD current results suggest that cytokines may be better markers for predicting a person's susceptibility for developing AD. In this regards a number of studies have demonstrated that polymorphisms in the regulatory regions of each of these inflammatory cytokines influence the risk of AD (91-96). Rather than altering the protein structure as is the case of other genes affecting the risk of AD such the amyloid precursor protein and apolipoprotein E (ApoE), it is significant that these genes influence the level of expression of inflammatory cytokines (51)

A recent investigation from the Framingham Study has provided some new and interesting evidence in showing that in contrast to circulating inflammatory cytokines that a two fold increase in the risk of developing AD seems to be related to an increased spontaneous production of IL-1 and TNF-α by peripheral blood mononuclear cells (PBMC)

(97). In addition to this investigation an increase in monocytes expressing cytokines have been reported in both AD and subjects with mild cognitive impairment (98). Both of these investigations are indeed of great interest as PBMC cross the blood brain barrier and therefore could have a direct effect on the brain.

There are reports that an increased production of CSF TNF-α accompanied by decreased production in TGF-β in persons with mild cognitive impairment (MCI) places them at risk for developing AD (99,100). These data suggests that measuring these cytokines in MCI could predict risks factors for developing AD and thereby could lead to early intervention.

Two areas where the determination of cytokines seems to hold a future as predictors for dementia are metabolic syndrome and depression. Advances in these fields need to be carefully observed as risk factors for dementia include both metabolic syndrome and depression. Furthermore monitoring cytokine levels in relationship to these disorders may have a future role in therapeutics as early intervention could reduce the risk of further inflammatory mediated damage to the brain.

Recent investigations highly suggest that risk factors associated with cardiovascular disorders such as hypertension, diabetes and metabolic syndrome need to be equally considered for dementia. Elegant work by Yaffe and collaborators (101,102) are to be highlighted. They reported that in three separate studies involving elders of different ethnicities, that the metabolic syndrome is a risk factor for accelerated cognitive aging. This was especially true for elders with the metabolic syndrome and with elevated serum levels of inflammation (101,102). The significance of the studies is related to their 5 year longitudinal study performed on healthy African and white Americans. This is important as it actually allowed the investigator to provide convincing information about the participation of elevated cytokines in persons with metabolic syndrome and their relation to cognitive decline. Their studies indicate a correlation between cognitive decline and increased levels of IL-6 and CRP. In this study TNF-α was not a factor in cognitive decline. (101,102).

In the 1990s observations that patients with severe depression displayed increased blood levels of proinflammatory cytokines produced a short lived "macrophage theory of depression" (103). This theory did not attract much attention because of lack of supporting evidence such as proof that an activated immune system could induce depression, that decreases in immune activation could decrease depression and links between cytokines and the brain. Today more attention due to increased supporting evidence is being given to the role of elevated cytokines and depression (104). As studies are beginning to demonstrate that depression may be a precursor for dementia it is timely to consider that cytokines may in fact be playing a role (105). Thus elevated levels of circulating cytokines in depression may be a warning of greater cognitive damage downstream. As described above the innate immune system is considered to play a major role in the pathogenesis of AD. In this respect administering the inflammatory agent lipopolysaccharide to old animals causes sickness or depression behavior, which was accompanied by full-blown immune response in the brain. The same treatment in younger animals fails to elicit the behavioral responses (106). Thus from a clinical prospective it is plausible that depending on the person's susceptibility that there is a risk factor link between depression accompanying innate immune activation and susceptibility to developing dementia. Further correlations of this nature may assist in understanding the growing observations that depression precedes dementia and in particular AD. As this is a new science there is still much to be learned about how cytokines influence the brain and whether early increases in these proteins actually trigger pathologies associated with dementia. For further information the reader is directed to three excellent reports on this new science (104, 107,108).

ANTIBRAIN ANTIBODIES

Though reports of immunoglobulins (IgGs) were first made in the early 70s (109) several follow up studies concluded that these IgGs did not rank as prominent features in the pathology. There is also a lack of B cells in the brain as well as T cells (33). With a paucity of supporting evidence the concept of autoimmunity in association with AD was shelved like a cold case. However emerging data is indicating that this concept needs to be reviewed and that autoimmune mechanisms could indeed be playing prominent roles in AD pathology. The recent examination of IgGs in AD brains is providing the basis for reconsidering autoimmune mechanisms (110-112). The novelty of these findings was the association of these positively stained neurons and other immune related components. Not only were IgG positive neurons found in AD, these were located to a specific population of degenerating pyramidal cells. The co-localization of complement proteins including the membrane attack complex in these IgG positive neurons together with nearby activated microglia highly suggests that neuronal death was the result of the antibody-induced classical complement pathway (110-112). The data implies auto-antibrain antibodies may indeed be participating at a greater frequency on the pathogenesis than presently being considered. The authors provided attractive hypotheses about the role of the IgGs in neuronal death. On one hand they suggested that the IgG binds to antigens on these specific neurons which subsequently degenerate. On the other hand it was suggested that IgG binding is subsequent to degeneration and binds to antigens involved in degeneration. The data reported by the authors supports that the IgG binding occurs before degeneration based on the fact that not all IgG positive neurons were degenerating and that degeneration possibly occurred after IgG binding which is common for numerous autoimmune disorders. The hypothesis that AD is an autoimmune disorder could provide a strong link between previous reports that an altered blood brain barrier BBB participates in AD (113-116). It is further implied that BBB dysfunction precedes neuronal death and dementia (110-112). These investigations have pointed out that neuronal antibrain antibodies in combination with an impaired blood brain barrier could gain entrance to brain target antigens thereby causing neuronal damage. Hence, these observations bring to the forefront the need to once again consider that antibrain antibodies could elicit an autoimmune response and contribute to cell death. In the midst of volumes published to the contrary it is enlightening that a revival of the concept of antibrain antibodies is on the horizon. (110-112).

The work concerning auto-antibrain antibodies has a long history, which is reviewed in the section below.

Antibrain antibodies: Overview

Of the long list of markers, antibrain antibodies may be considered as one of the 'grandfathers' with the earliest reports being in 1962 (117). One major drawback concerning antibrain antibodies is that the antibody-producing B-cells have not yet been demonstrated in the CNS (33). Otherwise, antibrain antibodies have been considered as an age-linked phenomenon (45, 46, 118) or not having any particular relationship to neurodegenerative disorders (119,120). However, efforts to identify antigens recognized by antibrain antibodies has definitely strengthened the concept that an IgG species could serve as a reflection of immune responses. One such investigation identified that sera from Huntington's Chorea recognized striatal neurons (121). The authors noted *"that damage to neurons and subsequent alteration of the native autologous neuronal antigens might be capable of inducing the synthesis of antibodies directed against neuronal structures"*. These observations were noted at least two decades before the actual demonstration of immunocompetent cells within the CNS. Based on the above hypothesis, information about antibodies in the serum and CSF of AD patients began to flourish in the late 80s. In a brief time span there were reports that anti-brain antibodies in AD CSF or serum recognized cholinergic neurons (122-125) ,neurofibrillary tangles (126), neurofilaments (127), thyroglobulin (125), vascular proteoglycans (128), and even pituitary cells (129). This suggests that CSF antibodies of AD patients may recognize antigens in other tissues than the brain, which in turn may be in harmony with previous observations showing that degenerative changes similar to those occurring in AD brain are also observed in other organs, including the thyroid and aorta (130,131). Pathological fibrillary lesions, similar to those occurring in the AD brain were also observed in several other organs including the thyroid (131). While it seemed logical to search for anti-brain antibodies associated with degenerating neurons and pathological elements these findings and others produced a repertoire of anti-brain antibodies associated with *but not selective* for AD.

A review, which extensively examined antibrain antibodies in the CSF and serum of patients with various neurological disorders, has further emphasized the complexity of correlating antigens with specific neurodegenerative disorders (132). Theoretically, a shower of new antigens may trigger the production of a number of brain-specific antibodies. Consequently, identifying a variety of antigens in the same neurodegenerative disorder may not be surprising. As a result, the search for antibrain antibodies, which display specificity for a given neurodegenerative disorder, may appear to be a Herculean task.

A recent publication has shed light on the significance of autobrain antibodies by projecting that one of the most vital contributions to this field will be the identification of the antigen to which the neuronal autoantibodies binds to (110-112). In view of our research which has aimed at identifying an antigen that binds to antibrain antibodies we fully agree with the conclusions of these investigators. Though this particular antibody may not have full international support as a marker for the differential diagnosis of dementia our work has demonstrated that there a consistent higher frequency of its presence in the CSF and serum in AD patients compared to its rare appearance in those diagnosed with other neurodegenerative disorders. The sections below will focus on the development of an antibody first discovered in the cerebrospinal fluid of AD and then later on in the serum.

CEREBROSPINAL FLUID AND SERUM ANTIBODIES IDENTIFICATION AND CHARACTERIZATION

Adult rat brain

Our initial approach to search for anti-brain antibodies began with the adult rat brain tissue. Our hypothesis was that cholinergic neurons in peril could release cholinergic–like antigens and antibodies against components of the cholinergic system would be produced. This approach demonstrated the presence of IgG type antibodies in AD CSF that recognized cholinergic in the medial septum area of the rat brain and the spinal motor neurons (123). After a couple of years it became obvious that this approach had serious limitations. One of the main being that it was not possible to discriminate between dementias (123). In spite of the limitations of this approach it had provided some interesting information such as the immunoreactivity produced by the CSF IgG species was possibly due to an IgG3 isotype (124) which further supports a role for immune responses in AD since this subclass initiates the classical complement pathway (55)

Embryonic brain tissue

The search for antibodies may have been short-lived had it not been for the serendipitous use of embryonic day 18 CNS tissue to further screen patient CSF. This tissue source definitely produced encouraging and supporting evidence that antibodies have a positive potential to be markers for AD. The first significant results were notable differences between structures recognized by AD CSF compared with CSF from other dementia patients. Such observations had not been possible using the adult rat CNS (133-135). Second, some AD CSF surprisingly recognized amoeboid microglial cells (133-135). The association between microglia and AD pathology was in its genesis at the time of these observations (31, 32, 136). We questioned whether CSF microglial antibodies had the potential to be harbingers of ongoing immune responses in AD. To gain answers, a number of issues would need to be established.

The possibility that the CSF antibody was nonspecifically binding to microglia needed consideration since amoeboid microglial cells contain high levels of the Fc receptor (137). Substantial evidence that AD CSF antibodies specifically recognized microglia was provided by negative reactions of control CSF towards the brain tissue .It should be mentioned that the control CSF in several patients had higher IgG levels than those of the AD CSF. Further examination revealed that the AD CSF immunoreactive cells exhibited all the structural features described previously for amoeboid microglia (12). An immunoelectron micrograph showed that AD CSF immunoreactivity was observed at the plasma membrane and its projecting filopodial and pseudopodial processes. All other organelles and inclusions, including vacuoles, phagosomes and lysosomes, were unreactive. Other glial types in the corpus callosum – astrocytes, oligodendrocytes, or glioblasts – were not reactive (133-135) Taken together, these results provided evidence that AD CSF contained an antibody, which could be considered specific for microglia.

Specificity of CSF microglia antibodies for AD

Once the antibody was characterized, the next challenge was be to examine whether or not it was specific to AD. During the course of these investigations, the associations between AD pathology and microglia were rapidly progressing (25-29, 34-39). Our initial study tested CSF from familial AD patients, their at-risk relatives (AR) and controls for microglia antibodies (133). Encouraging results revealed that the antibody had potential to distinguish AD patients from healthy aged-matched controls. This study also revealed that CSF from AR of affected patients with familial AD contained the antibody (133). Information provided to the investigators by the clinician revealed that 12% of the AR displaying the antibody subsequently developed AD (unpublished results). This preliminary investigation suggested that the antibody may have the potential to predict a person's susceptibility for developing AD before clinical manifestations.

To perform a more rapid screening of patients samples a cell culture system containing both cholinergic neurons and microglia was developed (138). This culture system provided the most significant means of screening microglial antibodies in patient samples. Though attempts have been made to use pure microglia cultures, cell lines and macrophages, the results have proven unsatisfactory. It should be mentioned that CSF and serum were obtained through collaborations with various centers in Europe and the USA. CSF was first used to test for the antibodies and this was soon followed by serum. The antibody was present in both samples with a much higher titer in serum. Thus further testing has been devoted to serum in clinically diagnosed patients. Subsequent testing of serum from a mixed population of dementia patients using the cell culture technique revealed that 35% of AD patients contained microglial antibodies. The antibodies were not found in other patient groups (139-144). Significantly preliminary data have shown that AD serum does not recognize proteins prepared from astrocyte cultures (139,140). These results agree with our earlier electron micrograph findings, which indicated that AD CSF did not stain astrocytes in the developing rat brain (133-135).

The use of the rodent CNS to ascertain the significance of human antibrain antibodies could be met with some reservations. First, the use of the cultures prepared from the developing rodent has demonstrated to a certain degree that serum and CSF microglial antibodies have the potential to distinguish AD patients from those diagnosed with other neurological disorders, including other types of dementia (139-145). Second, a report that AD serum antibodies recognized microglia in post mortem AD brains adds further support that the antibody is capable of recognizing microglia in both rodents and humans (146). Finally, we reported that CSF from a patient undergoing a ventricular peritoneal shunt when incubated against his own cortical biopsy recognized ramified and giant-sized microglia (140-142). In view that the patient did not respond to the shunt operation, he was considered to have AD. It should be noted that this same patient sample recognized microglia in the embryonic rat (140). Together, all these findings strengthen the reliability of using rodent CNS to screen human antibrain antibodies.

Reactive human leukocyte antigen DR antibody-positive microglia have been described in fixed CNS tissue from virtually every contemporary neurological disorder (27-29,147,148) To gain information about the association of the antibody with other neurodegenerative disorders, our investigation was extended to patients with Parkinson's disease dementia (PDD), multiple sclerosis (MS) and acute amyotrophic lateral sclerosis (ALS). In our hands, 12 CSF samples from ALS and MS patients tested negative for microglial antibodies

(144,145). There is a single case report of microglia antibodies in the CSF of an ALS patient with serious presenile dementia (149). Whether or not there could be a link between the dementia and the antibodies would need further investigation. Interestingly, PDD CSF displays antibodies towards microglia (unpublished results). This could be significant since pathological hallmarks in this disorder are considered to resemble those of AD. In view of the intimate relationship between microglia and AD pathology (27 for review), these serum and CSF anti-microglial antibodies most likely reflect an ongoing inflammatory process. This could be linked to the role that activated microglia play in the cascade of events leading to AD pathogenesis.

Observations that serum and CSF anti-microglial antibodies occur with a high frequency in AD basically relied on clinically diagnosed AD (145 for review). For a definite diagnosis of AD, histological confirmation of the pathological hallmarks of AD is needed. A further study was conducted to confirm the presence of CSF microglial antibodies in neuropathologically-confirmed AD cases compared with controls. In addition, the frequency of CSF anti-microglial antibodies was correlated with cortical Aβ levels (150 results described below are from this reference).

Based on a semi-quantitative analysis of Alzheimer's type cortical changes, 38 cases were divided into 4 groups: 7 controls without any Alzheimer's type pathology, 14 with mild Alzheimer's type Pathology (group AP1 with Braak stages I–II); 10 cases with moderate Alzheimer's type Pathology (group AP2 with Braak stage III–IV,) and 7 cases with severe AD pathology (group AD with Braak stages V–VI,). In the groups with mild and moderate Alzheimer's type cortical changes (AP1 and AP2), the accumulation of neurofibrillary tangles was restricted mainly to the entorhinal cortex and hippocampus. Severe accumulation of neurofibrillary tangles occurred in the associative frontal and parietal areas in the AD group. For each patient in this group, the criteria for the definite diagnosis of AD according to CERAD and the NIA-Reagan Institute were met. There were high numbers of senile plaques in the cerebral cortex in the group of definite AD cases (AD), as well as, in the AP2 group. In the group of definite AD cases all patients had dementia . There was no dementia recorded in any patients of the control group.

The results obtained confirm previous observations and show that CSF antimicroglial antibodies are present in a high percentage (71.5%) of neuropathologically-confirmed definite AD cases and, most importantly, the frequency of CSF antimicroglial antibodies was comparable (80%) in the group of cases with moderate AD-type cortical changes. These findings indicate that the presence of CSF microglial antibodies may be an early marker of AD which is in accord with previous observations showing that members at risk in familial AD exhibited CSF microglial antibodies more than two years before the clinical diagnosis of AD was made (133).

The frequency of anti-microglial antibodies increased with the severity of AD-type cortical changes. In the groups of patients where a high number of senile plaques accumulated in the cerebral cortex (groups AD2 and AD3), the percentage of cases with microglial antibodies was also very high. This association was further supported by a correlation between the cortical Aβ levels and the frequency of anti-microglial antibodies. Both were very high in the groups with moderate AD-type changes (AD2) and with definite AD.

We also analyzed whether the frequency of CSF anti-microglial antibodies was related to cerebrovascular lesions. The statistical analysis did not show a correlation between cerebrovascular pathology and CSF antimicroglial antibodies. When the correlation of CSF anti-microglial antibodies with age was analyzed in the three groups with AD-type changes there was no correlation between age and CSF anti-microglial antibodies.

The fact that the number of cases with CSF anti-microglial antibodies is very high, not only in the group of cases with definite AD, but also in the group of cases with moderate cortical changes, indicates that CSF microglial antibodies are present in preclinical stages of AD and may be early indicators of the evolution of the disease. The previous findings that at-risk family members with a history of familial AD contain microglial antibodies at least 2 years before clinical diagnosis provides further support for this concept. Reinforcing these implications, a recent study based on an in vivo positron emission tomographic (PET) marker for activated microglia demonstrated that their activity was increased in brain regions affected by AD pathology (151).

Antigen identification

More attention has been placed on attempting to determine the antigen associated with the microglia antibody. To gain insight into the microglial surface antigens recognized by AD CSF, blocking experiments were carried out. Preliminary results show that AD CSF immunoreactivity can be blocked by pre-incubating developing rat sections with OX-18 monoclonal antibody which detect MHC I antigens. These results suggest that the AD CSF and serum antibodies could be directed towards microglia expressing MHC I antigens. Pre-incubation with OX 42 antibody, which recognizes CR3 receptor antigen had no effect (145). These findings are further substantiated by a recent report, which quantified the expression of microglia in the early stages of AD brains. It was revealed that the increase in MHC antigens by microglia is correlated with early cognitive decline and the transition to AD (152) .The role of chronic inflammation, including the role of the MHC class 1 is well established in AD. Microglia as resident immune cells of the brain, play a pivotal role in immune surveillance, host defense mechanisms and tissue repair (29). They are consistently associated with senile plaques in AD (31-39,153). Therefore, the presence of CSF anti-microglial antibodies may contribute to the dysregulation of microglial function. Further investigations are important and are in course in order to establish the antigen or antigens recognized by CSF anti-microglial antibodies of AD patients.

Future Research

Our work showed that the serendipitous use of the developing rat CNS as a substrate for antibrain antibodies initiated an association between a cell that was rapidly evolving as a central feature of AD pathology and a possible marker for the disorder.

The linkage between microglial antibodies and active immune processes involved in AD remain to be elucidated. However, in view of the numerous associations between microglia as forerunners in the cascade of events leading to AD pathology, it seems to be more than a mere coincidence that AD CSF and serum contains antibodies directed against this cell (27). Their presence in preclinical stages of AD suggests that the detection of anti-microglial antibodies may be a potential biological marker for the early clinical diagnosis of AD. Even in the event that microglial antibodies do not achieve universal acceptance as a biomarker, their presence should be given consideration as they may be warnings of ongoing neurodegenerative processes. Thus, the presence of these antibodies may be a signal to administer therapeutic agents, which have the capacity to suppress chronic microglial activation. There is an extensive criterion for a biomarker and these antibodies certainly do not fulfill all the requirements (154). However, the fact that an antibody directed against a cell which is actively involved in the pathogenesis of AD is in the serum certainly deserves further consideration.

The next years should include studies aimed at establishing relationships among microglia, the hallmark lesions and neurons. Clarifying the interactions of microglia with substances, which lead to neurotoxicity need to be further examined. Studies of this nature may shed light on new therapeutic approaches or means to slow down the progression of AD. The results obtained from microglia antibodies have demonstrated that these antibodies have the potential to discriminate some AD patients from other types of dementia and that the antibodies are present in early stages of the disorder . Over the next few years a concerted effort needs to be made to capitalize on the ability of these antibodies to provide meaningful information about the disease process in AD patients. Their presence in patients 2 years before clinical manifestations and in patients with moderate AD suggests that further developing the assay may provide an improved means to relate the antibody to early events in AD.

As this report demonstrates the humble microglia has traveled a long and adventurous road.

It has been through the efforts of such distinguished investigators as Professors EA Ling, PL McGeer and WST Griffin that we are where we are today. Their work along with countless others has provided the basis for acceptance of inflammatory mechanisms in AD which could indeed provide novel therapeutics, diagnostics and creative means to retard the progression of this devastating disorder.

As the following sections will demonstrate, most of the current biomarkers for dementia rely on measuring levels of substances in the CSF and serum and then comparing these to control subjects. This is even true for the most recently reported test for AD. (155). An advantage to further developing the antimicroglial antibody assay is that a positive result alone appears sufficient to distinguish AD patients from other types of dementias. The presence of this antibody has been successfully employed to distinguish AD patients in European, North American and now recently in Caribbean populations (156) from other types of dementias.

GENETIC BIOMARKERS IN ALZHEIMER'S DISEASE

Genetic lesions that have been shown to contribute to at least some cases of AD occur on chromosomes 21, 19, 14, 12, and 1. These are generally seen in familial cases which tend to have an earlier age of onset- usually in the fourth to sixth decades. A defined pattern of inheritance accounts for only 5% to 10% of AD cases.

Over 80% of familial AD cases are associated with missense mutations in the presenilin 1 (PS1) gene on chromosome 14, which also result in the earliest onset. Less than 1% of cases are attributable to defects in the presenilin 2 gene on chromosome 1. Both genetic lesions ultimately result in increased beta amyloid production.

Genetic defects on chromosome 21 is seen in less that 1% of "early-onset" AD cases. These include those manifested in Down's syndrome patients surviving to middle age. The lesion involves amyloid precursor protein (APP) gene overexpression resulting in the neurotoxic deposits of beta amyloid characteristic of senile plaques. A small minority of individuals with Down's syndrome have partial trisomy of chromosome 21, and the subset that have only two copies of the APP gene do not develop AD neuropathology (157). A recent study has also shown that another genetic defect, the duplication of the APP gene, plays a role in some cases of familial AD (158). Mutations in APP surrounding the β- and γ-secretase sites are another rare cause of early-onset familial AD.

The role of genetic lesions in the more common "late-onset" cases of AD appears to be more complex. No deterministic genes have yet been identified. A cholesterol transporter – apolipoprotein E (apoE) is encoded on a genetic locus on chromosome 19. The ApoE protein binds to beta amyloid in cerebrospinal fluid, and is found in senile plaques in AD. An ε4 allele of apoE increases deposition of fibrillar beta amyloid and is seen in forty percent of AD patients. However, the ε2 allele is known to decrease susceptibility to AD. It has been shown however that the presence of apoEε4 is neither necessary nor enough for the pathogenesis of AD. Disease risk increases with the number of ε4 alleles, though some individuals with sporadic AD do not have any copies of ε4 and some individuals homozygous for this allele never develop AD (159). Seen in 30% of patients with AD, a genetic locus on chromosome 12 that encodes for alpha2 macroglobulin has also been implicated.

Under current scrutiny is the possible role of the cell division cycle (CDC2) gene located on chromosome 10q21. Polymorphism in this gene, designated Ex6 + 7I/D is associated with AD according to Johansson et al (160). Active CDC2 accumulates in neurons containing neurofibrillary tangles, a process that can actually precede tangle formation. Therefore, CDC2 is a promising candidate susceptibility gene for AD.

There is great interest in the utility of gene identification as a biomarker modality. There have been preliminary data which suggests a dose-dependent effect of the apoE ε4 allele on the CSF levels of beta amyloid in individuals with a family history of AD and a mean age in their late fifties(161). A lower CSF beta amyloid level generally correlates with senile plaque deposition. Nondemented individuals with a family history of AD who have no apoE ε4 allele have the highest levels of CSF beta amyloid, followed by persons with one allele, and then by individuals with two copies of apoE ε4.Usefulness of quantifying the apoE ε4 allele as an antecedent or diagnostic biomarker is currently limited. However, there is potential of incorporating this modality into a battery of measurements that may ultimately accomplish this goal.

Bertram et al undertook systematic meta-analyses of Alzheimer disease genetic association studies (162). In an article published in 2007 they described their publicly available, continuously updated online database *(http://www.alzgene.org)* that elaborately catalogs available genetic association studies pertaining to AD. They performed systematic meta-analyses for each polymorphism with available genotype data in at least three case-control samples. They acknowledged over a dozen potential AD susceptibility genes in addition to identifying the ε4 allele of apoE and its related effects. These included ACE, CHRNB2, CST3, ESR1, GAPDHS, IDE, MTHFR, NCSTN, PRNP, PSEN1, TF, TFAM and

TNF with statistically significant allelic summary odds ratios (ranging from 1.11-1.38 for risk alleles and 0.92-0.67 for protective alleles).

Gene sequencing of presenilin 1, presenilin 2 and APP could serve as antecedent and diagnostic biomarkers in the minority of individuals with early-onset AD. However, ethical issues may arise when early diagnosis is made in the absence of known preventive or curative interventions.

There is much optimism in using individuals identified (via genetic studies) as preclinical familial/early-onset AD in prospecting for antecedent biomarkers. This is due to the near certainty that these subjects will develop AD in the future The degree to which pathogenesis of familial AD bares relevance to that of late-onset AD remains uncertain and such approaches are borne on the assumption that substantial applicability exists.

At present, around fifty percent of AD patients have no identifiable genetic risk factors. There remains a great need to uncover the complex genetic basis of late-onset disease. Applying what has been learnt in cancer research, gene expression profiling may provide a means of biomarker identification. High-throughput, genomewide microarray analysis can be employed to discover genes that can be used as standalone screens (163). Quantitative trait analysis or the use of quantitative phenotypes in genetic analysis is an emerging modality which may serve to drive major advancements in the future (164).

BIOCHEMICAL BIOMARKERS IN ALZHEIMER'S DISEASE

Germane to the challenge of finding the ideal biomarker for AD is the uncertainty concerning the pathophysiology of the disease. Many have extrapolated that it would be most beneficial to first scrutinize the well-known histopathological fingerprints for their utility as antecedent, diagnostic or prognostic biomarkers. For this reason beta amyloid and tau protein levels have assumed some preeminence in research endeavors for many years.

Beta Amyloid Role in Pathophysiology

'Senile' plaques that are found in Alzheimer's disease can be either neuritic or diffuse. The typical neuritic plaques are composed of convoluted neuritic processes surrounding a central beta amyloid core. Diffuse plaques contain nonfibrillar beta amyloid. This 38-43 amino acid polypeptide is a result of the aberrant processing of the transmembrane amyloid precursor protein (APP). Extracellular deposition of amyloid depends on the proteolytic cleavage of APP by two proteases- beta secretase and gamma secretase. It is thought that over-expression of the gene that programs cells to make beta secretase results in an increase in the amount of beta secretase cleavage products and ultimately an increase in the amount of amyloid deposition. Amyloid plaques deposited in the brain of patients suffering from Alzheimer's disease, dementia with Lewy bodies and Parkinson's disease dementia mainly consist of carboxy-terminally elongated forms of beta amyloid peptides, such as beta amyloid 42 (Aβ42).

The beta amyloid senile plaques particularly affect the hippocampus, cerebral cortex and amygdala causing memory loss and behavioral changes typical of the clinical picture of AD. There is substantive evidence that the abnormal deposition of amyloid occurs many years before the onset of any characteristic symptoms. One series discovered that 28 percent of nondemented individuals had enough diffuse and neuritic plaques for postmortem diagnosis of AD in spite of absent symptomatology (165). This implies that plaque accumulation may delineate a preclinical population.

The precise mechanism by which beta amyloid contributes to AD pathophysiology is yet to be established. It is proposed that beta amyloid fragment deposition exceeds the phagocytic capacity of microglial cells and the persistence of these activated phagocytes instigates a protracted inflammatory response (166). The involvement of proinflammatory cytokines like interleukin-1β, apart from having a direct neurotoxic effect may facilitate a feed-forwarding cycle by increased processing of APP and the generation of even more beta amyloid fragments (166,167).

Wilkinson and Landreth posit that the juxtaposition of activated microglia to senile plaques contributes to the production of reactive oxygen species that mediate significant oxidative damage seen in the lesions of AD (168). Highlighting the role of inflammation, Aisen and Davis have demonstrated that acute phase proteins are elevated in the serum and are deposited in beta amyloid plaques. They also purport that activated microglia that stain for inflammatory cytokines accumulate around neuritic plaques and complement components including the membrane attack complex are present around dystrophic neurites and neurofibrillary tangles(169).

Hepler and Grimm et al produced evidence for soluble toxins being the responsible agent of disease progression (170). They suggested that a new form of amyloid – "amyloid beta derived diffusible ligands" or ADDLs – are the toxic species responsible for neurodegeneration associated with AD. These ADDLs have different properties compared to beta amyloid which kills a wide range of nerve cells including those that are not affected in Alzheimer's disease. However, ADDLs appear to affect only those types of neurons that are damaged in the disease. Notably, ADDLs are soluble and can therefore diffuse throughout the brain whereas beta amyloid fibrils are not found and the locations at which they are deposited do not always correlate with the site of lesions typical for AD.

A molecular mechanism of beta amyloid-mediated memory loss has also been proposed. Etcheberrigaray and Gibson et al found beta amyloid-induced dysfunction in potassium and calcium channels deemed critical in memory storage (171).

Beta Amyloid as a Biomarker

Studies have shown that mean CSF Aβ42 is lower in Alzheimer patients compared to controls. However there has been significant overlap in absolute values between the two groups (165, 172). This lack of mutual exclusion appears to preclude the use of CSF Aβ42 as an antecedent or diagnostic biomarker. It is important however, to recognize that meta-analyses of existing studies on CSF Aβ levels may be inherently compromised by methodological inconsistencies particularly as it pertains to Aβ measurement (173, 174). In the future more useful meta-analytic data can be gleaned if Aβ measurement methods are standardized.

A study published by Fagan et al in 2006 found an inverse relationship between in vivo brain amyloid load as measured by the amyloid-binding agent, 11C-Pittsburgh Compound-B (PIB) and CSF Aβ42 levels. Notably, there was no overlap between groups: all individuals with positive PIB binding had lower CSF Aβ42 than those who were negative for PIB binding. The study found no significant correlation between brain amyloid load and plasma

Aβ, CSF total or phoshorylated tau. Their results suggest that CSF Aβ42 alone could be an indicator of the amyloid status in the brain (175).

A recently-established quantitative urea-based Abeta-sodium-dodecylsulphate-polyacrylamide-gel-electrophoresis with Western immunoblot (Abeta-SDS-PAGE/immunoblot) has allowed the assay of various specific carboxy-truncated forms of beta amyloid in addition to the elongated forms like Aβ42. Bibl et al used the Abeta-SDS-PAGE/immunoblot to investigate disease-specific alterations of the Aβ peptide patterns between patients with AD, dementia with Lewy bodies(DLB) and Parkinson's disease dementia(PDD) versus nondemented controls (176). The study was able to evaluate the CSF Aβ peptide patterns for the differential diagnosis of the three neurodegenerative diseases. They found Aβ peptide patterns displayed disease-specific variations as did the ratio of differentially altered Aβ42 to Aβ37 levels. This was sufficient to discriminate all diagnostic groups from each other at a highly significant level, except DLB from PDD.

The researchers concluded that Aβ peptide patterns represent disease-specific pathophysiological pathways of different dementia syndromes as distinct neurochemical phenotypes. Despite the fact that Aβ peptide patterns were not able to fulfill the requirements for a sole biomarker, their combined evaluation with other biomarkers is promising in neurochemical dementia diagnosis.

An increasing amount of evidence shows that individuals with preclinical AD also have lower CSF Aβ42 levels. Furthermore, cognitively normal individuals in their late fifties with at least one ApoE ε4 allele have demonstrated lower levels of CSF Aβ42 than individuals without the allele (177). Moonis et al also found CSF Aβ42 levels in presymptomatic subjects with pathogenic mutations in the PS1 gene are also significantly lower than in an age-matched control group (178). This data supports the candidacy of CSF Aβ42 as an antecedent biomarker. However, longitudinal studies focusing on susceptible individuals in the preclinical age range is required to further explore and establish this finding.

Research has also been directed to investigate the utility of plasma Aβ as a biomarker of AD. Evidence has generally been less supportive of its candidacy as compared to its CSF counterpart. While at least one study showed no difference in plasma Aβ40 or Aβ42 levels in patients with sporadic AD compared to controls(179), Mayeux et al had findings on the contrary. In a longitudinal study of unrelated elderly individuals, those who eventually developed AD had higher plasma levels of Aβ42 at entry than did those who remained dementia-free (180).

Animal models of AD using PDGF promoter expressing Amyloid Precursor Protein (PDAPP) mice demonstrated that plasma levels of Aβ did not predict senile plaque load. This was attributable to the extremely short half-life of Aβ in serum. Consequently when an antibody (m266) which sequesters Aβ in the blood over an extended time is administered intravenously, levels of plasma Aβ began to correlate with amyloid burden in the hippocampus and cortex (181). Hence similar interventions to increase serum half-life of Aβ safely may significantly improve the utility of plasma Aβ as a biomarker in AD.

A cautious approach has been advocated regarding the use of plasma Aβ for diagnostic purposes in a population likely to have significant co-morbidity. Plasma levels of Aβ correlate with creatinine levels and may therefore be a nonspecific indicator of renal function (182). Furthermore, peripheral Aβ levels in particular may be affected by the general medical conditions that are often superimposed. Such confounds are not as readily seen using CSF Aβ levels.

Brettschneider et al have investigated the utility of serum autoantibodies against amyloid beta peptide found in patients with AD but which also occur naturally in the general population independently of the cognitive status (183). Analyses were done via a newly developed immunoprecipitation assay with radiolabeled Aβ42 peptide. The authors found a highly significant decrease of Aβ42 autoantibody levels in AD patients independently of age, cognitive status, and apolipoprotein E epsilon4 carrier status. Although the data indicated a potentially pathophysiologic decrease of serum Aβ42 autoantibodies in AD, serum quantification does not appear to be useful in pursuit of a standalone biomarker of AD.

Brain interstitial fluid has now become the target of Aβ assays in the search for potential biomarkers. Neurons may release soluble Aβ into the brain interstitial fluid in which conversion into toxic aggregates can occur. An in vivo microdialysis technique was developed to measure Aβ in this fluid compartment. Cirrito et al have proposed that when Aβ production is inhibited a new equilibrium is established between brain interstitial fluid Aβ and a loosely associated pool of docked, deposited Aβ that can reenter the soluble exchangeable Aβ pool (184). This now measurable in vivo pool offers some prospect for novel diagnostic strategies.

Tau Proteins Role in Pathophysiology

Tau proteins are a family of polypeptides made by alternative splicing of a single gene before translation. It has tandem repeats of a tubulin-binding domain and facilitates tubulin assembly. Tau proteins are major cytoskeletal components of neurons where they are predominantly associated with microtubules of the axon.

Another pathognomonic finding in AD is neurofibrillary tangles which result from the hyperphosphorylation of tau proteins. Hyperphosphorylation disengages the tau proteins from their associated microtubules. These liberated proteins accumulate as neuropil threads in axons and as neurofibrillary tangles in cell bodies. These lesions are believed to impair inter-neuronal communication (185). Ultimately neuronal processes degenerate, neurons die, and the neuropil thread and the neurofibrillary tangles are freed into the extracellular environment.

Neurofibrillary tangles are not unique to AD. They seem to be markers of neuronal injury and death. They are also found in nondemented persons with a predilection to certain areas of the brain, increasing markedly with age. Interestingly, in cognitively normal individuals who demonstrate senile plaques consistent with preclinical AD, there appears to be more neurofibrillary tangles as well as an increased rate of tangle development implying an interaction between plaque and tangle formation. Lewy bodies are often found in both familial and sporadic AD. The significance of this association is currently under study. However alpha synuclein, the main component of Lewy bodies have been shown to interact with tau proteins such that both proteins promote deleterious fibrillization of each other.

Tau proteins as a Biomarker

As with the findings for CSF beta amyloid, the prospect of singular use of CSF tau protein as a diagnostic modality for AD has been unfavorable thus far. Most studies have consistently shown elevated tau levels in the CSF of AD patients compared to controls. However, a significant amount of overlap in CSF tau protein levels also occurs between these two groups. Nonetheless, new evidence supports the superior candidacy of CSF tau proteins compared to CSF Aβ levels. This can also be attributed to the fact that CSF assays for tau are far more consistent across institutions than those for CSF Aβ.

Investigators have often cited that despite the aforementioned advantages, the utility of CSF tau may be limited to predicting clinical decline in AD. Since tau primarily enters and accumulates in CSF only after neuronal degeneration and death, it may have less merit as an antecedent biomarker compared to CSF Aβ levels. This is corroborated in the finding of a study of cognitively-normal fifty year-old subjects with a family history of AD that showed a relationship between ApoE ε4 and CSF Aβ (177, 186). There was no similar correlation with CSF tau levels.

In one study intra-vitam CSF hyperphosporylated tau at threonine 231 (p-tau (231)) was compared to post-mortem neuropathological data. The findings indicated that CSF p-tau (231) may serve as an in vivo surrogate biomarker of neurofibrillary pathology in AD (187).

Unlike its unphosphorylated counterpart, CSF phosphorylated tau protein has shown potential as an antecedent AD biomarker. Ewers et al looked at p-tau (231) for the prediction of AD in patients with mild cognitive impairment (188). Results revealed that the levels of p-tau (231) were a significant predictor of conversion to AD ,independent of age, gender, Mini-Mental State Examination and ApoE genotype. Using a priori-defined cutoff point of 27.32pg/ml, sensitivity ranged between 66.7% and 100% and specificity between 66.7% and 77.8% among participating study centers. The authors report that their findings suggests a good feasibility of a standard criterion of p-tau (231) for the prediction of AD. Indeed many researchers including Hampel et al have concluded that measurement of p-tau proteins significantly improves early and differential diagnosis, as well as disease prediction in subjects at risk for AD and comes closest to fulfilling proposed criteria of a biological marker for AD (189).

Recently, an improved test- the sensitive sandwich enzyme-linked immunosorbent assay has been developed which allows for quantitative tau measurements from 8 microl CSF/well. This assay has a sensitivity of 92% and a specificity of 97% (190). Using novel techniques Blasko et al, looking at thirteen CSF biomarker candidates concluded that the ratio P-tau181/Aβ42 could significantly distinguish AD patients from all other diagnostic subgroups (191).

Beta Amyloid /Tau Proteins Combination Biomarker

Hampel et al reported that CSF beta amyloid predicted AD in converted minimal cognitive impaired subjects with a sensitivity of 59% and a specificity of 100% compared to healthy controls (192). CSF tau protein levels yielded a greater sensitivity of 83% but a specificity of 90%. This necessitated the evaluation of a biomarker battery combining CSF beta amyloid and tau protein levels which may improve diagnostic accuracy. In one study involving 131 AD patients and 72 controls, this battery combining CSF Aβ and total tau produced 92% sensitivity and 82% specificity conferring utility of such a battery in diagnosing postsymptomatic individuals (193). The usefulness of this battery in the role of an antecedent biomarker is pending evaluation.

New Protein Markers

The AD-associated Neuronal Thread Protein (AD7c-NTP) was described in the scientific literature since the mid 1990's. This is an approximately 41 kD membrane-spanning phosphoprotein that causes apoptosis and neuritic sprouting seen in AD. The AD7c-NTP gene is over-expressed early in the subclinical phase of the disease. In the brain, increased AD7c-NTP immunoreactivity is associated with phospho-tau-immunoreactive cytoskeletal lesions, but not with beta amyloid deposits. The protein is believed to be released by dying cells into CSF. Of note, elevated levels of AD7c-NTP can be detected in both CSF and urine of patients with early or moderately severe AD, and the CSF and urinary levels of AD7c-NTP correlate with the severity of dementia. The newest version of the AD7c-NTP assay, termed "7c Gold", shows promise and the authors believe AD7c-NTP is an excellent biomarker that could be helpful in the routine clinical evaluation of elderly patients at risk for AD (194).

There remains a need for further investigation of not only the singular use of the biomarker candidates aforementioned but diagnostic batteries which would involve assay combinations of serum and CSF beta amyloid, total tau and phosphorylated tau proteins. The challenge is not only to establish a valid biomarker/battery with the ability to detect preclinical pathology but one that is reliable, safe, noninvasive, simple to perform inexpensive and acceptable both to patients and physicians.(195, 196)

Homocysteine

Homocysteine was discovered by Butz and Vigneaud in 1932. It is a sulpha-containing amino acid formed by the demethylation of methionine.Homocysteine has been implicated in coronary, cerebrovascular and peripheral atherosclerotic disease and is a risk factor for arterial and venous thrombosis. Associations have been reported between hyper homocysteinemia and stroke, deep vein thrombosis, vascular dementia, Alzheimer's disease as well as other conditions. There are many factors that affect the plasma levels of homocysteine: pathological conditions such as severe psoriasis, organ (especially kidney) transplant, dietary deficiencies of methionine, folate, vitamin B_{12} and B_6 and medications such as oral contraceptives, corticosteroids, cyclosporine and methotrexate all increase plasma levels. Physiological conditions like pregnancy as well as age, gender and ethnicity also affect plasma levels.

Results from the National Health and Nutrition Examination Survey (NHANES) have shown that homocysteine levels continue to rise as a person ages and that men have a higher mean concentration than women. Excess caffeine intake, smoking, a high alcohol intake and sedentary lifestyle tend to increase homocysteine levels. In addition, genetic factors are known to have an effect. Various mutations are known to exist such as the $T_{833}C$ and $G_{919}A$ mutations of the cystathionine-ß-synthase (CBS) gene the first case of which was reported in 1963, and the $C_{667}T$ mutation of the methylene tetrahydrofolate reductase (MTHFR) gene, the latter being clinically significant.

Mechanism of action of Homocysteine

Neurodegenerative diseases includes a number of conditions including Alzheimer's disease, Dementia, and Parkinson's disease among others. In 50% of the cases patients with Dementia usually present with mild cognitive impairment years earlier. The common feature of these disorders is the degeneration of certain nerve cells or neurons by mechanisms including neuronal death and oxidative stress.

Homocysteine and the vasculature

Hyperhomocysteinemia a known risk factor for cardiovascular disease is also implicated in neurodegenerative conditions. In the CNS hyperhomocysteniemia act at the vascular level the same as anywhere else in the body. The pathophysiologic mechanisms include endothelial dysfunction and injury followed by platelet activation and thrombus formation. Homocysteine also promotes atherothrombosis via several mechanisms including decreasing endothelial cell production of nitric oxide which is important for the detoxification of homocysteine (this detoxification takes place when nitric oxide combines with homocysteine to form S-nitroso-homocysteine), proliferation of vascular smooth muscle cells, lipid peroxidation and oxidation of LDL. The vascular effects in the CNS probably contributed to the findings in the Rotterdam Scan Study that total homocysteine levels are associated with silent brain infarcts and white matter lesions independent of each other and of other cardiovascular risk factors(197).

Homocysteine at the cell surface

At the cell surface homocysteine acts as an agonist at the N-methyl-D-aspartate (NMDA) receptor either directly or through effects on the sodium/potassium pumps. Research done by Lipton and colleagues shows that homocysteine not only acts as an agonist at the glutamate binding site ,but also as a partial antagonist of the glycine coagonist site. The relationship is complex, under normal physiological concentrations of glycine neurotoxic concentrations of homocysteine are in the milimolar range however when there is pathology such as stroke and head trauma and levels of glycine are increased, homocysteine becomes toxic at micromolar concentrations ,the agonist activity then outweigh the antagonist activity, homocysteine then becomes excitotoxic resulting in excessive Ca^{2+} influx and reactive oxygen generation oxidative damage and cell death.

Homocysteine at the cellular level

Hyperhomocysteinaemia causes apoptosis and affects the DNA of the cell. Research done in rats demonstrate that homocysteine causes DNA strand breaks as well as activation of poly-ADP-ribose polymerase (PARP) and NAD depletion. The DNA repair mechanisms are inhibited(198). Patients with Alzheimer's disease have a high level S-adenosylhomocysteine which inhibits methyltransferases, the levels of which are known to be decreased in brains with Alzheimer's disease. Methylation in the brain is important for maintaining normal DNA and neurotransmitter metabolism. The consequences of DNA hypomethylation include increase APP processing and Aß production (199).

Issues in the literature

Homocysteine, cognitive function and dementia

Dementia was reported in patients with B_{12} and Folic acid deficiency in 1956 and 1967 respectively. Elevated plasma homocysteine was demonstrated in primary degenerative dementia in 1990 and a hypothesis for a role for homocysteine in AD proposed in 1992.In the past ten years 1997-2007 there have been at least twenty major reports that investigated homocysteine and cognitive function. Mild cognitive impairment (MCI) is a risk factor for the development of dementia and Alzheimer's disease. Kim and colleagues studied 1215 individuals aged 60-85 years who were assessed for MCI based on the Mayo clinic criteria, plasma homocysteine levels were higher in individuals diagnosed with MCI than in normal elderly individuals, those with hyperhomocysteinemia greater than 15μmol per liter had a higher prevalence of MCI. The unadjusted odds ratio for MCI was greater in subjects with hyperhomocysteinemia than in normal subjects and increased according to the degree of hyperhomocysteinemia (200)

High levels of plasma homocysteine and low levels of plasma folate and /or vitamin B12 are associated with cognitive impairment in the elderly (201) but this may not be a direct relationship. An interesting study was done in a Chinese population that investigated whether homocysteine,folate or vitamin B12 have effects on cognitive function and if so on what aspects,Feng and collegues(202) studied 451 individuals aged greater than or equal to 55 years old who where fully independent based on Activities of Daily Living score with Mental Status Examination scores greater than or equal to 24 were studied with various cognitive test, log –transformed homocysteine was inversely associated with performance on Block Design and written Symbol Digit Modality Test. Log transformed folate was significantly associated with Rey Auditory Verbal Learning Test delayed recall, verbal learning, percentage of forgetting and categorical Verbal Fluency test and vitamin B12 was not associated with any cognitive test score. Since B12 and folate affect homocysteine levels these results probably reflect a complex relationship.

In a study that looked at the association between homocysteine and dementia and cognitive impairment without dementia (CIND) in 1779 Mexican Americans aged 60-101 years, plasma vitaminB-12 and red cell folate were measured at baseline and patients followed up over 4.5 years , diagnosis was made by neuropsychological and clinical examinations and expert adjudication. Not only was homocysteine found to be an independent risk factor for both dementia and CIND but higher plasma vitamin B-12 may reduce the risk of homocysteine-associated dementia or CIND(203).

It has long been postulated that lowering homocysteine levels would lead to improved cognitive performance and that plasma levels was inversely related to cognitive function. However in a double-blind, placebo-controlled, randomized two year clinical trial involving 276 healthy participants, 65 years of age or older with homocysteine levels higher than13μmol per liter the results were unexpected. When homocysteine levels were lowered by the administration of folate or vitamin B_{12} while monitoring cognitive performance the homocysteine levels were significantly lower (p<0.001) in the supplemented group compared to controls but there were no differences in the scores on tests of cognition. This finding suggested that supplementation does not lead to improved cogitative function. (204)

Some studies in the literature have reported that supplementation with vitamin B12 improves cognitive function in patients with hyperhomocysteinaemia and low B12 where as others have reported that it does not result in improved cognitive outcome. One possible explanation for the discrepancy is suggested by the work of Martin and colleagues (205). They investigated eighteen subjects with low serum cobalamin (less than 150pmol/L) who received a cyanocobalamin treatment regimen and was assessed based on the Mattis Dementia Rating Scale(DRS). Patients symptomatic for less than 12 months gained an average of 20 points significantly higher than those who had symptoms for more than twelve months who lost an average of three points; patients who were symptomatic for three months normalized their scores. This suggests that there may be an optimal time window during which therapy is most effective (206).

Many studies have identified homocysteine as an independent risk factor for dementia. However, work done by Tabet and colleagues(207) on a small group of patients suggest that the behavioral and psychological symptoms of Alzheimer-type dementia may not be correlated with plasma homocysteine concentration. Their study measured plasma homocysteine, serum vitamin B12 and folate in 23 Alzheimer's disease (AD) patients with behavioral and psychological symptoms of dementia (BPSD) and 27 AD patients without BPSD as determined through the use of the Neuropsychiatric Inventory (NPI). There was no significant difference between the mean plasma homocysteine levels in patients who had Alzheimer's disease with or without BPSD. This may suggest that the major role of hyper homocysteinemia is in cognitive impairment.

Studies reporting on the relationship between homocysteine and dementia have also be increasing in recent times. One of the larger studies was reported in 2002 when 1092 subjects without dementia from the Framingham Study was investigated. It involved 667 women and 425 men, with a mean age of 76 years .The relationship of total plasma homocysteine measured at baseline was correlated to the risk of newly-diagnosed dementia on follow-up over an eight-year period. After using multivariable proportional-hazards regression adjusting for factors that may have influence, including vascular risk factors other than homocysteine and plasma folate and vitamins B12 and B6, these subjects showed a risk of dementia that nearly doubled with a plasma homocysteine level greater than 14 μmol per liter. The relative risk of Alzheimer's disease was 1.8 (95%CI percent 1.3 -2.5) per increase of 1 SD at baseline and 1.6 (95% CI 1.2 - 2.1) per increase of 1 SD eight years before base line.

The development/causation of dementia and Alzheimer's disease and its relationship to hyperhomocystenemia, low levels of B12 and folate is an area that has been undergoing active research. The question arises- does hyperhomocysteniemia from renal impairment, age related decline in gastrointestinal absorptive function or some other non-vitamin cause result in mild cognitive impairment and then full dementia, which with its attendant behavioral and cogitative deficits leading to poor nutrition. In such cases it is possible to have patients with dementia or other neuropsychiatric disorders with the absence of macrocytic anemia. Such was the finding of Lindenbaun and colleagues (208) who concluded that neuropsychiatric disorders due to cobalamin deficiency occur commonly in the absence of anemia or an elevated mean cell volume. It is also possible that B12 deficiency is the primary pathology that leads to the disorder in homocysteine metabolism which then leads to mild cognitive impairment and dementia. Also B12 deficiency and Alzheimer's disease could quite likely coexist as separate entities.

Thus far a definitive diagnosis of Alzheimer's disease can only be made at autopsy when histology can be obtained. Only 70% of clinically-diagnosed AD cases have characteristic AD neuropathology. The number of cases of AD may therefore be over estimated. However one study that dispels this notion is that done by Clark and colleagues (206) who reported on 76 cases that were confirmed by autopsy, differences between serum homocysteine, serum and red cell folate between these cases and controls were significant.

Isoprostane

Isoprostane are prostaglandin-like compounds produced from esterified arachidonic acid (AA). They are a new class of lipids, isomers of conventional enzymatically derived prostaglandins. They are produced by free radical –catalyzed peroxidation of polyunsaturated fatty acids (209). These reactions do not involve enzymes and thus do not require cyclooxygenase (COX-1 and COX -2) for their formation.The Alzheimer's disease brain shows evidence of oxidative stress i.e. oxygen free radical-mediated damage. Isoprostanes is thus considered a candidate biomarker of oxidative stress.

Isoprostanes are known to exist both in the CSF as well as in the periphery. The source in the periphery is however different from that of the CSF. Work done by Montine and colleagues that investigated levels in plasma and urine found that they do not accurately reflect central nervous system levels and are not reproducibly elevated in body fluids outside the central nervous system of AD patients (210). Levels of peripheral isoprostanes are not increased in patients with AD (211). The measurement of the isoprostanes is more robust in the CSF which gives results that are consistent and correlate with pathology. Levels increase early in the course of the dementia. Quantification of isoprostanes in plasma and urine yields continue to yeld inconsistent results (212). The first longitudinal analysis of cerebrospinal fluid (CSF) F2-Isoprostanes in patients with mild Alzheimer's disease reported significant increases in patents followed for one year with correlation with clinical indices of dementia and were significantly lower in patients who used both alpha-tocopherol and vitamin C.

Elevated levels of isoprostanes occur both in patients with MCI as well as early AD. It may in fact play a role in the pathogenesis of the AD by stimulating Abeta generation and aggregation. Increased lipid peroxidation precedes amyloid plaque formation in an aminal model of Alzheimer's disease. However an early study that looked at the iosprostane levels in the lateral ventricular fluid of 23 AD and 12 age-matched controls showed that levels were significantly elevated in AD and were significantly correlated with reduction in brain weight, degree of cortical atrophy but were not related to density of neuritic plaques or neurofibillary tangles in some regions (213). Since AD is associated with increased CSF isoprostanes, the work of one group of researchers suggest that improving CSF drainage might enhance extracellular clearance of products of oxidative stress and lower brain lipid peroxidation (214). Elevated levels have also been found in other disease conditions such as Parkinson's disease and Huntington's disease.

An ongoing multicenter study of biomarkers of oxidative stress called BOSS from the National Institute of Health and Environment Studies (NIHES) found that F2 isoprostane was a sensitive and reliable iosprostane biomarker of lipid peroxidation. Measurement of isoprostanes has the potential to improve the diagnostic accuracy of AD. It may also be useful as a tool to assess antioxidant therapeutic intervention. Pathological changes typical of Alzheimer's disease have a long subclinical phase as previously alluded to. Studies have shown that isoprostane is increased in patients with MCI (215) however most reports relate to post-mortem brain examination so it is debatable whether elevated levels reflect early or late disease.

Sulfatide

Sulfatide is a lipid found mainly in the white matter in the brain, belonging in the class of sulfated galactosylceramide. They are sulfuric acid esters of galactocerebrosides synthesized from galactocerebrosides and activated sulfate, mainly in the ogoligodendrocytes. Sulfatide degradation takes place in two phases. First the sulfate group is cleaved by 3-Osulfogalactosyl cerebroside sulfatase then the ß-galactosyl group is cleaved from galactosylceramide. Alzheimer's disease has pathology in both the white and grey matter, it has been shown that sulfatides are depleted up to 93% in grey matter and 58% in white matter in AD patients with very mild dementia, other classes of lipids except plasmalogen are not altered when compared with normal individuals. Other significant findings was that the content of ceramides was more than three fold higher in white matter and peaked at the early stage of very mild dementia(216,217). When sulfatide levels were measured in the CSF of normal individuals and compared to subjects with MCI due to incipient dementia of the Alzheimer's type, the sulfatide to phosphatidylinositol ratio accurately differentiated very mild impaired subjects from controls (218,219). It is possible that the increase in ceramide content is related to sulfatide metabolism and early events in AD pathology. It has been proposed that alterations in apoE-mediated movement can lead to sulfatide depletion in the brain (220) also abnormal sulfatide metabolism can induce cell apoptosis due to endosome-mediated ceramide generation and the accumulation of cytotoxic levels of sulfatides in lysosomes(221).These interesting results reflect work done primarily by one research team, further investigations with larger populations and multiple centers may be necessary to fully realize the potential role of sulfatide in AD.

NEUROIMAGING AS A BIOMARKER IN ALZHEIMER'S DISEASE

In vivo structural computed tomography (CT) and magnetic resonance imaging (MRI) and functional brain imaging techniques including single photon emission computed tomography (SPECT) and positron emission tomography (PET) have been widely used to study the neuroanatomy and neurophysiology of Alzheimer's disease (AD) and to identify definite biological markers of the disease There is a need for non-invasive biomarkers associated with AD to aid early detection, diagnosis and as surrogate markers of disease progression and treatment.

Neuroimaging methods are an integral part of the diagnostic work-up of patients with suspected AD. Structural and functional imaging is being explored for potential use in the early detection of AD and as surrogate markers of treatment outcome. CT and MRI are recommended for routine evaluation, in order to exclude treatable causes of dementia and to exactly evaluate the degree of cerebral atrophy and the presence of parenchymal abnormalities. Functional imaging, including PET, SPECT and functional MR techniques, are able to investigate physiological cerebral function, such as blood perfusion, metabolism, activation, molecular composition and water diffusibility, and have the potential to detect subtle pathological changes earlier during the course of disease (222). More recently techniques such as diffusion tensor imaging (223) and newer PET techniques using fluorine-18-labelled-FDDNP and carbon-11-labelled-PIB to detect amyloid deposition and neurofibrillary tangles in the brains of patients with AD are also being explored as potential biomarkers (224).

According to *Chertkow and Black* (225) there are five potential major roles for neuroimaging with respect to dementia; (i) as a cognitive neuroscience research tool, (ii) for prediction of which normal or slightly impaired individuals will develop dementia and over what time frame, (iii) for early diagnosis of Alzheimer's disease (AD) in demented individuals, (sensitivity) and separation of AD from other forms of dementia (specificity), (iv) for monitoring of disease progression, and (v) for monitoring response to therapies (225).

In this section of the chapter, various forms of neuroimaging and their usefulness as biomarkers will be discussed.

Computed Tomography (CT)

Computed tomography (CT) is a first-line examination to rule out causes of surgical, and thus reversible, dementia such as subdural hematoma or normal pressure hydrocephalus. It, however, is not used as a biomarker and cannot be used as a true and reliable diagnostic tool for AD.

CT studies in AD have included assessment of cerebral surface atrophy, assessment of ventricular size and measurement of brain density. Mikko Laakso (226) reviewed previous CT studies that focused on the evaluation of gross brain atrophy in AD. These studies are based on assessing the dilatation of various ventricular and subarachnoidal spaces, and the enlargement of sulci, using linear measurements and indices, planimetry, or volumetry (227-232). In fact, few studies applying CT have been able to classify up to 90 % of AD patients and control subjects correctly. In these studies, the best results have been obtained by longitudinal follow-up, demonstrating an accelerated rate of volumetric atrophy (230, 231, 233).

Laaksoo (226) in his review concluded that "the face value of these measurements must be criticized as somewhat questionable, because gross brain atrophy may occur in normal elderly without any neurological or other deficits whatsoever, and may therefore be regarded as "physiological atrophy" (228, 229, 231,232).

Physiological differences in ventricular volumes, for example, may reach 200 % or more (231). Therefore, in early AD most CTs appear normal, or close to normal, and do not differentiate AD from normal aging or other neurodegenerative or neuropsychiatric disorders that might clinically resemble AD (231, 232). Also, the qualitative interpretation of these findings has often lacked reproducibility (231, 232). Moreover, detailed imaging of the temporal lobes in conventional axial CT images is virtually impossible due to beam hardening artifacts (231).

Cortical Atrophy in AD is usually greater than in normal aging, although some demented patients will have normal CT scans and some normal controls will have atrophic changes well into the range associated with dementia. These findings gathered strongly restrict the use of CT as a true and reliable diagnostic tool for AD. CT is useful in detecting vascular and some treatable causes of dementia (226).

Laakso (226) also reviewed papers regarding CT imaging of white matter pathology. He reported that imaging of white matter pathology had encountered similar obstacles as studies of common atrophy - studies reported these changes to be a normal phenomenon throughout life span (234) and appear in normal (at least nonsymptomatic) aging in 30-80 % of elderly individuals. Numerous well-controlled studies also failed to find differences in high signal foci (HSF) between normal subjects and AD patients (235, 229, 230, 236- 242). Their interpretation has been reported to suffer from poor intra- and interrater agreement, and they can be mixed with normal structures, such as Virchow-Robin spaces or deep gyri (229, 237, 243, 240).

Atrophic changes and incidental high signal foci (HSF) may be found in the elderly, whether symptomatic or not. Gross atrophy or large, confluent HSF may represent a more profound pathologic process but no reliable linkage of these incidental findings to support the diagnosis of AD, or any particular disease for that matter, have been confirmed (226).

Magnetic Resonance Imaging (MRI)

Magnetic Resonance Imaging (MRI) can provide both an accurate morphological assessment and a functional evaluation. Cross-sectional and longitudinal studies indicate that magnetic resonance-based volume measurements of atrophy are potential markers of the progression of Alzheimer's disease, starting from the preclinical stages. Other magnetic resonance techniques that are sensitive to the different aspects of Alzheimer's disease pathology, such as biochemical (proton magnetic resonance spectroscopy), microstructural (diffusion magnetic resonance imaging), functional (functional magnetic resonance imaging) and blood flow (perfusion magnetic resonance imaging) changes have not been as extensively studied longitudinally. Recent efforts of imaging amyloid plaques with magnetic resonance imaging generate the prospect for in vivo imaging of the pathologic substrate of Alzheimer's disease (244).

New MR techniques and image analysis software can detect subtle brain microstructural, perfusion or metabolic changes that provide new tools to study the pathological processes and detect pre-demented conditions(245). MRI (magnetic resonance imaging) is preferred for work-ups of dementia. In the neurodegenerative dementias, the topography of the atrophy provides information about the specific type: atrophy of the medial temporal lobe is predominant in Alzheimer disease, while atrophy of the frontal and anterior temporal lobes is seen in frontotemporal dementia, with less medial temporal atrophy than in Alzheimer disease for frontotemporal dementia; vascular dementia is marked by infarction, lacuna, and signal abnormalities in the white matter and sometimes microbleeding(246). MRI can detect predominantly left atrophic changes in the entorhinal cortex, amygdala and anterior hippocampus several years before the onset of clinical symptoms. (247).

Using magnetic resonance imaging, atrophy of the medial temporal lobe can be assessed volumetrically and visually, with a high correlation between the two methods. Medial temporal lobe atrophy is highly predictive of Alzheimer's disease, and correlates with neuropsychological performance and postmortem histologically measured volume. Cerebral volume changes over time seem to differentiate Alzheimer's disease and mild cognitive impairment progressing to Alzheimer's disease from controls with high accuracy(248). However, whilst atrophy rates are predictive under research conditions, they are not specific for AD and cannot be used as primary evidence for AD (249).

Jenkins and colleagues (250) from the Institute of Neurology, London, have reported that rates of atrophy could be used to diagnose AD, finding a 79% rate of sensitivity in patients who had 2 volumetric MRI scans with a 6-month interval that rose to 93% for patients who were scanned with a 12 month interval. Specificity was also high, but no other dementias were studied. This method therefore seems as accurate as other MRI measures of atrophy (i.e., hippocampal atrophy) but it requires 2 scans over a period of time.

Rombouts, from University Hospital VU, Amsterdam, The Netherlands (251) using the SPM method called voxel-based morphometry to compare normal individuals to AD patients has confirmed the presence of medial temporal atrophy in AD and has also reported symmetrical caudate atrophy in AD. Numerous MRI studies showed the same degree of hippocampal and amygdalar volume loss. MRI volumetry of the amygdala may be relevant as a marker of dementia severity in Alzheimer's disease. Asymmetry in amygdalar atrophy is useful in separating Alzheimer's disease and frontotemporal lobar degeneration. (252)

Functional MRI

Functional MRI (fMRI) makes use of the blood oxygen level-dependent technique, using the subject's blood as a natural contrast agent, to show signal intensity changes in areas that are active upon stimulation. fMRI is a relative newcomer in the field of neuroimaging but already shows great promise because of its non-invasiveness and repeatability

Functional MRI is a non-invasive imaging technology that can illuminate regional brain activity during the performance of a task, such as a memory paradigm, or at rest. (fMRI) can be used to study the neural correlates of complex cognitive processes, and the alterations in these processes that occur in the course of normal aging or superimposed neurodegenerative disease. fMRI data can be acquired during a session in which MRI data is also acquired to measure grey and white matter regional brain structure, and these measures can be analyzed together to investigate the relationships between altered regional brain function, structure, and cognitive task performance in neurologic illness.(253)

Sperling in his 2007 study (254) found that the specific regions of the hippocampus and prefrontal cortices are critical for successful memory in both young and healthy older subjects. His fMRI studies, as well as those of several other groups, have consistently demonstrated that, compared to cognitively intact older subjects, patients with clinical Alzheimer's disease (AD) have decreased fMRI activation in the hippocampus and related structures within the medial temporal lobe during the encoding of new memories. More recently, fMRI studies of subjects at risk for AD, by virtue of their genetics or evidence of mild cognitive impairment (MCI), have yielded variable results. Some of these studies, including Sperling's 2007 study (254), suggest that there may be a phase of paradoxically increased activation early in the course of prodromal AD. Further studies to validate fMRI in these populations are needed, particularly longitudinal studies to investigate the pattern of alterations in functional activity over the course of prodromal AD and the relationship to AD pathology. (254)

Magnetic Resonance Spectroscopy (MRS)

Magnetic Resonance spectroscopy has evolved as a tool for the diagnosis of different forms of degenerative dementia. (255). In vivo MRS studies of patients with AD have shown an elevations of percentage of phosphomonoesterase (PME) and phosphomonoesterase: phosphodiesterase (PME: PDE) ratio in the temporo parietal regions (256).

Single Photon Emission Computed Tomography (SPECT)

Single Photon Emission Computed Tomography (SPECT) is a non-invasive study of brain function. SPECT evaluates brain activity by tracing blood flow in the brain. Tracing blood flow allows us to observe the brain's actual metabolic process and its activities. The most commonly used tracers for studying cerebral perfusion with SPECT are Tc-99 m HMPAO (hexamethylpropylamine oxime, Cereteci), a lipid soluble macrocyclic amine, and Tc-99 m ECD (ethyl cysteinate dimer, Neurolitei). The characteristic SPECT finding in AD is bilaterally decreased regional cerebral blood flow (rCBF) in the parietal and posterior temporal lobes, with variable frontal lobe involvement in the later stages of illness (224). Research suggests that brain SPECT imaging can often identify the presence of Alzheimer's disease and it can be used as a screening tool several years before the onset of symptoms of this devastating disease.

Positron Emission Tomography (PET)

Positron emission tomography (PET) imaging of [18F]-2-fluoro-2-deoxy-D-glucose (FDG) is accurate in the early detection of Alzheimer's disease (AD) and in the differentiation of AD from the other causes of dementia. FDG-PET imaging is available widely and performed easily. Different patterns of abnormality with the various causes of dementia are well-described. Semiquantitative methods of image interpretation are available. In the United States Medicare covers FDG-PET imaging for the narrow indication of differentiation of possible AD from frontotemporal dementia. (257)

Fluoro-2-deoxy-D-glucose positron emission tomography (FDG-PET) imaging has revealed glucose metabolic reductions in the parieto-temporal association cortex, frontal and posterior cingulate cortices to be the hallmark of AD. Overall, the pattern of cortical metabolic changes has been useful for the prediction of future AD as well as in distinguishing AD from other neurodegenerative diseases. FDG-PET on average achieves 90% sensitivity in identifying AD, although specificity in differentiating AD from other dementias is lower. (258)

Glucose metabolic PET imaging with fluorodeoxyglucose (FDG) has the potential to detect very early neocortical dysfunction even before abnormal neuropsychological testing is obtainable. The implications are for the identification of minimally symptomatic patients that could benefit most from treatment strategies, as well as the monitoring of treatment response and possible therapeutic deceleration of the disease. FDG PET correlates with AD neuropathology and is able to indicate disease progression or severity, meeting both functional neuroimaging prerequisites in diagnosing AD. (259)

A PET scan can show the brain's biological changes attributable to Alzheimer's disease before any other diagnostic test. Alzheimer's disease can even be detected several years earlier than the onset of symptoms. The use of PET imaging to detect alterations in regional brain metabolism using [(18)F]FDG has enabled more sensitive and accurate early diagnosis of AD, especially in conjunction with traditional medical evaluation.

Newer PET studies

Newer PET markers allow for the evaluation of activated microglia in vivo, as well as for the study of amyloid deposition in the brain and the activity of enzymes such as acetyl-cholinesterase(260). Masdeau and his colleagues in their 2005 paper (224) looked at the regional density of AD-relevant substances measured with PET. The following excerpts from Masdeau's paper are highlighted:

Amyloid plaques and neurofibrillary tangles

Several compounds are now available to detect amyloid deposition and neurofibrillary tangles in the AD brain by means of PET. FDDNP binds in vitro amyloid fibrils and neurofibrillary tangles (224).

In a pilot study with clinical PET in 9 patients with AD and 7 controls, this compound was eliminated more slowly from the brain of patients with AD (224).

Its possible clinical use is yet to be clarified. More advanced is the testing of an uncharged derivative of thioflavin-T that has high affinity for Abeta fibrils and shows very good brain entry and clearance. 'Pittsburgh Compound B'' (PIB): it has been tested in 16 patients with early AD (261). Amyloid deposition was detected in all but 3 of the AD patients and in none of the controls. Amyloid was preferentially distributed in parietotemporaland frontal association cortex and posterior cingulate cortex, regions known to have heavy amyloid deposition in AD (262).

[11C]PIB was used in this study (224). Efforts are under way to commercialize an [18F] compound, with a longer half-life and easier use in a clinical setting.

Microglial activation

The brain of patients with AD contains activated microglia, which could mediate neuronal damage or simply contribute to cleaning neuronal debris, the result of the damage caused by other etiological agents. When cerebral microglia are activated, the expression of peripheral benzodiazepine receptors increases. Cagnin et al (263) measured the regional cerebral density of the activated microglia with PET and carbon 11, marked with (R) - PK11195, which has a great affinity for peripheral benzodiazepine receptors. In 15 normal people, the density did not change with age, except in the thalamus, where there was an increase with age. However, 8 patients with AD and one person with MCI had an increased density in the entorhinal, temporoparietal and cingulate cortex. (224)

Enzyme activity and receptor concentration

Several studies have shown that there is a loss of cortical acetylcholine esterase in AD (264, 265, 266). This loss is in proportion to the cognitive impairment and the duration of the disease. However, it is more important in patients with early-onset AD, who also tend to have a greater neuronal loss. Interestingly, in early AD binding to acetylcholine esterase receptors was decreased in cortex and amygdala, but not in the region of the nucleus basalis of Meynert (267). Acetylcholine esterase inhibition with drugs such as donepezil has also been studied with PET (268, 269).

Thus, it has been determined that inhibition in patients treated with the usual doses (5 and 10 mg) is only partial, and reaches approximately 27% of the enzyme activity with both doses, without a dose–response curve. There is a great interest in obtaining a marker for choline-acetyl-transferase, an enzyme that is directly related to the degree of cognitive impairment, without the floor effect observed with acetylcholine esterase (37% in advanced AD) (49,50). PET compounds that bind to neuronal receptors could be useful to detect regional neuronal loss in AD (224).

Diffusion tensor imaging

Diffusion tensor magnetic resonance imaging (DT-MRI) is a powerful quantitative technique with the ability to detect in vivo microscopic characteristics and abnormalities of brain tissue. It has been successfully applied to a number of neurological conditions, such as stroke, multiple sclerosis and brain tumors, providing information otherwise inaccessible on the pathological substrates. DT-MRI has also been used to study patients with cognitive decline, mainly those with Alzheimer's disease. Several image-analysis approaches have been employed, including region of interest, histogram, voxel-based analyses and DT-MRI-based tractography. Specific patterns of spatial distribution of tissue damage and correlations with neuropsychological measures have been reported (272). Molecular neuroimaging of the brain shows tremendous promise for clinical application (273)

Mild Cognitive Impairment

Mild Cognitive Impairment (MCI) refers to patients with significant but isolated memory impairment relative to subjects of identical age. Consistent with established histopathological data, structural imaging studies comparing patients with early probable AD to healthy aged subjects have shown that the most specific and sensitive features of AD at this stage are hippocampal and entorhinal cortex atrophy, especially when combined with a reduced volume of the temporal neocortex. MCI patients have significant hippocampal atrophy when compared to aged normal controls. When comparing patients with probable AD to MCI subjects, hippocampal region atrophy significantly extends to the neighboring temporal association neocortex. However, only longitudinal studies of MCI subjects are suited to assess (in a retrospective way) the predictive value of initial atrophy measurements for progression to AD. Few such studies have been published so far and for the most they were based on small samples. Furthermore, the comparison among studies is clouded by differences in both populations studied and MRI methodology used. Nevertheless, comparing the initial MRI data of at-risk subjects who convert to AD at follow-up to those of nonconverters suggests that a reduced association temporal neocortex volume combined with hippocampal or anterior cingulate cortex atrophy may be the best predictor of progression to AD. (274)

There is strong evidence that in mild cognitive impairments, AD-related volume losses can be reproducibly detected in the hippocampus, the entorhinal cortex (EC) and, to a lesser extent, the parahippocampal gyrus. Studies also indicate that lateral temporal lobe changes are becoming increasingly useful in predicting the transition to dementia. (275).

On functional MRI, activation paradigms activate a larger area of the parieto-temporal association cortex in persons at higher risk for AD, whereas the entorhinal cortex activation is lesser in MCI. Similar findings have been detected with activation procedures and water (H2150) PET. Regional metabolism in the entorhinal cortex, studied with FDG PET, seems to predict normal elderly who will deteriorate to MCI or AD. SPECT shows decreased regional perfusion in limbic areas, both in MCI and AD, but with a lower likelihood ratio than PET. (276)

It is now well known that MRI-determined hippocampal atrophy predicts the conversion from MCI to AD. The summarized studies have shown the conversion of NL subjects to MCI can also be predicted by reduced entorhinal cortex (EC) glucose metabolism, and by the rate of medial temporal lobe atrophy as determined by a semi-automated regional boundary shift analysis (BSA-R) (277).

Moreover, recent MRI-guided FDG-PET studies have shown that medial temporal lobe hypometabolism is the most specific and sensitive measure for the identification of MCI, while the utility of cortical deficits is controversial (258).

Current Practice

At this time structural and functional MRI as well as MRS, SPECT, PET, new types of PET imaging and diffuse tensor imaging are useful in predicting and diagnosing AD. These imaging tools are also useful for following the disease course over time and monitoring treatment effects. They provide a range of biomarkers that have been shown to correlate with the progression of AD.

De Leon (278) and his colleagues conclude that at this time the combined use of conventional imaging, that is MRI or FDG-PET, with selected CSF biomarkers incrementally, contributes to the early and specific diagnosis of AD. Moreover, selected combinations of imaging and CSF and/or serum biomarker measures are of importance in monitoring the course of AD and thus relevant to evaluating clinical trials.

CONCLUSION

The proposed criteria for effective biomarkers in AD have been described: "The ideal biomarker for AD should detect a fundamental feature of neuropathology and be validated in neuropathologically-confirmed cases; it should have a diagnostic sensitivity of more than 80 percent for detecting AD and a specificity of more than 80 percent for distinguishing other dementias; it should be reliable, reproducible, noninvasive, simple to perform and inexpensive" (279).

As our review describes, there have been numerous approaches which have attempted to meet the above criteria. To these requirements it has been recently added that a biomarker should also have the ability to predict preclinical pathology (279). Therefore, it may not be surprising that no candidate biomarker so far has satisfied all the aforementioned requirements. One then may ask the question: "Have the expectations of a biomarker been set at a standard which is out of reach?" This difficulty may be rooted in the complexity of the disease process itself. Though major advances have been made concerning the understanding of AD pathophysiology, it is still unclear as to when exactly does neuronal dysfunction and death begin. Indeed, many predict this can occur even decades before any clinical manifestation.

Although no candidate appears to qualify as a standalone biomarker, the prospect of formulating a biomarker battery or hybrid test combining the best genetic, immunological, biochemical and imaging modalities is promising. Perhaps this is the approach that would bring unprecedented success in this critical area of research.

REFERENCES

[1]   Metchnikoff E. *Lecons sur la pathologie compare' e de l inflammation*, Masson, Paris, 1892.

[2]   Holoborow, E.J, *An ABC of Modern Immunology,* 2nd edn. Little Brown and Co., Boston, 1973

[3]   Nissl, F., Ueber einige Beziehungen zwischen Nervenzellenerkrankungen und gliosen Erscheinungen bei verschiedenen Psychosen, *Arch. Psychiatry, 1899* 32 1-21.

[4]   Alzheimer, A. "Uber eine eigenartige Erkrankung der Hirnrinde.". *Allg. Z. Psychiat. Psych.-Gerichtl. Med* 1907. 64 (1-2): 146–148.

[5]   Alzheimer A. Uber Eigenartige Krankheitsfalle des spateren Alters. Zeitschr f d *Ges Neurol Psychiatr* 1911 ;4: 356–485.

[6]   Fischer O (1907) Miliare Nekrosen mit drusigen Wucherungen der Neurofibrillen, eine regelm€aassige Ver€aanderung der Hirnrinde bei seni- ler Demenz. Monatsch *Psychiat u Neurol* 1907 22: 361–372

[7]   Fischer O (1910) Die presbyophrene Demenz, deren anatomische Grundlage und klinische Abgrenzung. Z *Ges Neurol u Psychiat* 1910 3: 371–471

[8]   Simchowicz T Histologische student uber die senile *demenz Histol Histopathol Arb* 1911 4 267-444

[9]   Wisniewski HN and Terry AD Reexamination of the pathogenesis of the senile plaque *Prog Neuropathology* 1973 2 1-26

[10]   Kozlowski, P., Wisniewski, R.M., Moretz, R.C. and Lossinsky, A.S., Evidence of induction of localized amyloid deposits in neuritic plaques by an infectious agent, *Ann. Neurol.,* 1981 10 517-523.

[11]   Probst A Brunnschweiler H Lautenschlager C Ulrich J A special type of senile plaque possibly an initial stage *Acta Neuropathol* 198774 133-141

[12]   Ling, E.A. and Wong, WC. The origin and nature of ramified and ameoboid microglia: A historical review and current concepts. *Glia* 1993 7: 9-18.

[13]   Rio-Hortega, P. del. (1932) Microglia. In: *Cytology and Cellular Pathologv of the Nervous System, Vol.* 2. Penfield, W (ed) Paul B. Hoeber, New York, pp. 481-584.

[14]   Rio-Hortega P. del and Penfield, W (Cerebral cicatrix: the reaction of neuroglial and microglia to brain wounds. *Johns Hopkins Hosp. Bull.* 1927 41: 278-313.

[15]   Mori S and Leblond CP Identification of microglia in light and electron microscopy *J Comp Neurology* 135 57-80 1969

[16]   Santha K and Juba A *Arch Psychiat Nervenkr* 1933 98: 598-613

[17]   Ling EA   Transformation of monocytes into amoeboid microglia in the corpus callosum of postnatal rats as shown by labeling monocytes with carbon particles *J Anat* 1979 128 847-858

[18]   Ling, E.A., Penney, D. and Leblond, C.P. Use of carbon labeling to demonstrate the role of blood monocytes as the precursors of the ameboid cells" in the corpus callosum of postnatal rats. *J.Comp Neurol* 1980 193:631~57.

[19]   Kaur C , Ling EA and Wong WC Transformation of amoeboid microglial cells into microglia in the corpus callosum of the postnatal rat brain An electron microscopic study *Arch Histol Jpn* 1985 48 17-25

[20]   Guilian, D., Ameboid microglia as effectors of inflammation in the central nervous

system, *J. Neurosci. Res.*, 18 (1987) 155-171.

[21]   Streit, W.J., Graeber, M.B. and Kreutzbcrg, G. W. Functional plasticity of microglia: A review. *Glia* 1988 I: 301-307.

[22]   Ling, E.A., Kaur, C., Vide, T. and Wong, WC. Immunocytochemical localizationof CR3 complement receptors with OX 42 in amoeboid microglia in postnatal rats. *Anat. Embryol.* 1990 182: 481-486.

[23]   Ling, E.A., Kaur, C. and Wong, WC. Expression of major histocompatibility complex antigens and CR3 complement receptors in activated microglia following an injection of ricin into the sciatic nerve in rats. *Histol. Histopathol.* 1992 7: 93-100.

[24]   Streit WJ, Walter SA, Pennell NA Reactive microgliosis *Progressive in Neurobiology* 1999 57 563-581

[25]   McGeer PL, Akiyama H, Itagaki S, McGeer EG. Immune system response in Alzheimer's disease. *Can J Neurol Sci* 1989; 16: 516-527.

[26]   Giulian D. Neurogenetics'99 . Microglia and the immune pathology of Alzheimer's disease. *Am. J. Hum. Genet.* 1999 65, 13–18

[27]   Neuroinflammation Working Group: Inflammation and Alzheimer's disease. *Neurobiol. Aging* 2000 21, 383–421

[28]   McGeer E, McGeer P. Chronic inflammation in Alzheimer's disease offers therapeutic opportunities. *Expert Rev. Neurotherapeutics* 1, 53–60 (2001).

[29]   McGeer PL, McGeer EG. Inflammation, autotoxicity and Alzheimer's disease *Neurobiol. Aging* 2001 22, 799–809 .

[30]   Welkle, He., Linington, H., Lassmann, H. and Meyermann, R Cellular immune reactivity within the CNS. *TINS* 1986 9: 271-277.

[31]   McGeer P, Itagaki S, Tago H, McGeer E. Reactive microglia in patients with senile dementia of the Alzheimer's type are positive for the histocompatibility glycoprotein HLA-DR. *Neurosci Lett* 1987; 79: 195-200.

[32]   Rogers, J., Lubcr-Narod, J., Styren, S. and Civin, H. Expression of Immune system-associated antigens by cells of the human central nervous system: relationship to the pathology of Alzheimer's disease. *Neurobiol. Aging* 1988 9: 339-349.

[33]   Rogers, J. and Rovigatti, U., Immunologic and tissue culture approaches to the neurobiology of aging, *Neurobiol. Aging,* 1988 9 759-762.

[34]   Haga, S.; Akai, K.; Ishii, T. Demonstration of microglial cells in and around senile (neuritic) plaques in the Alzheimer brain: An immunohistochemical study using a novel monoclonal antibody. *Acta Neuropathol* 1989. 77:569-575.

[35]   Wiegiel, J. and Wisniewski, H.M., The complex of microglial cells and amyloid star in three dimensional reconstruction *Acta Neuropathol.,* 1990 81 116-124.

[36]   Cras, P.; Kawai, M.; Siedlak, S.; Mulvihill, P.; Gambetti, P.; Lowery, D.; Gonzalez-DeWhitt, P.; Greenberg, B.; Perry, G, Neuronal and microglial involvement in Beta-amyloid protein deposition in Alzheimer's disease. Am. J. Pathol. 1990 137:241-246.

[37]   Mattice, L. A.; Davies, P.; Yen, S. H.; Dickson, D. W. Microglia in cerebellar plaques in Alzheimer's disease. *Acta Neuropathol.* 1990 80:493-498

[38]   Shigematsu, K.; McGeer, P. L.; Walko, D. G.; Ishii, T.; McGeer, E. G. Reactive microglia/macrophages phagocytose amyloid precursor protein produced by neurons following neuronal damage. *J. Neurosci. Res.* 1992 31:443-453.

[39]   Haga, S.; Ikeda, K.; Sato, M.; Ishii, T. Synthetic Alzheimer amyloid beta/A4 peptides enhance production of complement C3 component by cultured microglial cells. *Brain*

Res. 1993. 601:88-94

[40]   Ikeda S, Allsop D, Glenner GG Morphology and distribution of plaque and related deposits in the brains of Alzheimer's disease and control cases. An immunohistochemical study using amyloid beta-protein antibody. *Lab Invest.* 1989 60:113-122.

[41]   Mackenzie IRA., Hao C. Munoz D G Role of Microglia in Senile Plaque Formation *Neurobiology of Aging*, 1995 16: 797-804.

[42]   El Khoury J, Toft M, Hickman SE, Means TK, Terada K, Geula C, Luster AD Ccr2 deficiency impairs microglial accumulation and accelerates progression of Alzheimer-like disease. *Nat Med* 2007 13 432-438

[43]   Burnet PM. An immunological approach to aging. *Lancet* 1970; ii: 358-360.

[44]   Lennon, V.A. and Carnegie, P.R, Immunopharmacological disease: a break in tolerance to receptor sites, *Lancet,* 1971 1 630-634.

[45]   Threatt J, N andy K, Fritz R. Brain reactive antibodies in serum of old mice demonstrated by immunofluorescence. *J Gerontol* 1971 26: 316-323.

[46]   Nandy K. Brain reactive antibodies in mouse serum as a function of age. *J Gerontol* 1972; 27: 173-177.

[47]   Ingram, C.R, Phegan, K.J. and Blumenthal, H.T, Significance of an age linked neuron binding gamma globulin fraction of human sera, *J. Gerontol.,* 29 (1974) 20-27.

[48]   Mayer, P.P., Chughtai, M.A. and Cape, RD.T. An immunological approach to dementia in the elderly, *Age and Aging, 5* (1976) 164-170.

[49]   Torack, R.M., *The Pathological Physiology of Dementia,* Springer Verlag, Wien, 1978.

[50]   Lal, H. and Forster, M.J., Autoimmunity and age associated cognitive decline, *Neurobiol. Aging, 9* (1988) 733-742.81: 591-596.

[51]   McGeer PL and McGeer EG Local neuroinflammation and the progression of Alzheimer's disease *Journal of NeuroVirology*, 8: 529–538, 2002

[52]   Yasojima, K., Schwab, C., McGeer, E.G., and McGeer, P.L. Upregulated production and activation of the complement system in Alzheimer's disease brain. *Am. J. Pathol.* 154, 927- 936 (1999).

[53]   Eikelenboom P, Stam FC. Immunoglobulines and complement factors in senile plaques. An immunoperoxidase study. *Acta Neuropathol* 1982; 57: 239-242.

[54]   Ishii T, Haga S. Immunoelectron microscopic localization of complement in amyloid fibrils of senile plaques. *Acta Neuropathol* 1984; 63: 296-300.

[55]   McGeer P, Akiyama H, Itagaki S, McGeer EG. Activation of the classical complement pathway in brain tissue of Alzheimer's patients. *Neurosci Lett* 1989; 197: 341- 346

[56]   Eikelenboom P, Hack CE, et al (1989). Complement activation in amyloid plaques in Alzheimer's dementia. *Virchows Arch Cell Pathol* 56: 259–262.

[57]   Webster S, Bonnell B, et al. Charge-based binding of complement component C1q to the Alzheimer's amyloid beta-peptide. *Am J Pathol* 1997 150: 1531–1536.

[58]   Itagaki S, Akiyama H, et al Ultrastructural localization of complement membrane attack complex (MAC)-like immunoreactivity in brains of patients with Alzheimer's disease. *Brain Res* 1994 645: 78–84.

[59]   Webster S, Lue LF, et al Molecular and cellular characterization of the membrane attack complex, C5b-9, in Alzheimer's disease. *Neurobiol Aging 1997* 18: 415–

[60] Yasojima K, McGeer EG, et al. Complement regulators C1 inhibitor and CD59 do not significantly inhibit complement activation in Alzheimer's disease. *Brain Res* 1999 833: 297–301.

[61] Rogers J, Cooper NR, et al Complement activation by β -amyloid in Alzheimer's disease. *Proc Natl Acad Sci* USA 1992 89: 10016–10020.

[62] Yasojima K, Schwab C, et al Human neurons generate C-reactive protein and amyloid P: upregulation in Alzheimer's disease. Brain Res 2000 887: 80– 89.

[63] Yasojima K, Schwab C, et al. Generation of C-reactive protein and complement components in atherosclerotic plaques. *Am J Pathol* 2001 158: 1039–1051. 169–176.

[64] McGeer PL, McGeer EG. The inflammatory response system of brain: implications for therapy of Alzheimer and other neurodegenerative diseases. *Brain Res Rev* 1995;21:195–218.

[65] Ricklin D_& John D Lambris JD_Complement-targeted therapeutics *Nature Biotechnology* 2007 25, 1265 - 1275

[66] Mulder C, Schoonenboom SN, Wahlund LO, Scheltens P, van Kamp GJ, Veerhuis R, Hack CE, Blomberg M, Schutgens RB, Eikelenboom PCSF markers related to pathogenetic mechanisms in Alzheimer's disease.. *J Neural Transm.* 2002 109 :1491-1498

[67] Finehout EJ , Franck Z , Kelvin H. Lee KH Complement protein isoforms in CSF as possible biomarkers for neurodegenerative disease *Disease Markers* 2005 21 93 – 101

[68] Enabling Technologies for Alzheimer's Disease Research Sixth Bar Harbor Workshop, 2006 Alz Forum Gabrielle Strobel http://www.alzforum.org/res/enab/workshops/2006.asp

[69] Pietila K, Harmoinen AP, Jokinitty J, Pasternack AI. Serum C-reactive protein concentration in acute myocardial infarction and its relationship to mortality during 24 months of follow-up in patients under thrombolytic treatment. *Eur Heart J* 1996;17: 1345–1349.

[70] Griffin WST, Stanley LC, Ling C, White L, MacLeod V, Perrot LJ, White CL 3rd, Araoz C. Brain interleukin 1 and S-100 immunoreactivity are elevated in Down syndrome and Alzheimer's disease. *Proc Soc Natl Acad Sci* USA 1989; 86: 7611–7615.

[71] Griffin WST, Sheng JG, Roberts GW, Mrak RE. Interleukin-1 expression in different plaque types in Alzheimer's disease: significance in plaque evolution. J *Neuropathol Exp Neurol* 1995; 54: 276 – 281.

[72] Sheng JG, Mrak RE, Griffin WS. Neuritic plaque evolution in Alzheimer's disease is accompanied by transition of activated microglia from primed to enlarged to phagocytic forms *Acta Neuropathol.* 1997 94:1-5

[73] Mrak RE and Griffin WST Potential Inflammatory biomarkers in Alzheimer's disease *Journal of Alzheimer's Disease* 2005 8 369–375)

[74] Bauer J, Strauss S, Schreiter–Gasser U, et al. IL-6 and alpha-2-macroglobulin indicate an acute-phase state in Alzheimer's disease cortices. *FEBS Lett* 1991; 285:111– 114.

[75] Bauer J, Ganter U, Strauss S, Stadtmuller G, Frommberger U, Bauer H, Volk B, Berger M, The participation of interleukin-6 in the pathogenesis of Alzheimer's disease. Forty-fifth forum in *Immunology, Res. Immunol.* 143 1992 650–657.

[76] Huell M, Strauss S, Volk B, Berger M, Bauer J Interleukin-6 is present in early stages of plaque formation and is restricted to the brains of Alzheimer's disease patients. *Acta*

Neuropathol. 1995;89: 544-551.

[77]   Giulian, D., Young, D.G. , Lachman, L.B. Interleukin I of the central nervous system. Production by amoeboid microglia. *J. Exp. Med.* 1986 164: 594- 604.

[78]   Giulian, D. Microglia, cytokines, and cytotoxines: Modulation of cellular responses after injury to the central nervous system. 1. *Immunol. Immunopharmaco*l. 1990 10: 15-21.

[79]   Szczepanik AM, Funes S, Petko W and. Ringheim GE IL-4, IL-10 and IL-13 modulate Aβ(1–42)-induced cytokine and chemokine production in primary murine microglia and a human monocyte cell line *Journal of Neuroimmunology* 2001 113 49-62

[80]   Del Villar K, Miller CA. Down-regulation of DENN/MADD, a TNF receptor binding protein, correlates with neuronal cell death in Alzheimer's disease brain and hippocampal neurons. *Proc Natl Acad Sci* USA 2004;101: 4210–4215.

[81]   van der Wal, E. A., Gomez-Pinilla F, and Cotman CW. Transforming growth factor-B is in plaques in Alzheimer and Down pathologies. *Neuroreport* 1993 4:69-72.

[82]   Peress NS, Perillo E. Differential expression of TGF-beta 1, 2 and 3 isotypes in Alzheimer's disease: a comparative immunohistochemical study with cerebral infarction, aged human and mouse control brains. *J Neuropathol Exp Neurol* 1995 54: 802–811

[83]   Wyss-Coray T, Masliah E, Mallory M, et al. Amyloidogenic role of cytokine TGF-beta1 in transgenic mice and in Alzheimer's disease. *Nature.* 1997;389: 603-605.

[84]   Hyoung-gon Lee, Masumi Ueda, Xiongwei Zhu George Perry, Mark A. Smith Ectopic expression of phospho-Smad2 in Alzheimer's disease: Uncoupling of the transforming growth factor- pathway? *Journal of Neuroscience Research* 2006 1856 – 1861

[85]   Ravaglia G , Forti P , Maioli F , Chiappelli M , Montesi F , Tumini E , Mariani E , Licastro F , Patterson C Inflammatory markers and risk of dementia: The Conselice Study of Brain Aging *Neurobiology of Aging* 2007 28 1810–1820

[86]   Luterman JD, Haroutunian V, Yemul S, Ho L, Purohit D, Aisen PS Mohs R , Giulio Pasinetti M Cytokine Gene Expression as a Function of the Clinical Progression of Alzheimer Disease Dementia *Arch Neurol.* 2000; 57:1153-1160

[87]   A De Luigi , C Fragiacomo,U Lucca P Quadri , M Tettamanti , MG De Simoni Inflammatory markers in Alzheimer's disease and multi-infarct dementia *Mechanisms of Ageing and Development* 2001 122 1985-1995

[88]   Dik MG, Jonker C, Hack CE, Smit JH, Comijs HC, Eikelenboom P Serum inflammatory proteins and cognitive decline in older persons. *Neurology.* 2005 64:1371-1377

[89]   Schram MT, Euser SM, de Craen AJ, Witteman JC, Frölich M, Hofman A, Jolles J, Breteler MM, Westendorp RG. Systemic markers of inflammation and cognitive decline in old age. *J Am Geriatr Soc.* 2007 55: 708-716

[90]   Rafnsson SB, Deary IJ, Smith FB, Whiteman MC, Rumley A, Lowe GD, Fowkes FG Cognitive decline and markers of inflammation and hemostasis: the Edinburgh Artery Study. *J Am Geriatr So*c. 2007 55:700-707

[91]   Nicoll JAR, Mrak RE, Graham D, Stewart J, Wilcock G, MacGowan S, Esiri MM, Murray LS, Dewar D, Love S, Moss T, Griffin WS. Association of interleukin-1 gene polymorphisms with Alzheimer's disease. *Ann Neurol* 2000; 47:365–368.

[92]   Papassotiropoulos A, Bagli M, Jessen F, Nayer TA, Maier W, Rao ML, Heun R. A

genetic variation of the inflammatory cytokine interleukin-6 delays the initial onset and reduces the risk for sporadic Alzheimer's disease. *Ann Neurol* 1999; 45:666 – 668.

[93]   Rebeck GW. Confirmation of the genetic association of interleukin-1A with early onset sporadic Alzheimer's disease. *Neurosci Lett* 2000; 293:75–77.

[94]   Collins JS, Perry RT, Watson B, Harrell LE, Acton RT, Blacker D, Albert MS, Tanzi RE, Bassett SS, McInnis MG, Campbell RD, Go RCP. Association of a haplotype for tumor necrosis factor in siblings with late-onset Alzheimer disease: The NIMH Alzheimer disease genetics initiative. *Am J Med Genet* 2000; 96:823–30.

[95]   Licastro F, Pedrini S, Bonafe M, Grimaldi LME, Olivieri F, Cavallone L, Giovannetti S, Franceschi C. Polymorphisms of the IL-6 gene increase the risk for late onset Alzheimer's disease and affect IL-6 plasma levels. *Neurobiol Aging* 2000; 21(1S):S38.

[96]   Luedecking EK, DeKosky ST, Mehdi H, Ganguli M and Kamboh MI, Analysis of genetic polymorphisms in the transforming growth factor-beta1 gene and the risk of Alzheimer's disease, *Hum. Genet.* 106 (2000), 565–569.

[97]   ZS. Tan, AS. Beiser, RS. Vasan, R. Roubenoff, CA. Dinarello, TB. Harris, EJ. Benjamin, R. Au, D. P. Kiel, P. A. Wolf and S. Seshadri Inflammatory markers and the risk of Alzheimer disease: The Framingham Study *Neurology* 2007;68; 1902-1908

[98]   Guerreiro RJ, Isabel Santana I, Brás JM, Santiago B, Paiva A, Oliveira C Peripheral Inflammatory Cytokines as Biomarkers in Alzheimer's Disease and Mild Cognitive Impairment *Neurodegenerative Diseases* 2007; 4:406-412

[99]   Tarkowski E, Andreasen N, Tarkowski A,Blennow K Intrathecal inflammation precedes development of Alzheimer's disease *J Neurol Neurosurg Psychiatry* 2003;74:1200–1205

[100]   Alvarez A , Cacabelos R , Sanpedro C , Garcia-Fantini M , Aleixandre M Serum TNF-alpha levels are increased and correlate negatively with free IGF-I in Alzheimer disease *Neurobiology of Aging* 2007 28 533–536

[101]   Yaffe K, Kanaya A, Lindquist K, Simonsick E, Harris T, Shorr R, Tylavsky F, Newman A The metabolic syndrome, inflammation, and the Risk of Cognitive Decline *JAMA* 2004 292 2237- 2242.

[102]   Yaffe K. Metabolic syndrome and cognitive disorders: is the sum greater than its parts? *Alzheimer Dis Assoc Disord.* 2007 211 67-71

[103]   Smith RS The macrophage theory of depression *Medical Hypothesis* 1991 35 298-305

[104]   Dantzer R, O'Connor J, Freund G, Johnson R, Kelly K From Inflammation to sickness and depression when the immune system subjugates the Brain *Nature Reviews Neuroscience* 2008 9 46-56

[105]   Baboolal NS Prescribing Practices In The Treatment Of Depression: A Survey Among Psychiatrists and Other Doctors Providing Psychiatric Care in Trinidad and Tobago. *The Internet Journal of Third World Medicine.* 2004. Volume 1 Number 1

[106]   Godbout JP, Moreau M, Lestage J, Chen J, Sparkman NL, Connor JO, Castanon N, Kelley KW, Dantzer R, Johnson RW. Aging exacerbates depressive- like behavior in mice in response to activation of the peripheral innate immune system *Neuropsychopharmacology* (in press)

[107]   CL. Raison, L Capuron and A H. Miller Cytokines sing the blues: inflammation and the pathogenesis of depression *TRENDS in Immunology* 2006 27 24-31

[108]   Irwin MR, Miller AH Depressive disorders and immunity: 20 years of progress and discovery Brain, *Behavior, and Immunity* 2007 21 374–383

[109]   Ishii, T and Haga, S., Immunoelectron microscopic localization of immunoglobulines in amyloid fibrils of senile plaques, *Acta Neuropathol.,* 1976 *36* 243-249.

[110]   D'Andrea MR Evidence linking neuronal cell death to autoimmunity in Alzheimer's disease *Brain Research* 2003 982 19–30

[111]   D'Andrea MR. Add Alzheimer's disease to the list of autoimmune diseases. *Med Hypotheses.* 2005 64: 458-463

[112]   D'Andrea MR antibody-dependent complement pathway Evidence that immunoglobulin-positive neurons in Alzheimer's disease are dying via the classical *Am J Alzheimers Dis Other Demen* 2005; 20; 144

[113]   Wisniewski HM, Kozlowski PB. Evidence for blood brain barrier changes in senile dementia of the Alzheimer type. *Ann NY Acad Sci* 1982; 396: 119-127.

[114]   Alafuzoff I, Adolfsson G, Bucht G, Winblad B. Albumin and immunoglobuline in plasma and cerebrospinal fluid and blood cerebrospinal barrier function in patients with dementia of Alzheimer type and Multiinfarct Dementia. *J Neurol Sci* 1983; 60: 465-472.

[115]   Hardy JA, Mann DMA, Wester P, Winblad B. An integrative hypothesis concerning the pathogenesis and progression of Alzheimer's disease. *Neurobiol Aging* 1986; 7: 489-502.

[116]   Blennon K, Wallin A, Fredman P, Karlsson I, Gottfries CG, Svennerholm L. Blood-brain barrier disturbance in patients with Alzheimer's disease is related to vascular factors. *Acta Neurol* Scand 1990; 81: 323-326.

[117]   Skalickova 0, Jezkova Z, Slavickova V. Immunological aspects of psychiatric geronotology. *Czechoslovak Psychiatry* 1962; 58: 1-10.

[118]   Nandy K. Alzheimer's disease: Senile dementia and related disorders. In: Aging (Vol.7). Katzman RD, Terry RD, Bick KL (Eds). Raven Press Publisher, New York, NY, USA, 503–512 (1978).

[119]   Whittingham S, Lennon V, Mackay IE, VernonDavies G, Davies B. Absence of brain antibodies in senile dementia. *Br J Psychiat* 1970; 116: 447-48.

[120]   Watts H, Kennedy PGE, Thomas M. The significance of anti-neuronal antibodies in Alzheimer's disease. *J Neuroimmunol* 1981; 1: 107-116.

[121]   Husby G, Li L, Davis LE, Wedege E, Kokmen E, Williams RC Jr. Antibodies to human caudate nucleus neurons in Huntington's chorea. *J Clin Invest* 1977; 59: 922-932.

[122]   Chapman J, Korczyn AD, Hareuveni M, Michaelson DM. Antibodies to cholinergic cell bodies in Alzheimer's disease. In: Alzheimer's and Parkinson's diseases: Strategies for Research and Development. Fisher A, Hanin I, Lachman C (Eds). Plenum Press, New York, NY, USA, 329–333 (1986).

[123]   McRae-Degueurce A, Booj S, Haglid K etal. Antibodies in the cerebrospinal fluid of some Alzheimer's diseases patients recognize cholinergic neurons in the rat central nervous system. *Proc. Natl Acad. Sci.* 1987 USA 84, 9214–9218

[124]   McRae-Degueurce, A, Haglid, K., Rosengren, L., Wallin, A, B1ennow, K., Gotffries, C.G. and Dahlstrom, A Antibodies recognizing cholinergic neurons and

Throglobuline are found in thc cerebrospinal fluid of a subgroup of patients with Alzheimer's disease. *Drug Devel. Res.* 198815:153-163

[125] Foley P, Bradford H, Docherty M etal. Evidence for the presence of antibodies to cholinergic neurons in the serum of patients with Alzheimer's disease. *J. Neurol.* 1988 235 466–471

[126] Gaskin F, Kingley BS, Fu SM. Autoantibodies to neurofibrillary tangles and brain tissue in Alzheimer's disease. Establishment of Epstein-Barr virus transformed antibody-producing cell lines. *J Exp Med* 1987; 165: 245-250.

[127] Chapman J, Bachar O, Korczyn etal. Alzheimer's disease antibodies bind specifically to neurofilament protein in Torpedo cholinergic neurons *J. Neuroscience* 1989 9, 2710–2717

[128] Fillit HM, Kemeny E, Luine V, Weksler ME, Zabriskie JB. Antivascular antibodies in the sera of patients withsenile dementia of the Alzheimer's type. *J. Geronotol.* 1987 42, 180–184

[129] Pouplard P, Emile J. New immunological fmdings in senile dementia. Pituitary autoantibodies as a marker for Alzheimer's disease. *Interdiscipl Topics Geront* 1985;19: 62-71.

[130] Joachim, C.L., Mori, H., Selkoe, D.J., . Amyloid beta-protein deposition in tissues other than brain in Alzheimer's disease. *Nature.* 1989 341, 226-230.

[131] Miklossy J, Kraftsik R, Pillevuit O, Lepori D, Genton C, Bosman FT. Curly fiber and tangle-like inclusions in the ependyma and choroid plexus--a pathogenetic relationship with the cortical Alzheimer-type changes? *J Neuropathol Exp Neurol.* 1998 57:1202-12.

[132] Terryberry JW, Thor G, Peter JB. Autoantibodies in neurodegenerative intrathecal analysis. *Neurobiol. Aging* 1998 19, 205–216 .

[133] McRae,A., Ling , E.A., Polinsky,R., Gotffries, C.G., Dahlström, A. Antibodies in the cerebrospinal fluid of some Alzheimer's disease patients recognize amoeboid microglial cells in the developing rat central nervous system. *Neuroscience* 1991 41: 739-752

[134] McRae A, Blennon K, Gottfries CG, Walin A, Dahlström A: Brain specific antibodies in the CSF of patients with Alzheimer's disease and other types of dementias. in: Fowler CJ, Carlson LA,Gottfries CG,Winblad B.(eds): Biological Markers in Dementia of Alzheimer Type. London, Smith-Gordon, 1990; p135-148.

[135] Ling E.A., Dahlström A. , Polinsky R., Nee L McRae, A. Studies of activated microglia cells and macrophages using Alzheimer's disease cerebrospinal fluid in adult rats with experimentally induced lesions. *Neuroscience* 1992 51: 815-825.

[136] Rogers J, Luber-Narod J, Styren S , Civin H: Expression of Immune system-associated antigens by cells of the human central nervous system: relationship to the pathology of Alzheimer's disease. *Neurobiol. Aging* 1988 9: 339-349

[137] Raff MC, Fields KL, Hakomori S, Mirsky R, Pruss RM, Winter J. Cell-type specific markers for distinguishing and studying neurons and the major class of glial cells in culture *Brain Res.* 1979 174, 283–308.

[138] Wigander A., Lundmark K., McRae A. et al. Survival of rat fetal cholinergic neurons co-cultured with human midgut carcinoid tumour cells. *Acta Scand Physiol* 1989 136: 291-292

[139] Dahlström A , Wigander A , Lundmark K , Gottfries CG, McRae, A. Investigations on autoantibodies in Alzheimer's and Parkinson's diseases, using defined neuronal cultures. *J. Neural Trans.* 1990 29: (suppl) 195-206

[140] Dahlström A, McRae A, Polinsky R, et al. Microglia investigations with cell cultures and human cortical biopsies. *Molecular Neurobiology* 1994 9: 41-54

[141] McRae A and Dahlstrom Immune responses in brains of Alzheimer's and Parkinson' disease patients : Hypothesis and Reality *Reviews in the Neurosciences* 1992 3 79-97

[142] McRae A, Dahlstrom A, Polinsky R, Ling EA. Cerebrospinal fluid antibodies: potential diagnostic markers for immune mechanisms in Alzheimer's disease. *Behavioural Brain Res.* 1993 57, 225–234.

[143] McRae A, Ling EA. Microglia; an antigen for Alzheimer's cerebrospinal fluid antibodies In: Topical Issues in Microglia Research. Ling EA, Tan CK, Tan CBS (Eds). Goh Bros Enterprise Humanities Press Publisher, Singapore, 109–117 1996

[144] McRae A Dahlstrom A and Ling EA Microglia in Neurodegenerative disorders Emphasis on Alzheimer 's disease *Gerontology* 1997 43 93-108

[145] McRae A and Ling EA Cerebrospinal fluid and serum anti microglia antibodies prospects for early diagnosis of Alzheimer' disease *Expert Review Neurotherapeutics* 2003 3 247-257

[146] Lemke MR, Glatzel M, Henneberg AE. Antimicroglia antibodies in sera of Alzheimer's disease patients. Biol. Psychiatry 45, 508–511 (1999).

[147] Giulian D. Microglia and diseases of the nervous system In: Current Issues in Neurology 1992 Vol .12. Mosby Year Book Inc., MO, USA, 23–54 (1992).

[148] Thomas WE. Brain macrophages: evaluation of microglia and their function. Brain Res. Rev. 17, 61–74 (1992).

[149] Banati RB, Gehrmann J, Kellner M, Holsboer F. Antibodies against microglia/ brain macrophages in the cerebrospinal fluid of a patient with acute amyotrophic lateral sclerosis and presenile dementia. *Clin. Neuropathol.* 14, 197–200 (1995).

[150] McRae A, Martins RN, Fonte J, Kraftsik R, Hirt L, Miklossy J, Cerebrospinal fluid anti microglial antibodies in Alzheimer Disease,: a Putative marker of an ongoing inflammatory process, *Exp. Gerontol.* 2007 42 355 - 363.

[151] Cagnin A, Brooks DJ, Gunn RN et al. In vivo measurement of activated microglia in dementia *Lancet* 2001 358, 461–467

[152] Parachikova A , M.G. Agadjanyan MG, Cribbs DH, Blurton-Jones M , Perreau V , J. RogersJ , T.G. Beach TG , Cotman CW Inflammatory changes parallel the early stages of Alzheimer disease *Neurobiology of Aging* 2007 28 1821–1833

[153] D'Andrea MR, Cole GM Ard MD The microglial phagocytic role with specific plaque types in the Alzheimer disease brain *Neurobiology of Aging* 2004 25 675–683

[154] Anonymous. Consensus report of the Working Group on: 'Molecular and Biochemical Markers of Alzheimer's disease.' The Ronald and Nancy Reagan Research Institute of the Alzheimer's Association and the National Institute on Aging Working Group. *Neurobiol. Aging* 19, 109–116 (1998).

[155] Ray S, Britschgi M, Herbert C, Takeda-Uchimura Y, Boxer A, Blennow K, Friedman LF, Galasko DR, Jutel M, Karydas A, Kaye JA, Leszek J, Miller BL, Minthon L, Quinn JF, Rabinovici GD, Robinson WH, Sabbagh MN, So YT, Sparks DL, Tabaton M, Tinklenberg J, Yesavage JA, Tibshirani R, Wyss-Coray T. Classification and prediction of clinical Alzheimer's diagnosis based on plasma signaling proteins. *Nat*

Med. 2007 13:1359-1362.

[156]   Davis GK, Baboolal NS, Seales D, Ramchandani J, McKell S, McRae A. Potential biomarkers for dementia in Trinidad and Tobago. *Neurosci Lett.* 2007; 424: 27-30.

[157]   Prasher VP, Farrer MJ, Kessling AM, Fisher EM, West RJ, Barber PC, Butler AC. Molecular mapping of Alzheimer-type dementia in Down's syndrome. *Ann Neurol.* 1998 Mar; 43(3):380-3.

[158]   Rovelet-Lecrux A, Hannequin D, Raux G, Le Meur N, Laquerriere A, Vital A, Dumanchin C, Feuillette S, Brice A, Vercelletto M, Dubas F, Frebourg T, Campion D. APP locus duplication causes autosomal dominant early-onset Alzheimer disease with cerebral amyloid angiopathy. *Nat Genet.* 2006 Jan; 38(1):24-6. Epub 2005 Dec 20.

[159]   Selkoe DJ, Podlisny MB. Deciphering the genetic basis of Alzheimer's disease. *Annu Rev Genomics Hum Genet.* 2002; 3:67-99. Epub 2002 Apr 15

[160]   Johansson A, Zetterberg H, Hampel H, Buerger K, Prince JA, Minthon L, Wahlund LO, Blennow K. Genetic association of CDC2 with cerebrospinal fluid tau in Alzheimer's disease. *Dement Geriatr Cogn Disord.* 2005; 20(6):367-74. Epub 2005 Sep 29.

[161]   Sunderland T, Mirza N, Putnam KT, Linker G, Bhupali D, Durham R, Soares H, Kimmel L, Friedman D, Bergeson J, Csako G, Levy JA, Bartko JJ, Cohen RM. Cerebrospinal fluid beta-amyloid1-42 and tau in control subjects at risk for Alzheimer's disease: the effect of APOE epsilon4 allele. *Biol Psychiatry.* 2004 Nov 1;56(9):670-6.

[162]   Bertram L, McQueen MB, Mullin K, Blacker D, Tanzi RE. Systematic meta-analyses of Alzheimer disease genetic association studies: the AlzGene database. *Nat Genet.* 2007 Jan; 39(1):17-23.

[163]   Welsh JB, Sapinoso LM, Kern SG, Brown DA, Liu T, Bauskin AR, Ward RL, Hawkins NJ, Quinn DI, Russell PJ, Sutherland RL, Breit SN, Moskaluk CA, Frierson HF Jr, Hampton GM. Large-scale delineation of secreted protein biomarkers overexpressed in cancer tissue and serum. *Proc Natl Acad Sci U S A.* 2003 Mar 18; 100(6):3410-5. Epub 2003 Mar 6.

[164]   Souto JC, Blanco-Vaca F, Soria JM, Buil A, Almasy L, Ordonez-Llanos J, Martin-Campos JM, Lathrop M, Stone W, Blangero J, Fontcuberta J. A genomewide exploration suggests a new candidate gene at chromosome 11q23 as the major determinant of plasma homocysteine levels: results from the GAIT project. *Am J Hum Genet.* 2005 Jun; 76(6):925-33. Epub 2005 Apr 22.

[165]   Price JL, Morris JC. Tangles and plaques in nondemented aging and "preclinical" Alzheimer's disease. *Ann Neurol.* 1999 Mar 1; 45(3):358-68.

[166]   Bayer TA, Buslei R, Havas L, Falkai P (1999). Evidence for activation of microglia in patients with psychiatric illnesses. *Neurosci Lett* 271: 126–128.

[167]   Heneka MT, O'Banion MK (2007). Inflammatory processes in Alzheimer's disease. *J Neuroimmunol* 184: 69–91.

[168]   Wilkinson BL, Landreth GE (2006). The microglial NADPH oxidase complex as a source of oxidative stress in Alzheimer's disease. *J Neuroinflamm* 3: 30–42.

[169]   Aisen PS, Davis KL. Inflammatory mechanisms in Alzheimer's disease: implications for therapy. *Am J Psychiatry.* 1994 Aug; 151(8):1105-13.

[170]   Hepler RW, Grimm KM, Nahas DD, Breese R, Dodson EC, Acton P, Keller PM, Yeager M, Wang H, Shughrue P, Kinney G, Joyce JG. Solution state characterization

of amyloid beta-derived diffusible ligands. *Biochemistry.* 2006 Dec 26;45(51):15157-67. Epub 2006 Dec 6.

[171]   Etcheberrigaray E, Gibson GE, Alkon DL. Molecular mechanisms of memory and the pathophysiology of Alzheimer's disease. *Ann N Y Acad Sci.* 1994 Dec 15; 747:245-55.

[172]   Rumble B, Retallack R, Hilbich C, Simms G, Multhaup G, Martins R, Hockey A, Montgomery P, Beyreuther K, Masters CL. Amyloid A4 protein and its precursor in Down's syndrome and Alzheimer's disease. *N Engl J Med.* 1989 Jun 1;320(22):1446-52.

[173]   Sunderland T, Gur RE, Arnold SE. The use of biomarkers in the elderly: current and future challenges. *Biol Psychiatry.* 2005 Aug 15;58(4):272-6.

[174]   Sunderland T, Linker G, Mirza N, Putnam KT, Friedman DL, Kimmel LH, Bergeson J, Manetti GJ, Zimmermann M, Tang B, Bartko JJ, Cohen RM. Decreased beta-amyloid1-42 and increased tau levels in cerebrospinal fluid of patients with Alzheimer disease. *JAMA.* 2003 Apr 23-30; 289(16):2094-103. Erratum in: JAMA. 2007 Oct 3; 298(13):1516.

[175]   Fagan AM, Mintun MA, Mach RH, Lee SY, Dence CS, Shah AR, LaRossa GN, Spinner ML, Klunk WE, Mathis CA, DeKosky ST, Morris JC, Holtzman DM. Inverse relation between in vivo amyloid imaging load and cerebrospinal fluid Abeta42 in humans. *Ann Neurol.* 2006 Mar; 59(3):512-9.

[176]   Bibl M, Mollenhauer B, Esselmann H, Lewczuk P, Klafki HW, Sparbier K, Smirnov A, Cepek L, Trenkwalder C, Rüther E, Kornhuber J, Otto M, Wiltfang J. CSF amyloid-beta-peptides in Alzheimer's disease, dementia with Lewy bodies and Parkinson's disease dementia. *Brain.* 2006 May;129(Pt 5):1177-87. Epub 2006 Apr 6.

[177]   Fagan AM, Younkin LH, Morris JC, Fryer JD, Cole TG, Younkin SG, Holtzman DM. Differences in the Abeta40/Abeta42 ratio associated with cerebrospinal fluid lipoproteins as a function of apolipoprotein E genotype. *Ann Neurol.* 2000 Aug; 48(2):201-10.

[178]   Moonis M, Swearer JM, Dayaw MP, St George-Hyslop P, Rogaeva E, Kawarai T, Pollen DA. Familial Alzheimer disease: decreases in CSF Abeta42 levels precede cognitive decline. *Neurology.* 2005 Jul 26;65(2):323-5.

[179]   Fukumoto H, Tennis M, Locascio JJ, Hyman BT, Growdon JH, Irizarry MC. Age but not diagnosis is the main predictor of plasma amyloid beta-protein levels. *Arch Neurol.* 2003 Jul; 60(7):958-64.

[180]   Mayeux R, Tang MX, Jacobs DM, Manly J, Bell K, Merchant C, Small SA, Stern Y, Wisniewski HM, Mehta PD. Plasma amyloid beta-peptide 1-42 and incipient Alzheimer's disease. *Ann Neurol.* 1999 Sep; 46(3):412-6.

[181]   Mehta PD, Pirttilä T, Mehta SP, Sersen EA, Aisen PS, Wisniewski HM. Plasma and cerebrospinal fluid levels of amyloid beta proteins 1-40 and 1-42 in Alzheimer disease. *Arch Neurol.* 2000 Jan; 57(1):100-5.

[182]   Arvanitakis Z, Lucas JA, Younkin LH, Younkin SG, Graff-Radford NR. Serum creatinine levels correlate with plasma amyloid Beta protein. *Alzheimer Dis Assoc Disord.* 2002 Jul-Sep;16(3):187-90.

[183]   Brettschneider S, Morgenthaler NG, Teipel SJ, Fischer-Schulz C, Bürger K, Dodel R, Du Y, Möller HJ, Bergmann A, Hampel H. Decreased serum amyloid beta(1-42) autoantibody levels in Alzheimer's disease, determined by a newly developed

immuno-precipitation assay with radiolabeled amyloid beta(1-42) peptide. *Biol Psychiatry.* 2005 Apr 1; 57(7):813-6.

[184]   Cirrito JR, May PC, O'Dell MA, Taylor JW, Parsadanian M, Cramer JW, Audia JE, Nissen JS, Bales KR, Paul SM, DeMattos RB, Holtzman DM. In vivo assessment of brain interstitial fluid with microdialysis reveals plaque-associated changes in amyloid-beta metabolism and half-life. *J Neurosci.* 2003 Oct 1;23(26):8844-53.

[185]   Mi K, Johnson GV (2006). The role of tau phosphorylation in the pathogenesis of Alzheimer's disease. *Curr Alzheimer Res* 3: 449–463.

[186]   Arai H, Terajima M, Miura M, Higuchi S, Muramatsu T, Matsushita S, Machida N, Nakagawa T, Lee VM, Trojanowski JQ, Sasaki H. Effect of genetic risk factors and disease progression on the cerebrospinal fluid tau levels in Alzheimer's disease. *J Am Geriatr Soc.* 1997 Oct;45(10):1228-31.

[187]   Buerger K, Ewers M, Pirttilä T, Zinkowski R, Alafuzoff I, Teipel SJ, DeBernardis J, Kerkman D, McCulloch C, Soininen H, Hampel H. CSF phosphorylated tau protein correlates with neocortical neurofibrillary pathology in Alzheimer's disease. *Brain.* 2006 Nov; 129(Pt 11):3035-41. Epub 2006 Sep 29.

[188]   Ewers M, Buerger K, Teipel SJ, Scheltens P, Schröder J, Zinkowski RP, Bouwman FH, Schönknecht P, Schoonenboom NS, Andreasen N, Wallin A, DeBernardis JF, Kerkman DJ, Heindl B, Blennow K, Hampel H. Multicenter assessment of CSF-phosphorylated tau for the prediction of conversion of MCI. *Neurology.* 2007 Dec 11;69(24):2205-12.

[189]   Hampel H, Mitchell A, Blennow K, Frank RA, Brettschneider S, Weller L, Möller HJ. Core biological marker candidates of Alzheimer's disease - perspectives for diagnosis, prediction of outcome and reflection of biological activity. *J Neural Transm.* 2004 Mar; 111(3):247-72. Epub 2003 Dec 3.

[190]   Yamamori H, Khatoon S, Grundke-Iqbal I, Blennow K, Ewers M, Hampel H, Iqbal K. Tau in cerebrospinal fluid: a sensitive sandwich enzyme-linked immunosorbent assay using tyramide signal amplification. *Neurosci Lett.* 2007 May 17;418(2):186-9. Epub 2007 Mar 14.

[191]   Blasko I, Lederer W, Oberbauer H, Walch T, Kemmler G, Hinterhuber H, Marksteiner J, Humpel C. Measurement of thirteen biological markers in CSF of patients with Alzheimer's disease and other dementias. *Dement Geriatr Cogn Disord.* 2006; 21(1):9-15. Epub 2005 Oct 21.

[192]   Hampel H, Teipel SJ, Fuchsberger T, Andreasen N, Wiltfang J, Otto M, Shen Y, Dodel R, Du Y, Farlow M, Möller HJ, Blennow K, Buerger K. Value of CSF beta-amyloid1-42 and tau as predictors of Alzheimer's disease in patients with mild cognitive impairment. *Mol Psychiatry.* 2004 Jul;9(7):705-10.

[193]   Sunderland T, Linker G, Mirza N, Putnam KT, Friedman DL, Kimmel LH, Bergeson J, Manetti GJ, Zimmermann M, Tang B, Bartko JJ, Cohen RM. Decreased beta-amyloid1-42 and increased tau levels in cerebrospinal fluid of patients with Alzheimer disease. JAMA. 2003 Apr 23-30; 289(16):2094-103. Erratum in: *JAMA.* 2007 Oct 3; 298(13):1516.

[194]   De La Monte SM, Wands JR. The AD7c-NTP neuronal thread protein biomarker for detecting Alzheimer's disease. *J Alzheimers Dis.* 2001 Jun; 3(3):345-353.

[195]   Patricia G. McCaffrey. Antecedent Biomarkers for the Early and Preclinical Detection of Alzheimer's Disease- 5th Leonard Berg Symposium. Alzheimer Research Forum.

Updated March 29, 2006. Available at: http://www.alzforum.org/res/enab/workshops/ biomarkers3.asp. Accessed December 19, 2007.

[196]   Gila Z. Reckess. Antecedent Biomarkers in Alzheimer's Disease: Uses, Limitations, and Future Directions for Research. Alzheimer Research Forum. Posted 7 November 2003. Available at: http://www.alzforum.org/res/enab/workshops/biomarkers.asp. Accessed December 19, 2007.

[197]   Vermeer SE, van Dijk EJ, Koudstaal PJ, Oudkerk M, Hofman A, Clarke R, Breteler MM. Homocysteine, silent brain infarcts, and white matter lesions: The Rotterdam Scan Study. *Ann Neurol.* 2002 Mar; 51(3):279-81

[198]   Kruman II, Culmsee C, Chan SL, Kruman Y, Guo Z, Penix L, Mattson MP. Homocysteine elicits a DNA damage response in neurons that promotes apoptosis and hypersensitivity to excitotoxicity. *J Neurosci.* 2000; 20:6920-6

[199]   Kennedy BP, Bottiglieri T, Arning E, Ziegler MG, Hansen LA, Masliah E. Elevated S-adenosylhomocysteine in Alzheimer brain: influence on methyltransferases and cognitive function. *J Neural Transm.* 2004; 111:547-67

[200]   Kim J, Park MH, Kim E, Han C, Jo SA, Jo I. Plasma homocysteine is associated with the risk of mild cognitive impairment in an elderly Korean population. *J Nutr.* 2007; 137:2093-7

[201]   Dimopoulos N, Piperi C, Salonicioti A, Psarra V, Gazi F, Nounopoulos C, Lea RW,Kalofoutis A. Association of cognitive impairment with plasma levels of folate, vitamin B12 and homocysteine in the elderly. *In Vivo* 2006; 20:895-9.

[202]   Feng L, Ng TP, Chuah L, Niti M, Kua EH. Homocysteine, folate, and vitamin B-12 and cognitive performance in older Chinese. *Am J Clin Nutr.* 2006; 84:1506-12.

[203]   Haan MN, Miller JW, Aiello AE, Whitmer RA, Jagust WJ, Mungas DM, Allen LH, Green R. Homocysteine, B vitamins, and the incidence of dementia and cognitive impairment:results from the Sacramento Area Latino Study on Aging. *Am J Clin Nutr.* 2007; 85:511-7.

[204]   McMahon JA, Green TJ, Skeaff CM, Knight RG, Mann JI, Williams SM. A controlled trial of homocysteine lowering and cognitive performance. *N Engl J Med.* 2006; 29;354:2764-72.

[205]   Martin DC, Francis J, Protetch J, Huff FJ. Time dependency of cognitive recovery with cobalamin replacement: report of a pilot study. *J Am Geriatr Soc.* 1992 Feb; 40(2):168-72

[206]   Clark R,Smith AD,Jobst KA,et al.Folate ,vitamin B12 and serum total homocysteine levels in confirmed Alzheimer`s disease. *Arch Neurol* 1998; 55:1449-55

[207]   207.Tabet N,Rafi H,Weaving G,Lyons B,Iversen SA.Behavioral and psychological symptoms of Alzheimer type dementia are not correlated with plasma homocysteine concentration.*Dement Geriatr Cogn Disord.*2006;22:432-8

[208]   208.Lindenbaum J, Healton EB, Savage DG, Brust JC, Garrett TJ, Podell ER, Marcell PD,Stabler SP, Allen RH. Neuropsychiatric disorders caused by cobalamin deficiency in the absence ofanemia or macrocytosis. *N Engl J Med.* 1988; 318:1720-8.

[209]   209.Praticò D, Rokach J, Lawson J, FitzGerald GA. F2-isoprostanes as indices of lipid peroxidation in inflammatory diseases. *Chem Phys Lipids.* 2004 Mar; 128(1-2):165-71.

[210]   210.Montine TJ, Quinn JF, Milatovic D, Silbert LC, Dang T, Sanchez S, Terry E,Roberts LJ 2nd, Kaye JA, Morrow Peripheral F2-isoprostanes and F4-

neuroprostanes are not increased in Alzheimer's disease.JD.*Ann Neurol*. 2002 Aug;52(2):175-9.

[211]   211. Bohnstedt KC, Karlberg B, Wahlund LO, Jönhagen ME, Basun H, Schmidt S. Determination of isoprostanes in urine samples from Alzheimer patients using porous graphitic carbon liquid chromatography-tandem mass spectrometry. *J Chromatogr B Analyt Technol Biomed Life Sci*. 2003 Oct 25; 796(1):11-9.

[212]   212. Montine TJ, Neely MD, Quinn JF, Beal MF, Markesbery WR, Roberts LJ, Morrow JD. Lipid peroxidation in aging brain and Alzheimer's disease. *Free Radic Biol Med*. 2002 Sep 1; 33(5):620-6.

[213]   213.Montine TJ, Markesbery WR, Zackert W, Sanchez SC, Roberts LJ 2nd, Morrow JD. The magnitude of brain lipid peroxidation correlates with the extent of degeneration but not with density of neuritic plaques or neurofibrillary tangles or with APOE genotype in Alzheimer's disease patients. *Am J Pathol*. 1999 Sep; 155(3):863-8.

[214]   214. Praticò D, Yao Y, Rokach J, Mayo M, Silverberg GG, McGuire D J Reduction of brain lipid peroxidation by CSF drainage in Alzheimer's disease patients. *Alzheimers Dis*. 2004 Aug; 6(4):385-9; discussion 443-9.

[215]   215. Markesbery WR, Kryscio RJ, Lovell MA, Morrow JD. Lipid peroxidation is an early event in the brain in amnestic mild cognitive impairment. *Ann Neurol*. 2005 Nov; 58(5):730-5.

[216]   216. Han X, M Holtzman D, McKeel DW Jr, Kelley J, Morris JC.Substantial sulfatide deficiency and ceramide elevation in very early Alzheimer's disease: potential role in disease pathogenesis.*J Neurochem*. 2002 Aug; 82(4):809-18.

[217]   217.Gottfries CG, Karlsson I, Svennerholm L. Membrane components separate early-onset Alzheimer's disease from senile dementia of the Alzheimer type.*Int Psychogeriatr*. 1996 Fall;8(3):365-72.

[218]   Han X, Fagan AM, Cheng H, Morris JC, Xiong C, Holtzman DM. Cerebrospinal fluid sulfatide is decreased in subjects with incipient dementia. *Ann Neurol*. 2003 Jul; 54(1):115-9.

[219]   Fredman P, Wallin A, Blennow K, Davidsson P, Gottfries CG, Svennerholm L.Sulfatide as a biochemical marker in cerebrospinal fluid of patients with vascular dementia.*Acta Neurol Scand*. 1992 Feb;85(2):103-6.

[220]   Han X. Potential mechanisms contributing to sulfatide depletion at the earliest clinically recognizable stage of Alzheimer's disease: a tale of shotgun lipidomics. *J Neurochem*. 2007 Nov; 103 Suppl 1:171-9.

[221]   Zeng Y, Cheng H, Jiang X, Han X. Endosomes and lysosomes play distinct roles in sulfatide-induced neuroblastoma apoptosis: Potential mechanisms contributing to abnormal sulfatide metabolism in related neuronal diseases. *Biochem J*. 2007 Oct 17 [Epub ahead of print]

[222]   Gualdi GF, Colaiacomo MC, Bertini L, Melone A, Rojas M, Di Biasi C . Neuroimaging of Alzheimer disease: current role and future potential. *Clin Ter*. 2004 Oct; 155(10):429-38

[223]   Bozzali M, Cherubini A. Diffusion tensor MRI to investigate dementias: a brief review. Magn Reson Imaging. 2007 Jul; 25(6):969-77. *Epub* 2007 702Apr 23.

[224] Jose C. Masdeua,d,*, Jose L. Zubietab, Javier Arbizuc. Neuroimaging as a marker of the onset and progression of Alzheimer's disease *Journal of the Neurological Sciences* 236 (2005) 55 – 64.

[225] Chertkow H, Black S. Imaging biomarkers and their role in dementia clinical trials. *Can J Neurol Sci.* 2007 Mar; 34 Suppl 1:S77-83.

[226] Mikko Laakso MRI of Hippocampus In Incipient Alzheimer's Disease. *Neurologian klinikan julkaisusarja*, No 37, 1996 Series of Reports, Department of Neurology

[227] LeMay M, Stafford JL, Sandor T, Albert M, Haykal H, Zamani A. Statistical assessment of perceptual CT scan ratings in patients with Alzheimer type dementia. *J Comput Assist Tomography* 1986; 10:802-809.

[228] Nagata K, Basugi N, Fukushima T, Tango T, Suzuki I, Kaminuma T, Kurashina S. A quantitative study of physiological cerebral atrophy with aging: a statistical analysis of the normal range. *Neuroradiology* 1987; 29:327-332

[229] Drayer BP. Imaging of the aging brain, part I. Normal findings. *Radiology* 1988; 166:785-796.

[230] Drayer BP. Imaging of the aging brain, part II. Pathologic conditions. *Radiology* 1988; 166:797-806.

[231] DeCarli C, Kaye JA, Horwitz B, Rapoport SI. Critical analysis of the use of computer assisted transverse axial tomography to study human brain in aging and dementia of the Alzheimer type. *Neurology* 1990; 40:872-883

[232] DeCarli C, Haxby JV, Gillette JA, Teichberg D, Rapoport SI, Schapiro MB. Longitudinal changes in lateral ventricular volume in patients with dementia of the Alzheimer type. *Neurology* 1992; 42:2029-2036

[233] Shear PK, Sullivan EV, Mathalom DH, Lim KO, Davis LF, Yesavage JA, Tinklenberg JR, Pfefferbaum A. Longitudinal volumetric computed tomograpgic analysis of regional brain changes in normal aging and Alzheimer's disease. *Arch Neurol* 1995; 52:392-402

[234] Autti T, Raininko R, Vanhanen SL, Kallio M, Santavuori P. MRI of the normal brain from early childhood to middle age. I. Appearances on T2- and proton density-weighted images and occurrence of incidental high-signal foci. Neuroradiology 1994;36:644-648

[235] Fazekas Fazekas F, Chawlug JB, Alavi A, Hurtig HI, Zimmerman RA. MR signal abnormalities at 1.5 T in Alzheimer's dementia and normal aging. AJR 1987;149:351-356

[236] W. E. Kozachuk, C. DeCarli, M. B. Schapiro, E. E. Wagner, S. I. Rapoport and B. Horwitz. White matter hyperintensities in dementia of Alzheimer's type and in healthy subjects without cerebrovascular risk factors. A magnetic resonance imaging study. Vol. 47 No. 12, December 1990

[237] Leys D, Soetaert G, Petit H, Fauquette A, Pruvo J-P, Steinling M. Periventricular and white matter magnetic resonance imaging hyperintensities do not differ between Alzheimer's disease and normal aging. Arch Neurol 1990; 47:524-527

[238] Harrel LE, Duvall E, Folks DG, Duke L, Bartolucci A, Conboy T, Callaway R, Kerns D. The relationship of high intensity signals on magnetic resonance images to cognitive and psychiatric state in Alzheimer's disease. Arch Neurol 1991;48:1136-1140

[239] Kumar A, Yousem D, Soulder E, Miller D, Gottlieb G, Gur R, Alavi A. High-intensity signals in Alzheimer's disease without cerebrovascular risk factors: a magnetic resonance imaging evaluation. Am J Psychiatry 1992; 149:248-250

[240] Yetkin FZ, Haughton VM, Fischer ME, Papke RA, Daniels DL, Mark LP, Hendrix LE, Asleson RJ, Johansen J. High signal foci on MR images of the brain: observer variability in their quantification. AJR 1992;159:185-188

[241] Erkinjuntti T, Fuqiang G, Lee DH, Eliasziw M, Merskey H, Hachinski VC. Lack of difference in brain hyperintensities between patients with early Alzheimer's disease and control subjects. Arch Neurol 1994; 51:260-268

[242] Wahlund L-O, Basun H, Almkvist O, Andersson-Lundman G, Julin P, Sääf J. White matter hyperintensities in dementia: does it matter? Magn Reson Imaging 1994;12:387-394

[243] Davis PC, Gray L, Albert M, Wilkinson W, Hughes J, Heyman A, Gado M, Kumar AJ, Destian S, Lee C, Duvall E, Kido D, Nelson MJ, Bello J, Weathers S, Jolesz F, Kikinis R, Brooks M. The Concortium to Establish a Registry for Alzheimer's Disease (CERAD). Part III. Reliability of standardized MRI evaluation of Alzheimer's disease. Neurology 1992; 42:1676-1680

[244] Kantarci K. Magnetic resonance markers for early diagnosis and progression of Alzheimer's disease. Expert Rev Neurother. 2005 Sep;5(5):663-70.

[245] Lehéricy S, Marjanska M, Mesrob L, Sarazin M, Kinkingnehun S. Magnetic resonance imaging of Alzheimer's disease. Eur Radiol. 2007 Feb; 17(2):347-62. Epub 2006 Jul 25.

[246] Lehéricy S, Delmaire C, Galanaud D, Dormont D. Neuroimaging in dementia. Presse Med. 2007 Oct;36(10 Pt 2):1453-63. Epub 2007 Jul 3.

[247] Henry-Feugeas MC.J Neuroradiol. 2007 Oct;34(4):220-7. Epub 2007 Aug 24.

[248] 248.   Scheltens P, Korf ES. Contribution of neuroimaging in the diagnosis of Alzheimer's disease and other dementias. Curr Opin Neurol. 2000 Aug; 13(4):391-6.

[249] de Leon MJ, DeSanti S, Zinkowski R, Mehta PD, Pratico D, Segal S, Clark C, Kerkman D, DeBernardis J, Li J, Lair L, Reisberg B, Tsui W, Rusinek H.

[250] Jenkins R, Fox NC, Rossor MN. MRI and CSF studies in the early diagnosis of Alzheimer's disease.Registration of serial MRI scans in Alzheimer's disease: sensitivity and specificity of rates of atrophy. J Intern Med. 2004 Sep;256(3):205-23.Neurobiol Aging. 2000; 21(suppl 1):S39. Abstract 176.

[251] Rombouts SARB, Barkhof F, Witter MP, et al. Unbiased detection of atrophy in mild to moderate Alzheimer's disease. Neurobiol Aging. 2000; 21(suppl 1):S106. Abstract 479.

[252] Horínek D, Varjassyová A, Hort J. Magnetic resonance analysis of amygdalar volume in Alzheimer's disease. Curr Opin Psychiatry. 2007 May; 20(3):273-7.

[253] 253.   Dickerson BC. Functional MRI in the early detection of dementias. Rev Neurol (Paris). 2006 Oct; 162(10):941-4.

[254] Sperling R. Functional MRI studies of associative encoding in normal aging, mild cognitive impairment, and Alzheimer's disease.Ann N Y Acad Sci. 2007 Feb;1097:146-55.

[255] Felber SR. Magnetic resonance in the differential diagnosis of dementia. J Neural Transm. 2002 Jul; 109(7-8):1045-51.

[256] Gray KF, Cummings L chapter 21. Neurimaging in dementia. Localization and neuroimaging in neuropsychology edited by Andrew Kertesz

[257] Positron emission tomography diagnosis of Alzheimer's disease.*Neuroimaging Clin N Am*. 2005 Nov; 15(4):837-46,

[258] Mosconi L. Brain glucose metabolism in the early and specific diagnosis of Alzheimer's disease. FDG-PET studies in MCI and AD.*Eur J Nucl Med Mol Imaging*. 2005 Apr;32(4):486-510.

[259] Demetriades AK. Functional neuroimaging in Alzheimer's type Dementia.*J Neurol Sci*. 2002 Nov 15; 203-204:247-51.

[260] Masdeu J. Neuroimaging in Alzheimer's disease: an overview *Rev Neurol*. 2004 Jun 16-30; 38(12):1156-65.

[261] Klunk WE, Engler H, Nordberg A, Wang Y, Blomqvist G, Holt DP, et al. Imaging brain amyloid in Alzheimer's disease with Pittsburgh Compound-B. Amyloid deposition was detected. *Ann Neurol* 2004; 55:306–19.

[262] Brun A, Englund E. Brain changes in dementia of Alzheimer's type relevant to new imaging diagnostic methods. *Prog NeuropsychopharmacolBiol Psychiatry* 86;10:297–308.

[263] Cagnin A, Brooks DJ, Kennedy AM, Gunn RN, Myers R, TurkheimerFE, et al. In-vivo measurement of activated microglia in dementia.*Lancet* 2001;358:461–7.

[264] Kuhl DE, Koeppe RA, Minoshima S, Snyder SE, Ficaro EP, Foster NL, et al. In vivo mapping of cerebral acetylcholinesterase activity in aging and Alzheimer's disease. *Neurology* 1999;52:691–9.

[265] Shinotoh H, Namba H, Fukushi K, Nagatsuka S, Tanaka N, Aotsuka A, et al. Progressive loss of cortical acetylcholinesterase activity in association with cognitive decline in Alzheimer's disease: a positron emission tomography study. *Ann Neurol* 2000;48:194–200.

[266] Tanaka N, Fukushi K, Shinotoh H, Nagatsuka S, Namba H, Iyo M, etal. Positron emission tomographic measurement of brain acetylcholinesteraseactivity using N-[(11)C]methylpiperidin-4-yl acetate without arterial blood sampling: methodology of shape analysis and its diagnostic power for Alzheimer's disease. *J Cereb Blood Flow Metab* 2001;21:295–306.

[267] Herholz K, Weisenbach S, Zundorf G, Lenz O, Schroder H, Bauer B, et al. In vivo study of acetylcholine esterase in basal forebrain,amygdala, and cortex in mild to moderate Alzheimer disease. *Neuroimage* 2004;21:136–43.

[268] Kuhl DE, Minoshima S, Frey KA, Foster NL, Kilbourn MR, Koeppe RA. Limited donepezil inhibition of acetylcholinesterase measured with positron emission tomography in living Alzheimer cerebral cortex. *Ann Neurol* 2000; 48:391–5.

[269] Shinotoh H, Aotsuka A, Fukushi K, Nagatsuka S, Tanaka N, Ota T, et al. Effect of donepezil on brain acetylcholinesterase activity in patientswith AD measured by PET. *Neurology* 2001;56:408–10.

[270] Shinotoh H, Namba H, Fukushi K, Nagatsuka S, Tanaka N, Aotsuka A, et al. Progressive loss of cortical acetylcholinesterase activity in association with cognitive decline in Alzheimer's disease: a positron emission tomography study. *Ann Neurol* 2000; 48:194–200.

[271] Tanaka N, Fukushi K, Shinotoh H, Nagatsuka S, Namba H, Iyo M, et al. Positron emission tomographic measurement of brain acetylcholinesterase activity using N-

[(11)C]methylpiperidin-4-yl acetate without arterial blood sampling: methodology of shape analysis and its diagnostic power for Alzheimer's disease. *J Cereb Blood Flow Metab* 2001;21:295–306.

[272]   Bozzali M, Cherubini A. Diffusion tensor MRI to investigate dementias: a brief review. *Magn Reson Imaging.* 2007 Jul;25(6):969-77. Epub 2007 Apr 23.

[273]   Hammoud DA, Hoffman JM, Pomper MG. Molecular neuroimaging: from conventional to emerging techniques.*Radiology.* 2007 Oct;245(1):21.

[274]   Chetelat G, Baron JC. Early diagnosis of Alzheimer's disease: contribution of structural neuroimaging. *Neuroimage.* 2003 Feb;18(2):525-41.

[275]   Mosconi L. Brain glucose metabolism in the early and specific diagnosis of Alzheimer's disease. FDG-PET studies in MCI and AD. *Eur J Nucl Med Mol Imaging.* 2005 Apr;32(4):486-510.

[276]   J. Masdeu, J. Zubieta, J. Arbizu. Neuroimaging as a marker of the onset and progression of Alzheimer's disease. *Journal of the Neurological Sciences,* Volume 236, Issue 1-2, 55-64

[277]   Scheltens P, Korf ES. Contribution of neuroimaging in the diagnosis of Alzheimer's disease and other dementias *Curr Opin Neurol.* 2000 Aug;13(4):391-6.

[278]   de Leon MJ, Mosconi L, Blennow K, DeSanti S, Zinkowski R, Mehta PD, Pratico D, Tsui W, Saint Louis LA, Sobanska L, Brys M, Li Y, Rich K, Rinne J, Rusinek H. Imaging and CSF studies in the preclinical diagnosis of Alzheimer's disease.*Ann N Y Acad Sci.* 2007 Feb;1097:114-45.

[279]   www.alzforum.org/res/enab/workshops/biomarkers.asp

In: Alzheimer's Disease in the Middle-Aged
Editor: Hyun Sil Jeong, pp. 315-323

ISBN: 978-1-60456-480-8
© 2008 Nova Science Publishers, Inc.

Chapter 13

EVALUATION OF THE PROGRESSION OF EARLY-ONSET ALZHEIMER DISEASE BY USING DIFFUSION TENSOR IMAGING

Chen Shaoqiong, He Bingjun and Kang Zhuang

Zhang, jiansheng; Department of Radiology, the Third Affiliated Hospital,
Sun Yat-Sen University, Guangzhou 510630, P.R.China
Hu, Xiquan; Department of Rehabilitation, the Third Affiliated Hospital,
Sun Yat-Sen University, Guangzhou 510630, P.R.China

BACKGROUND

Early-onset dementia (EOD) refers to those patients with dementia onset before the age of 65 years. In most, but not all, studies the most frequent EOD of AD accounts for 20–34% of the patients, Despite a plurality of AD, the proportion of EOD patients with AD is far less than for late-onset dementia (LOD). AD accounts for about two thirds of all dementias for LOD, but only about one third of all patients with an early age of onset. [1]

In China, there is no detailed data about the frequency of early-onset AD. The patients were very rare in clinical activity. We followed up a patient with early-onset AD for twenty-two months, and used diffusion tensor imaging (DTI) to study the brain of the patient to assess the progression of the disease.

Diffusion tensor imaging (DTI) is a magnetic resonance imaging (MRI) technique that can be used to characterize the orientational properties of the diffusion process of water molecules [2]. Application of this technique to the brain has been demonstrated to provide exceptional information on white matter architecture. Usually, the information is conveyed into two types of parameters: mean diffusivity (D) which is a measure of the average molecular motion independent of any tissue directionality and is affected by cellular size and integrity [3,4], and the fractional anisotropy (FA), which is one of the most used measures of deviation from isotropy and reflects the degree of alignment of cellular structures within fiber tracts, as well as their structural integrity [5]. There are no articles available about using DTI in a longitudinal study of AD. We investigated the dynamic change of the D value and FA value in the brain of this patient.

MATERIALS AND METHODS

The patient and her husband gave their informed consent prior to their inclusion in this study. The patient, a 53-year-old female with primary school education, was a kitchener before retiring.

The National Institute of Neurological and Communicative Disorders and Stroke/Alzheimer's Disease and Related Disorders Association (NINCDS/ADRDA) criteria were used for the diagnosis of clinically probable AD. Major systemic, psychiatric, and other neurological illnesses were carefully investigated and excluded in this patient.

NEUROPSYCHOLOGICAL TESTS

Mini-mental state examination (MMSE), activities of daily living (ADL), and Barthel Index (BI) were used to assess cognitive function for the patient. The MMSE score of the patient was 3 and the ADL score was 90 in the first examination during the patient's first hospitalization. Twenty-two months later, the MMSE score of the patient was 2 and the ADL score was 75.

MRI ACQUISITION

MRI was obtained by using a 1.5-T Vision MRI system (GE Signa Twinspeed, USA). A standard (8HRBRAIN) head coil was used. Prior to DTI, all subjects underwent T2 FLAIR (fluid-attenuated inversion recovery) sequence: repetition time (*TR*) 8802 ms, echo time (*TE*) 120 ms, matrix 512×512, field of view (FOV) 240 mm, 5 mm thickness, and 1 mm gap. DTI data were acquired by using a single-shot, diffusion weighted echo-planar imaging sequence (*TR*=8000 ms, *TE*=80 ms). The imaging matrix was 128×128, with a field of view of 246 mm×246 mm. Transverse sections of 3-mm thickness were acquired parallel to the anterior commissure-posterior commissure line. Coronal sections were angulated, perpendicular to the anterior commissure-posterior commissure line. Scan sections covered the entire hemisphere and brainstem without gaps. Diffusion weighting was encoded along 25 independent orientations, and the *b* value was 1000 s/mm^2. The acquisition time per dataset was approximately 9 minutes.

The DTI datasets were transferred to a workstation and processed using functool LX software. *D* and *FA* were measured in different regions which were carefully selected on the dual echo scans to avoid partial volume averaging from the CSF (cerebrospinal fluid). Regions of interest (ROIs) were range 20~60 mm^2. The following areas were measured bilaterally: the anterior, middle and posterior cingulate gyrus; hippocampus, parahippocampal gyrus and amygdale; lentiform nucleus; caudate nucleus; dorsal medial thalamus and middle cerebellar peduncle (figure.1a~1c).

The area of the body of bilateral lateral cerebral ventricle was measured on the T2 FLAIR image.(figure.2)

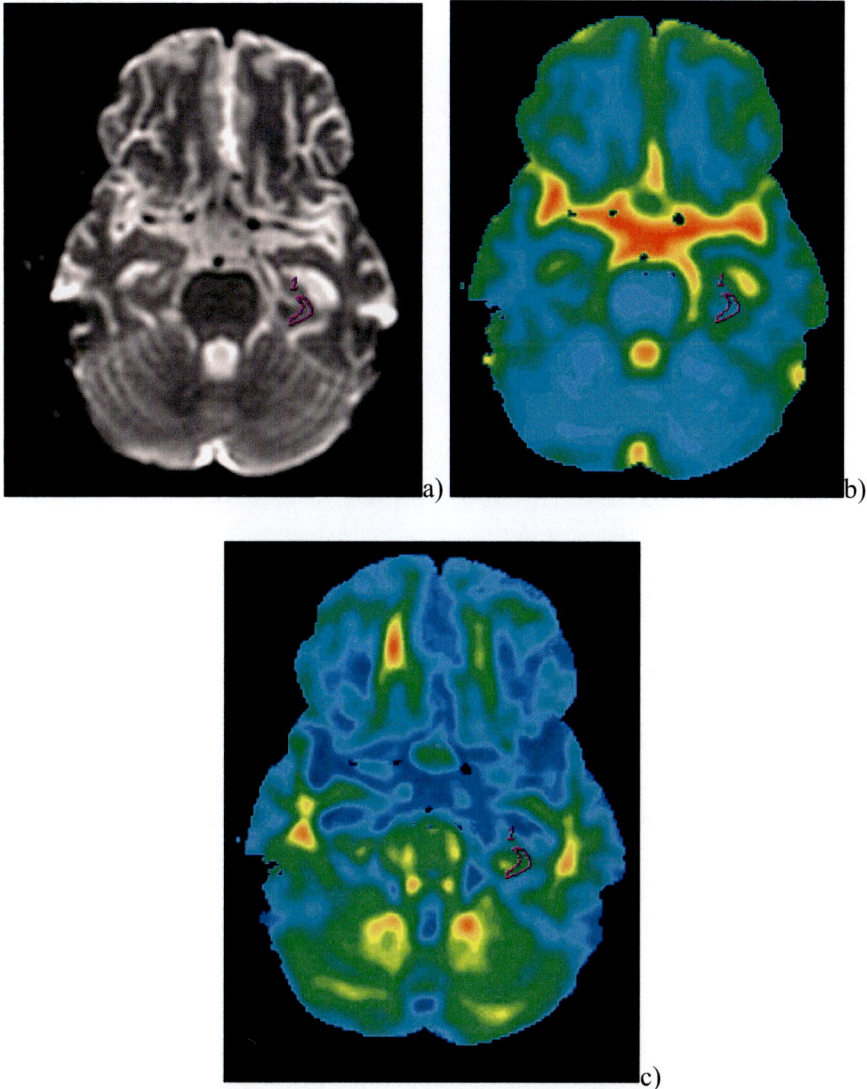

Figure 1. b=0 s/mm2 image from the echo planar imaging (EPI) sequence for DTI (a), apparent diffusion coefficient (ADC) (b) and FA images (c).ROIs for measurement of D and FA indices: 1=hippocampus.

RESULTS

The patient's brain showed no abnormal signal but atrophy of the whole brain on T2 FLAIR image. The area of the body of bilateral lateral cerebral ventricle apparently increased during 22 months' follow-up (table1). The ventricular dilatation was more apparent on the left side than that on the right side. The rate of change was 24.4% on the left side and 19.9 on the right side.

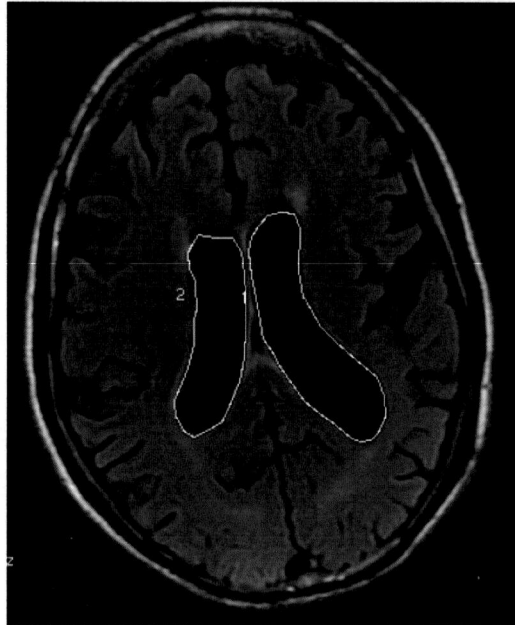

Figure 2. Measure the areas of the body of bilateral lateral cerebral ventricle from the patient.

Table 1. Area (mm^2) of the body of bilateral lateral cerebral ventricle from the patient

Date	2005/11/2	2007/9/10
Left side	1347	1676
Right side	1029	1234

Note: Left side: left lateral cerebral ventricle. Right side:right lateral cerebral ventricle.

During the 22 months, D value apparently increased in bilateral anterior, middle and posterior cingulate gyrus; hippocampus, parahippocampal gyrus; amygdale; caudate nucleus; dorsal medial thalamus. The structures with the most discriminating power were right hippocampus, right posterior cingulate gyrus, left middle cingulate gyrus, right middle cingulate gyrus, left amygdale, left posterior cingulate gyrus, left hippocampus, left parahippocampal gyrus. However, there was little increase in D value in bilateral middle cerebellar peduncle and lentiform nucleus (table2 and figure 3).

FA value apparently decreased in the some structures except left caudate nucleus, bilateral lentiform nucleus, bilateral middle cingulate gyrus and bilateral middle cerebellar peduncle. The structures with the most discriminating power were left hippocampus, right hippocampus, right posterior cingulate gyrus, left posterior cingulate gyrus, left parahippocampal gyrus, left anterior cingulate gyrus. However, FA value was elevated in bilateral lentiform nucleus and middle cingulate gyrus, and didn't change much in left caudate nucleus and bilateral middle cerebellar peduncle (table2 and figure 4).

Table 2. Mean (*SD*) *D* values and FA value of the selected areas from the patient

Date	D value		FA value	
	2005/11/2	2007/9/10	2005/11/2	2007/9/10
Lefe Hippocampus	8.31	11.8	0.295	0.104
Right Hippocampus	7.88	12.6	0.295	0.118
Left amygdale	7.82	11.3	0.145	0.0859
Right amygdale	7.85	8.88	0.155	0.119
Left parahippocampal gyrus	8.30	11.3	0.347	0.197
Right parahippocampal gyrus	9.97	10.4	0.265	0.244
Left caudate nucleus	6.87	8.60	0.191	0.195
Right caudate nucleus	7.05	9.16	0.208	0.186
Left lentiform nucleus	6.42	7.36	0.170	0.198
Right lentiform nucleus	6.38	7.40	0.147	0.217
Left dorsal medial thalamus	7.05	8.12	0.232	0.230
Right dorsal medial thalamus	6.64	7.90	0.269	0.242
Left anterior cingulate gyrus	7.37	9.25	0.419	0.275
Right anterior cingulate gyrus	6.95	8.39	0.384	0.285
Left middle cingulate gyrus	6.61	9.78	0.476	0.586
Right middle cingulate gyrus	6.37	9.40	0.548	0.650
Left posterior cingulate gyrus	8.43	12.0	0.319	0.171
Right posterior cingulate gyrus	6.89	10.7	0.349	0.151
Left middle cerebellar peduncle	5.86	6.61	0.632	0.644
Right middle cerebellar peduncle	5.77	6.49	0.607	0.658

D, mean diffusivity, expressed in units of $m^2 s^{-1} \times 10^{-10}$. FA, fractional anisotropy.

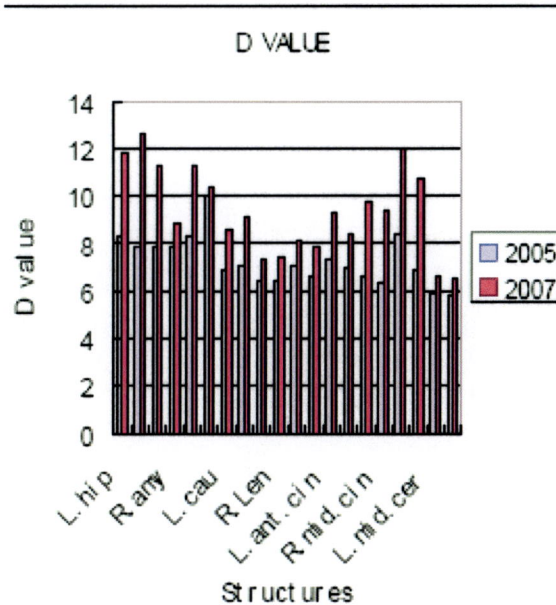

Figure 3.

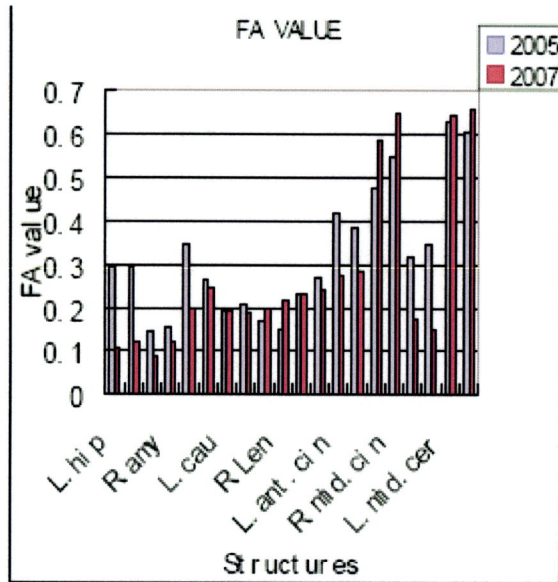

Figure 4.

DISCUSSION

A prior study on lateral ventricle expansion showed that annualized expansion rates in normal young people (age 22-55 years) were 4.8% on the left side and 4.15 on the right side [6]. Our data showed the apparent dynamic change rates in this early-onset AD patient.

The ventricular dilated at a relatively fast rate on the left side. This might be due to the relatively apparent atrophy in the left hemisphere which involves language ability that induced the decline of the MMSE score.

This feature is consistent with prior studies of late-onset AD patients that showed the greatest dynamic change rates were found in the inferior ventricular horns which expanded at a striking rate (L: +18.1% +/- 3.8% per year; R: +12.8% +/- 4.7% per year), significantly more rapidly than in controls (P < 0.0005). Annualized expansion rates correlated with rates of cognitive decline, as measured by MMSE scores (L: P < 0.017, R: P < 0.029); those with faster ventricular expansion declined faster. Larger temporal horn volume at the baseline was also associated with a larger annualized percent change in temporal horn volume (L: P < 0.03; R: P < 0.0001) [7].

In comparison with the prior studies, we found a faster brain atrophy rate in this early-onset AD patient than that of late-onset AD patients.

Previous studies including our prior data have showed that there were higher D values in the hippocampi, the temporal stem, the cingulum, the corpus callosum, the centrum semiovale, and the frontal, temperal, occipital and parietal white matter of AD patients than in controls [8].There were lower FA values in the hippocampus, the corpus callosum, the cingulum, the white matter of the frontal, temporal and parietal lobes of AD patients than in controls [8].

There were no articles available about using DTI in a longitudinal study of AD. Our data demonstrated there was a striking rate of change in the D value and FA values in the limbic system. A prior study found there was no change in D value or FA value in health control (age 25-68 years) during a 15-month follow-up [9]. The dynamic elevated D value in our AD patient meant the increase of the mean diffusivity of water molecules of the structures, and the reduced FA value indicated disturbed integrity of white matter tracts in this region. The explanation for these results might be related to pathological damage in the brain. Pathological changes of AD originate in the medial temporal region, in the entorhinal cortex and hippocampus, subsequently spreading over the entire limbic cortex and then into neocortical association areas [10]. Damage is believed to occur due to mechanisms outside the neuron, as well as inside the neuron, and is characterized by the appearance of extracellular senile (amyloid) plaques and intracellular neurofibrillary tangles. The large plaques that form then damage brain cells and attract reactive cells, microglia and astrocytes, which cause further damage. From inside the cell, tau proteins, which normally stabilize microtubules in brain cells, undergo abnormal chemical changes and assemble into spirals called paired helical filaments, thus creating tangles that disrupt cell functions and lead to cell death [11]. Neuron death and reactive cell accumulation might be expected to enlarge the extracellular spaces, and also the anterograde degeneration of the neurofibril with disruption of myelin and axons might be expected to increase the mean diffusivity of water molecules. A reduced FA value might be due to the breakdown of the myelin sheath and disintegration of axonal microfilaments which damage the structural integrity of fiber tracts, and also due to accumulation of extracellular senile (amyloid) plaques and intracellular neurofibrillary tangles which disrupt the isotropy and alignment of cellular structures within fiber tracts. Thus, DTI would be sensitive to the detection of changes of the degenerative aspects of early-onset AD pathology. The most discriminating measures pertain to hippocampus, cingulate gyrus, amygdale and parahippocampal gyrus. These results further confirmed that these regions were the most damageable structures in AD progression. Furthermore, the greatest change rate of the FA value was 64.7% in the left hippocampus, and that of the D value was 59% in the right hippocampus which were much higher than the atrophy rate(24.4 and 19.9%), thus DTI was much more sensitive to detection of the progression of the disease than that of structure measure as atrophy rate.

However there was less change in the D value and FA values in the middle cerebellar peduncle which involves the extrapyramidal system. The result might explain the lack of extrapyramidal signs in this patient. Researchers found that extrapyramidal signs (EPSs) at initial assessment are associated with the presence of Lewy bodies (LBs), and EPSs and LBs are independently associated with shorter survival. Furthermore, the presence of EPSs and LBs in the same individual is associated with a poorer survival rate than either finding alone [12].

Change in the FA value in bilateral lentiform nucleus and middle cingulate gyrus differed from that of other structures involving AD pathology. Lentiform nucleus usually involving the extrapyramidal system might be less damaged in AD pathology. A lot of studies showed that anterior cingulate gyrus and posterior cingulate gyrus involve cognitive function [13, 14]. However, middle cingulate gyrus was less mentioned in prior reports about brain function. Might it be involved in more complicated functions or remain relatively still in cognitive activity? Might it be less involved in AD pathology? Another consideration was that change of FA value had proved to be not always consistent with age-related cognitive change [15]. Further research needs to be done to clear up these problems.

CONCLUSION

Dynamic expansion of lateral ventricle in early-onset AD is more rapid than in late-onset AD. Dynamic increase of the D value and decline of the FA value in the limbic system of the patient supported that DTI was much more sensitive to the detection of the progression of AD than that of structure measure as atrophy rate in early-onset AD patient.

REFERENCES

[1]   McMurtray A, Clark DG, Christine D, Mendez MF(2006). Early-onset dementia: frequency and causes compared to late-onset dementia. *Dement Geriatr. Cogn. Disord*, 21(2), 59-64.

[2]   Basser, P.J., Mattiello, J., Le Bihan, D (1994a). MR diffusion tensor spectroscopy and imaging. *Biophys. J.*, 66(1),259-267.

[3]   Basser, P.J., Mattiello, J., Le Bihan, D (1994b). Estimation of the effective self-diffusion tensor from the NMR spin-echo. *J. Magn. Reson.* B, 103(3),247-254.

[4]   Pierpaoli, C., Jezzard, P., Basser, P.J., Blarnett, A., Di Chiro, G(1996). Diffusion tensor MR imaging of the human brain. *Radiology*, 201(3),637-648.

[5]   Basser, P.J., Pierpaoli, C(1996). Microstructural features measured using diffusion tensor imaging. *J. Magn. Reson.* B, 111(3),209-219.

[6]   Daniel H. Mathalon, PhD, MD; Edith V. Sullivan, PhD; Kelvin O. Lim, MD; Adolf Pfefferbaum, MD(2001). Progressive Brain Volume Changes and the Clinical Course of Schizophrenia in Men A Longitudinal Magnetic Resonance Imaging Study. *Arch Gen Psychiatry* ,58, 148-157.

[7]   Thompson PM, Hayashi KM, De Zubicaray GI, Janke AL, Rose SE, Semple J, Hong MS, Herman DH, Gravano D, Doddrell DM, Toga AW (2004). Mapping hippocampal and ventricular change in Alzheimer disease. Neuroimage, 22(4),1754-66.

[8]   CHEN S.Q, KANG Z, HU X.Q, HU B, ZOU Y (2007). Diffusion tensor imaging of the brain in patients with Alzheimer's disease and cerebrovascular lesions.*J. Zhejiang Univ Sci B*, 8(4),242–247.

[9]   Marco Rovaris, Antonio Gallo, Paola Valsasina, Beatrice Benedetti, Domenico Caputo, Angelo Ghezzi, Enrico Montanari, Maria Pia Sormani, Antonio Bertolotto, Gianluigi Mancardi, Roberto Bergamaschi, Vittorio Martinelli, Giancarlo Comi and Massimo Filippi (2005). Short-term accrual of gray matter pathology in patients with progressive multiple sclerosis: an in vivo study using diffusion tensor MRI. *NeuroImage*, 24(4), 1139-1146

[10] Braak, H., Braak, E (1998). Evolution of neuronal changes in the course of Alzheimer's disease. *J. Neural. Transm. Suppl*, 53,127-140.

[11] Jeffrey R. Petrella, MD, R. Edward Coleman, MD and P. Murali Doraiswamy, MD 2003.Neuroimaging and Early Diagnosis of Alzheimer Disease: A Look to the Future. *Radiology*, 226,315-336

[12] Mary N. Haan; William J. Jagust; Douglas Galasko; Jeffrey Kaye (2002). Effect of Extrapyramidal Signs and Lewy Bodies on Survival in Patients With Alzheimer Disease. *Arch Neurol*, 59,588 - 593

[13] Mulert C, Juckel G, Brunnmeier M, Leicht SK, Mergl R, Möller HJ, Hegerl U, Pogarell O (2007). Rostral anterior cingulate cortex activity in the theta band predicts response to antidepressive medication. *Clin EEG Neurosci*, 38(2), 78-81

[14] Wang L, Hosakere M, Trein JC, Miller A, Ratnanather JT, Barch DM, Thompson PA, Qiu A, Gado MH, Miller MI, Csernansky JG(2007). Abnormalities of cingulate gyrus neuroanatomy in schizophrenia. *Schizophr Res*, 93(1-3),66-78.

[15] David J. Madden, Julia Spaniol, Wythe L. Whiting, Barbara Bucur, James M. Provenzale, Roberto Cabeza, Leonard E. White, and Scott A. *Huette*l (2007).

[16] Adult age differences in the functional neuroanatomy of visual attention: A combined fMRI and DTI study, Neurobiol Aging, 28(3),459–476.

In: Alzheimer's Disease in the Middle-Aged
Editor: Hyun Sil Jeong, pp. 325-328

ISBN: 978-1-60456-480-8
© 2008 Nova Science Publishers, Inc.

Chapter 14

THE PSYCHOSOCIAL NEURAL SENSORIAL ALTERNATIVE ALZHEIMER´S THEORY

Luis María Sánchez de Machado[*]
Alzheimer´s; Project Argentina

The Chronic Progressive Dementization, (CPD), the scientific name of that vulgarly called Alzheimer, is a quite different question than depression, different types of psychosis and obviously of sometimes surprising behaviors of the normal aging, and in the long run much more serious.

Although the final phase of cerebral disintegration is similar, there are two types of processes: the one that occurs in young adults or greater adults, and another different one that it happens in very greater adults, around 80 years or more. In these, at the final phase the problem it is "*simply*" the loss of the vital motivation, the exhaustion of desire to continue living. Abandonment of dreams, as Miguel de Unamuno would say on the cession of such dreams that Don Quixote in favor of Sancho did, and then, obviously, dying.

Persons with risk for a CPD (Alzheimer) are those that generally have an introverted personality, few and restricted social relations, with and isolation tendency, coping deficit for difficulties and losses, tendency to depend on others, to had constructed their personal identity in the shade of another one (the woman of the doctor, the husband of…) or some other equivalent transference, tendency to be obstinate to proper painful events or of the other's life, which is diagnosed in general like depression.

Then, in any way it touches to anyone.

There is nothing of chance's dependence, neither suddenly nor no magician in it. Logically with advance into years the probability that these people suffer a painful loss increases, obviously, like everybody. With its coping deficit the risk increases enormously when they have a painful loss, for example her husband who gave or lent the personal identity, or a son or daughter who gave sense to their life, of their work that justified the existence to him, of their corporal and mental capacity to which he had bet or concentrated,

---

[*] TE 0054 3442 431442;stopalz@gmail.com; www.stopalz.org

and when not counting on a familiar network and a social network that stopped its fall after the duel impossible to elaborate and to go on, the person collapses.

It is the beginning of the aim. It can have 40 years old (the younger case than we have was a woman of 38 years), or 80 years old. It does not related to aging, but only that when they advance the years is more probable that we suffer painful losses. Until this moment its brain is totally normal, does not show absolutely anything abnormal and is totally useless to want to see something in images or less even in electroencephalograms, that it is something so coarse and inadequate as a toad arrives of a luxurious piano of tail.

The landslide of the person, its "delivery" as much in the dictionary of the Real Spanish Academy like in the original dictionaries of all the languages, is expressed in the idea to wish to die, in the fixation of the attention in its own one and wished death. Then the abnormal thing begins, the unnatural thing, the destructive thing, because in fact we are programmed biologically, ancestrally, for all the opposite, as it is to explore, to fight, to defend to us, to hunt (in the literal sense and the symbolic sense), to attack, to ask to us, to inquire to us, and our attention concentrated in each objective part of a basic alert status that we never lose, except for when we slept very well. We are not programmed to give to us tamely, as it is not it in any animal.

HOW TAKES PLACE THEN THE CEREBRAL DAMAGE THAT LEADS TO THE DEATH?

To understand this we need to explain some very basic things, although surprising little known. In the first place that we have nine senses: vision, hearing, equilibrium, tact, space perception/orientation, taste, sense of smell, sense of strange it (or familiarity sense) and of the corporal perception. All these senses, and perhaps others more, are active in the basic alert status and they have two components: an automatic one of immediate reaction (one falls in love a light and blinking, it smells hydrosulfuric vapors, the substance that is put to the gas tubes to detect a loss immediately, and I separate, etc.), and another component of recognition, in which the stimuli are sent to the brain and there it is collated if that information has been loaded. They are the sensorial recognition systems we have.

Then, everything what we do, everything what we thought, by more banal or insignificant than is, is recorded in the brain in form of neuronal network in which participate neurons of the sensorial recognition's systems of the nine channels, inexorably.

And those networks that are armed in our brain also were reinforced when we return to make the same act or the same thought.

But in addition because in fact all is connected with all, which we are going to do was connected in more or less straight forward form with which already we have done and loaded like neuronal networks in our brain.

Some of those connections have a great importance in the every day actions and others very remotely: although the door seems to be very heavy, already we know that the force that we must make to open it isn't so high. Or for example the natural attraction by rhythm that are multiple or sub multiple of the heart rate (that we listened for the first time in our mother's uterus), seems like related with this indeed. That is to say, to live means to be stimulating everything somehow what we have done, lived and thought. It seems exhausting, but it is a fascinating question.

However, when a person fix attention to death, that is something abstract that does not required any motor or cognitive reply, and resorting to the natural and available mechanism disposed in all persons they to block the reception of other stimuli when we concentrated the attention in something intensively attracted, these people happen to block, at the outset in oscillating form, with variations throughout a day or of days, the sensorial stimuli of the different channels. It is a biological basic mechanism since we must be concentrated in the tiger that attacks to us and we cannot disperse with the colored birds that are jumping back: it's a survival principle. Who know more the utility of this principle are the pickpockets of the human agglomerates: one of them produces a smaller but clear aggression on the victim. In reaction the victim is put in guard and concentrates its attention on the aggressor, while his companion removes the wallet or cuts the portfolio's strap, because we have blocked the tact and the corporal perception when putting to us in guard in front of the aggressor and concentrating the attention in him.

The displacement of the attention towards different objectives is a normal and a routinely task, but in the people who enter CPD process they are persistently blocking the reception of stimuli by the different sensorial channels and the consequent arrived to the brain, so that the neurons of the sensorial recognition systems that comprise of the sensorial networks doesn't receive stimuli, with which in the long run lose the synaptic connections and the networks are disarmed. Something equivalent to the atrophy of a muscle we never use. This avoid progressively all the recognition tasks. No longer they recognize, no longer have capacity of recovery of recent events (weak neuronal networks, with low sensorial stimulation), and however still can recover events of the past. But not anyone, but those in which the lived events (SENSORIAL NETWORKS ARMED IN THE PAST) were possible with a great stimulation (emotional), prolonged reinforced and connected with multiple other sensorial networks, like the door of our home at our childhood, by where we did not shelter, by where we shook to arrive all smeared, by where we arrived to eat, etc.

Thus, those faults of the sensorial recognition systems were the more consistent biological indicators to detect that a person is in a dementia of this type. Chemicals or physical parameters aren't the unique biological indicators

The progressive disintegration of the neuronal networks in our brain by stimulation deficit of the recognition sensorial systems is the essence of the dementization process, and leads to the death because an automatic essential system has connections with sensorial networks, that when also they get to be affected, causes the death.

Then isn't properly a disease *("signs and symptoms that responds to a well-known cause")*, isn't genetic, it doesn't have relation with aging (frequent confusion comes from that to greater age is the probability of suffering painful losses, that are a very frequent trigger one, since we have already said), does not begin with any damage in the brain but that concludes in the long run in this, isn't a problem of the memory but of the attention, and before this one of the desire, and before this one of the satisfaction search, and before this one of the biological and psychological impulsions arranged by the will, and even before the basal state of alert that characterizes to us. One of the last forms of the expression of the process is the problem with the memory, but in fact the difficulty to recover events is the last link of a very long chain, and to have concentrated in it and not in the attention's deficit of can be the reason of the delayed to understand the process, and the habitual confusion with several behaviors proper of aging.

And finally, isn't irreversible, since it is possible and it gives clear and forceful result, to elevate to those people the self-esteem and the attention to him, and to permute the abstract idea of wished death by the one of a real life that surrounds it, the shade by the light that surrounds us to all to little that we lend a little attention, taken care of and love, and inserting it in a new extolling routine for the dairy life. It is not easy, is an abyss of difference with giving a tablet, but it is tremendously positive as much for the affected ones as for which we worked with the protocols derived from the psycho-social neural sensorial disintegrative theory of the chronic progressive dementization.

FEW REFERENCES

Sanchez de Machado LM et al., *Rev. Neurol.* 2007; 44(4): 198-202.
Sanchez de Machado LM, I *J. World Health and Societal Politics* 2005, Vol. 2 (1)
Sanchez de Machado LM, *Rev. Esp. Geriatr. Gerontol.* 2004; 39(6):371-80.
Sanchez de Machado LM, *Geriatrianet* 2004, Vol. 6(1)

Chapter 15

EARLY ONSET DEMENTIA: ROLE OF GENETICS IN THE PATHOGENESIS OF ALZHEIMER'S DISEASE AND FRONTOTEMPORAL LOBAR DEGENERATION

Daniela Galimberti, Chiara Fenoglio and Elio Scarpini*

Department of Neurological Sciences, "Dino Ferrari" Center, University of Milan,
Fondazione Ospedale Maggiore Policlinico IRCCS, Via F. Sforza 35, 20122, Milan, Italy

ABSTRACT

Despite most cases of Alzheimer's disease (AD) are sporadic, about 3-5% are inherited in an autosomal dominant fashion, and are characterized by an early onset. It has become clear from phenotypic analyses of familial AD forms versus sporadic cases that these two forms are phenotypically highly similar and often indistinguishable, except for the earlier age at onset. Autosomal dominant forms are characterized by mutations in three genes: Amyloid β precursor protein (β-*APP*), Presenilin 1(*PSEN1*) and Presenilin 2 (*PSEN2*) genes. The mutations in Amyloid Precursor Protein (APP) occur at its cleavage sites, thus altering APP processing such that more pathogenetic Aβ42 peptide is produced. *PSEN1* and *PSEN2* represent a central component of γ-secretase, the enzyme responsible for liberating the C-terminal fragment of APP. Mutations in presenilins also alter APP, leading to an increased production of Aβ42. Another degenerative dementia with an onset about 50-60 years is Frontotemporal Lobar Degeneration (FTLD). In 1994 an autosomal dominantly inherited form of Frontotemporal Dementia (FTD) with parkinsonism was linked to chromosome 17q21.2. Subsequently, other familial forms of FTD were found to be linked to the same region, resulting in the denomination "frontotemporal dementia and parkinsonism linked to chromosome 17" (FTDP-17) for this class of diseases. All cases of FTDP-17 have so far shown a filamentous pathology made of hyperphosphorylated tau protein. Although many FTD families exhibit *MAPT* mutations, in some cases these mutations did not occur suggesting that other, related genes on chromosome 17 also cause FTD in an autosomal-dominant manner.

---

* Corresponding Author . Phone ++ 39.2.55033858; Fax ++ 39.2.50320430; E-mail: daniela.galimberti@ unimi.it

Subsequently, region within the 3.53 centimorgan critical region defined by haplotype analysis in reported families was examined. Several pathogenic mutations were therefore found in progranulin gene (*PGRN*), harbouring a new causative gene in FTLD pathology. *PGRN* is a widely expressed growth factor, which plays a role in multiple processes including development, wound repair and inflammation by activating signalling cascades that control cell cycle progression and cell motility. Its role in neurodegeneration is at present under investigation.

As regards sporadic forms, genetic factors play a role in determining the age at disease onset. The gene mainly related to the sporadic forms of AD is *APOE*, which is located in chromosome 19 and was initially identified in 1991 as a risk factor for AD. In addition, the *APOE 4/4* genotype seems to correlate with an earlier onset of the disease.

In this chapter, these genetic studies recently carried out will be described and discussed in detail.

1. ALZHEIMER'S DISEASE

Alzheimer's disease (AD), originally described by Alois Alzheimer and Gaetano Perusini in 1906, is clinically characterized by a progressive cognitive impairment, including impaired judgment, decision-making and orientation, often accompanied, in later stages, by psychobehavioural disturbances as well as language impairment. The two major neuropathologic hallmarks of AD are extracellular beta-amyloid (Aβ) plaques and intracellular neurofibrillary tangles (NFTs). The production of Aβ, which represents a crucial step in AD pathogenesis, is the result of cleavage of Amyloid precursor protein (APP), which is overexpressed in AD (Griffin, 2006). Aβ forms highly insoluble and proteolysis resistant fibrils known as "senile plaques".

Neurofibrillary tangles are composed of the tau protein. In healthy controls, tau is a component of microtubules, which are the internal support stuctures for the transport of nutrients, vesicles, mitochondria and chromosomes whithin the cell. Microtubules also stabilize the growing axons, which are necessary for the development and growth of neurites (Griffin, 2006). In AD, tau protein is abnormally hyperphosphorilated and forms insoluble fibrils, which originate deposits within the cell.

Despite AD is the most common cause of dementia in the elderly, with a prevalence of 5% after 65 years of age, a number of cases are characterized by an early-onset and by familiarity (EOFAD). It has been known for at least several decades that clinically typical AD can cluster in families and be inherited in an autosomal dominant fashion. Estimates of the prevalence of inherited forms of AD have varied widely from as little as 2-3% to as high as 30% or more. Despite the uncertainty about the degree to which AD is accounted for by genetic factors, it has become clear from phenotypic analyses of EOFAD versus apparently non-familial ("sporadic") cases (SAD) that these two forms are phenotypically highly similar and often indistinguishable, except for the earlier age at onset of the known autosomal dominant forms.

Autosomal dominant EOFAD forms are characterized by mutations in three genes: *β–APP* (Goate et al., 1991), *PSEN1* (Sherrington et al., 1995) and *PSEN2* (Levy Lahad et al., 1995) (Table 1).

In contrast to EOFAD, in SAD no causal genes have been identified to date, but there is a growing body of evidence suggesting that a large proportion of these cases are also significantly influenced by genetic factors. Risk genes are likely to be numerous, displaying intricate patterns of interaction with each other as well as with non-genetic variables, and-unlike classical Mendelian ("simplex") disorders- exhibit no simple mode of inheritance. Mainly due to this reason, the genetics of SAD has been labeled "complex" (Bertram and Tanzi, 2005). The gene mainly related to SAD is *APOE*, which is located in chromosome 19 and was initially identified in 1991 as a risk factor for AD. In addition, the *APOE* gene likely influence the age at onset of the disease.

1.1. EOFAD

In 1987, EOFAD linkage was reported on the long arm of chromosome 21, which encompassed a region harboring the *β–APP* gene, a compelling candidate for AD (Tanzi et al., 1987). The gene is located at chromosome 21q21.22 and encodes for a transmembrane protein that is normally processed into amyloid fragments. In 1991, the first missense mutation in APP was reported (Goate et al., 1991). Since then, 27 different mutations have been described in the *β–APP* gene in 75 families (http://molgen-www.uia.ac.be). All these mutations cause amino acid changes in putative sites for the cleavage of the protein, thus altering the APP processing, such that more pathological Aβ42 is produced (Hardy and Selkoe 2002). Interestingly, the chromosome 21, in which *β–APP* resides, is triplicated in Down syndrome and most of the cases manifest also AD by the age of 50. Post-mortem analyses of Down's patients who die young show diffuse intra-neuronal deposits of Aβ, suggesting that its deposition is an early event in cognitive decline. The recent discovery of an extra copy of the *β–APP* gene in FAD (Rovelet-Lecrux et al., 2006) provides further support that increased Aβ production can cause the disease.

Table 1. Causative genes of EOFAD

Gene (Protein)	Chromosomal location	Mode of inheritance	Relevance to AD pathogenesis
APP (β Amyloid Precursor Protein	21q21.3	Autosomal-dominant	Increase in Aβ (Aβ42/Aβ40 ratio; mutations close to γ-secretase site
PSEN1 (presenilin 1)	14q24.3	Autosomal-dominant	Increase in Aβ (Aβ42/Aβ40 ratio; essential for γ-secretase activity
PSEN2 (presenilin 2)	1q31-42	Autosomal-dominant	Increase in Aβ (Aβ42/Aβ40 ratio; essential for γ-secretase activity (?)

The other two genes causing EOFAD are *PSEN1* (14q24.3) and *PSEN2* (1q31-q42), both representing a central component of γ-secretase, the enzyme responsible for originating Aβ from the C-terminal fragment of the APP protein. Mutations in presenilins also alter APP cleavage, leading to an increased production of Aβ42. So far, more than 150 EOFAD causing mutations in *PSEN1* have been identified and approximately 10 additional mutations have been found in the homologous gene *PSEN2* (http://molgen-www.uia.ac.be).

Most variants in *PSEN1* are missense mutations resulting in single amino-acid substitutions. Some are more complex, for example, small deletions or splice mutations. The most severe mutation in *PSEN1* is a donor-acceptor splice mutation that causes a two-aminoacid substitution and an in-frame deletion of exon 9. However, the biochemical consequences of these mutations for γ-secretase assembly seem to be limited (Steiner et al., 1999; Bentahir et al., 2006). All these clinical mutations are likely to cause a specific gain of toxic function for *PSEN1*, determined by an increase of the ratio between Aβ42 and Aβ40 amyloid peptides, thus indicating that presenilins might modify the way in which γ-secretase cuts APP.

Mutations in presenilins occur in the catalytic subunit of the protease responsible for determining the length of Aβ peptides therefore generating toxic Aβ fragments. However, presenilins have also non-proteolytic functions (Baki et al., 2004; Huppert et al., 2005), the disruption of which might also contribute to familial AD pathogenesis.

1.2. SAD

The gene mainly related to the sporadic forms of AD is the Apolipoprotein E (*APOE*; Corder et al., 1993), which is located at chromosome 19q13.32 and was initially identified by linkage analysis (Pericak-Vance et al., 1991). The relationship between APOE and AD has been confirmed in more than 100 studies conducted in different populations. The gene has three different alleles, *APOE*2, APOE*3* and *APOE*4*. The *APOE*4* allele is the variant associated with AD. Longitudinal studies in Caucasian populations have shown that carriers for one *APOE*4* allele have a two-fold increase in the risk for AD (Raber et al., 2004). The risk increases in homozygous for the *APOE*4* allele, and this allelic variant is also associated with an earlier onset of the disease.

Recently, several linkage studies have been performed, giving rise to additional candidate susceptibility loci at chromosomes 1, 4, 6, 9, 10, 12 and 19. In particular, the most promising loci have been found at chromosome 9 and 10 (Grupe et al., 2006; Li et al., 2006).

Also, a large number of candidate genes studies have been performed in order to search a robust risk factor for the sporadic form of the disease. Several studies were mainly focused in genes clearly involved in the pathogenesis of AD such as genes encoding for inflammatory molecules or involved in the oxidative stress cascade, both considered major factors in AD pathology (Table 2). One of the strongest evidence of the role played by genetic variants in inflammatory molecules to increase the risk of AD involves the Interleukin-1 (IL1) complex, which is located at chromosome 2q14-21 and includes *IL1-α, IL1-β,* and IL1R antagonist protein (*IL-1Ra*), all of which have significant polymorphisms found to be associated with AD in several case- controls studies carried out in different populations (Du et al., 2000; Grimaldi et al., 2000; Nicoll et al., 2000). Several polymorphisms in *IL-6,* which is a potent inflammatory cytokine but has also regulatory functions, have been investigated as well. The *IL6* gene is located at chromosome 7p21 and polymorphisms exist in the -174 promoter region and in the region of a variable number of tandem repeats (VNTR), which is located in the 3'untraslated region. Both of them have been found associated with AD in case-controls studies (Papassotiropoulos et al., 1999; Licastro et al., 2003). Investigation of Tumor Necrosis Factor-α (*TNFα*) polymorphisms was initiated because genome screening suggested a putative association of AD with a region on chromosome 6p21.3, which lies within 20 centimorgans of the *TNFα* gene. Furthermore, other polymorphisms located in the promoter region of *TNFα* have been associated with autoimmune and inflammatory diseases (Collins et al., 2000). *α*1-Antichymotrypsin (*ACT*) is an acute-phase reactant produced by activated astrocytes and is elevated in brains affected with AD. A combined effect of *ACT* and *IL1β* polymorphisms has been hypothesized (Licastro et al., 2003).

As with *TNFα*, investigations of the role of α-2macroglobulin (*A2M*) were initiated as a result of screening studies of the genome. In this case, linkage was found in the region of chromosome 1p, where *A2M* and its low-density lipoprotein receptor are found. Blacker et al. (1998) tested for association of polymorphisms with AD showing a strong involvement of this gene in AD.

Very recently, polymorphisms in chemokines have been investigated with regard of susceptibility of AD. In particular, Monocyte Chemoattractant Protein-1 (*MCP-1*) and *RANTES* genes have been widely screened in different neurodegenerative diseases (Huerta et al. 2004). The distribution of the *A-2518G* variant was determined in different AD populations with concordant results (Fenoglio et al., 2004; Combarros et al., 2004a) showing no evidence for association of this variant in AD compared with controls. Moreover, Fenoglio et al. (2004) found a significant increase of MCP-1 serum levels in AD carrying at least one *G* mutated allele. Therefore, the *A-2518G* polymorphism does not seem to be a risk factor for the development of AD, but its presence correlates with higher levels of serum MCP-1.

RANTES promoter polymorphism *-403 A/G*, found to be associated with several autoimmune diseases, was examined in AD population, failing to find significant differences between patients and controls (Huerta et al., 2004).

CCR2 and *CCR5* genes, encoding for the receptors of MCP-1 and RANTES respectively, have been also screened for association with AD. The most promising variants involve a conservative change of a valine with an isoleucine at codon 64 of *CCR2* (*CCR2-64I*) and a 32-bp deletion in the coding region of *CCR5* (*CCR5Δ32*), which leads to the expression of a non-functional receptor. A decreased frequency and an absence of homozygous for the polymorphism *CCR2-64I* were found in AD, thus suggesting a protective effect of the mutated allele on the occurrence of the disease (Galimberti et al., 2004); conversely, no different distribution of the *CCR5Δ32* deletion in patients compared with controls were shown (Galimberti et al., 2004; Combarros et al., 2004b).

Another chemokine recently tested for susceptibility with AD is IP-10. A mutation scanning of the gene coding region has been performed in AD patients searching for new variants. The analysis demonstrated the presence of two previously reported polymorphisms in exon 4 (*G/C* and *T/C*), which are in complete linkage disequilibrium, as well as a novel rare one in exon 2 (*C/T*). Subsequently these SNPs have been tested in a wide case-control study but no differences in haplotype frequencies were found (Venturelli et al., 2006).

Other genes under investigation are related to oxidative stress, a process closely involved in AD pathogenesis. In this regard, genes coding for the nitric oxide synthase (NOS) complex have been screened. The common polymorphism consisting in a *T/C* transition (*T-786C*) in *NOS3*, previously reported to be associated with vascular pathologies, has been tested in AD, but no significant differences with controls were found. Nevertheless, expression of *NOS3* in PBMC either from patients or controls seems to be influenced by the presence of the *C* mutated allele, and is likely to be dose dependent, being mostly evident in homozygous for the mutated variant. The influence of the polymorphism on *NOS3* expression rate supports the hypothesis of a beneficial effect exerted in AD by contributing to lower oxidative damage (Venturelli et al., 2005).

Table 2. Genes claimed to be potential susceptibility or modifier factors for SAD

Gene	Chromosome	Reference
APOE	19q13.32	Corder et al., 1993
IL1-α	2q14-q21	Grimaldi et al., 2000
IL1-β	2q14-q21	Nicoll et al., 2000
IL-1R	2q14-q21	Du et al., 2000
IL-6	7p21	Grimaldi et al., 2000
TNF-α	6p21.3	Collins et al., 2000
ACT	14q32.1	Licastro et al., 2003
A2M	12p13.3-p12.3	Blacker et al., 1998
MCP-1	17q11.2-q12	Fenoglio et al., 2004
RANTES	17q11.2-q12	Huerta et al., 2004
CCR2	3p21.31	Galimberti et al., 2004
CCR5	3p21	Galimberti et al., 2004
IP-10	4q21	Venturelli et al., 2006
NOS3	7q36	Venturelli et al., 2005
NOS1	12q22	Galimberti et al. 2004

An additional variant in *NOS3* gene has been extensively investigated in AD patients, although the results are still controversial. It is a common polymorphism consisting in a single base change (*G894T*), which results in an aminoacidic substitution at position 298 of *NOS3* (Glu298Asp). Dahiyat et al. (1999) determined the frequency of the Glu298Asp variant in a two-stage case-control study, showing that homozygous for the wild-type allele were more frequent in late onset AD. However, studies in other populations failed to replicate these results (Crawford et al.,2000; Sánchez-Guerra et al., 2001; Tedde et al., 2002; Monastero et al., 2003).

Recently Guidi et al (2005) correlated this variant with total plasma homocysteine (tHcy) levels in 97 patients and 23 controls, on the basis of a previous study from Brown et al. (2003) who demonstrated, in two independent healthy populations, that subjects homozygous for the mutation tend to have higher tHcy concentrations compared with Glu/Asp and Glu/Glu subjects.

The Glu/Glu genotype was correlated with higher levels of tHcy, which represent a known risk factor for AD (Seshadri et al., 2002), and its frequency was increased in AD patients (Guidi et al., 2005). Thus the mechanism by which this genotype contributes to increase the risk in developing AD could be mediated by an increase of tHcy.

However, *NOS-1* is the isoform most abundantly expressed in the brain. Recent genetic analyses demonstrated that the double mutant genotype of the synonymous *C276T* polymorphism in exon 29 of the *NOS1* gene represents a risk factor for the development of early onset AD (Galimberti et al., 2005), whereas the dinucleotide polymorphism in the 3'UTR of *NOS1* is not associated with AD (Liou et al., 2002). To date, the promoter region of *NOS1*, located approximately 200 kb upstream of these polymorphism, has not been investigated for susceptibility to AD. Due to this reason and to further explore a possible association of *NOS1* polymorphisms with AD, the distribution of a functional polymorphisms and a variable number of tandem repeats (VNTR) was analyzed very recently in a case-control study, which tested 184 AD patients as well as 144 healthy subjects (Galimberti et al., in press). The functional variant considered is located in exon 1c, which is one of the nine alternative first exons (named 1a-1i), resulting in *NOS1* transcripts with different 5'-untraslated regions (Wang et al., 1999). Three SNPs have been identified in exon 1c, but only the *G-84A* variant displays a functional effect, as the *A* allele decreases the transcription levels by 30% in in-vitro models (Saur et al., 2004). Regarding exon 1f, a variable number of tandem repeats (VNTR) polymorphism has been recently reported in its putative promoter region, termed *NOS1* Ex1f-VNTR. This VNTR is highly polymorphic and consists of different numbers of dinucleotides (B-Q), which, according to their bimodal distribution, have been dichotomized in short (B-J) and long (K-Q) alleles for association studies (Reif et al., 2006). Both Ex1c *G-84A* and Ex1f-VNTR are associated with psychosis and prefrontal functioning in a population of patients with schizophrenia (Reif et al., 2006). Notably, both Ex1c and Ex1f transcripts are found in the hippocampus and the frontal cerebral cortex (Reif et al., 2006), i.e. brain regions implicated in the pathogenesis of schizophrenia as well as AD. The presence of the short *(S)* allele of *NOS1* Ex1f-VNTR represents a risk factor for the development of AD. The effect is cumulative, as in *S/S* carriers the risk is doubled. Most interestingly, the effect of this allele is likely to be gender specific, as it was found in females only. In addition, the *S* allele was shown to interact with the APOE*4 allele both in males and females, increasing the risk to develop AD by more than 10 fold (Galimberti et al., in press). Thus, *NOS1* seems to be a risk factor for AD, but only in female population. This could be explained by a possible interaction with other genes or with additional environmental factors present in females but not males. Epidemiological data indicate that the prevalence of AD is increased in females compared with males. Therefore, it is conceivable that different factors contribute to the development of the pathology in females rather than males, including genetic ones.

2. FRONTOTEMPORAL LOBAR DEGENERATION

Frontotemporal Lobar Degeneration (FTLD) occurs most often in the presenile period, and age at onset is typically 45-65 years, with a mean in the 50s. Distinctive features in FTLD concern behaviour, including disinhibition, loss of social awareness, overeating and impulsiveness. Despite profound behavioural changes, memory is relatively spared (Hou et al., 2004). Conversely to AD, which is more frequent in women, FTLD has an equal distribution among men and women. The current consensus criteria (Neary et al., 1998) identify three clinical syndromes: FTD, Progressive nonfluent Aphasia (PA) and Semantic Dementia (SD), which reflect the clinical heterogeneity of FTLD (Table 3). Frontotemporal dementia is characterized by behavioural abnormalities, whereas PA is associated with progressive loss of speech, with hesitant, nonfluent speech output (Scarpini et al., 2006), and SD is associated with loss of knowledge about words and objects. This variability is determined by the relative involvement of the frontal and temporal lobes, as well as by the involvement of right and left hemispheres (Rosen et al., 2002).

Frontotemporal Lobar Degeneration is a heterogeneous disease characterized by a strong genetic component in its aetiology as up to 40% of patients report a family history of the disease in at least one extra family member (Snowden et al., 2002). In 1994 an autosomal dominantly inherited form of FTD with parkinsonism was linked to chromosome 17q21.2 (Wilhelmsen et al., 1994). Subsequently, other familial forms of FTD were found to be linked to the same region, resulting in the denomination "frontotemporal dementia and parkinsonism linked to chromosome 17" (FTDP-17) for this class of diseases. All cases of FTDP-17 have so far shown a filamentous pathology made of hyperphosphorylated tau protein.

Up to now, seven chromosomal loci have been identified using mainly linkage analysis on chromosomes 3, 9p (two loci), 9q, 17q, 21 (two loci) and 17q24 (Wilhelmsen et al., 1994; Brown et al., 1995; Lendon et al., 1998; Hosler et al., 2000; Wilhelmsen et al., 2004; Vance et al., 2006; Morita et al., 2006). Currently several causal genes mapping in these susceptibility loci have been identified (Table 3).

2.1. Chromosome 17q21

Approximately 15-20% of familial FTLD results from mutations in *MAPT* gene on chromosome 17q21, which encodes the microtubule associated protein tau (Hutton et al., 1998; Poorkaj et al., 1998; Spillantini et al., 1998).

Table 3. Causative genes of familial forms of FTD

Gene	Chromosome	Reference
MAPT	17q21.1	Hutton et al., 1998
PSEN1	14q24.3	Dermaut et al., 2004
PGRN	17q21.31	Baker et al., 2006

Currently, 41 different mutations in the *MAPT* gene have been described in totally 117 families (http://molgen-www.uia.ac.be). *MAPT* mutations are either non-synonimous or deletion, or silent mutations in the coding region, or intronic mutations located close to the splice-donor site of the intron after the alternatively spliced exon 10 (Rademakers et al., 2004).

Mutations are mainly clustered in exons 9-13, except for two recently identified mutations in exon 1 (Rademakers et al., 2002). As regards possible effects on *MAPT* mutations, different mechanisms are involved, depending on the type and location of the mutation. Many of them disturb the normal splicing balance, producing altered ratios of the different isoforms. A number of mutations promote the aggregation of tau protein, whereas others enhance tau phosphorylation (Goedert and Jakes, 2005). Besides pathogenic mutations, several polymorphisms have been reported to date, mostly in intronic regions.

An association between Progressive Supranuclear Palsy (PSP) and a dinucleotide repeat polymorphism in the intron between exons 9 and 10 was described in 1997 (Conrad et al., 1997). The alleles at this locus carry 11 to 15 repeats. Subsequently, two common *MAPT* haplotypes, named H1 and H2, were identified (Baker et al., 1999). They differ in nucleotide sequence and intron size, but are identical at the amino acid level. Homozygosity of the more common allele H1 predisposes to PSP and Corticobasal Degeneration (CBD), but not to AD or Pick Disease (Baker et al., 1999; Di Maria et al., 2000).

Interestingly, there have been reports of numerous families with autosomal dominant FTLD that are genetically linked to the same region of chr17q21 that contains *MAPT* but in which no pathogenic mutations can be identified, despite extensive analysis of this gene (Lendon et al., 1998; Rosso et al., 2001; van der Zee et al., 2006). The neuropathological phenotype in these families was similar to the microvacuolar-type observed in a large proportion of idiopathic FTD cases with ubiquitin immunoreactive neuronal inclusions. Moreover, clinically, the disease in these families was consistent with diagnostic criteria for FTLD (Neary et al., 1998). Sequence analysis of the whole *MAPT* region failed to find a mutation and tau protein appeared normal in these families (Cruts et al., 2005). Moreover the minimal region containing the disease gene for this group of families was approximately 6.2 Mb in physical distance. This region defined by markers D17S1787 and D17S806 is particularly gene rich, containing around 180 genes. Collectively, these data strongly argued against *MAPT* and pointed to another gene. Systematic candidate gene sequencing of all remaining genes within the minimal candidate region was performed and after sequencing 80 genes, including those prioritized on known function, the first mutation in progranulin gene (*PGRN*) was identified. It consists in a 4-bp insertion of *CTGC* between coding nucleotides 90 and 91, causing a frameshift and premature termination in progranulin (C31LfsX34) (Baker et al., 2006). Subsequently, these results have been replicated and improved by Cruts and colleagues (2006), who analyzed other families with a FTLD-U disease without *MAPT* pathology, finding a mutation five base pairs into the intron following the first non coding exon of the *PGRN* gene (IVS0+5G-C). This is predicted to prevent splicing out of the intron 0, leading the mRNA to be retained within the nucleus and subjected to nuclear degradation (Cruts et al., 2006). At present there is no obvious mechanistic link between the mutations in *MAPT* and *PGRN*, currently assuming that their proximity on chromosome 17 is simply a coincidence. Progranulin is known by several different names including granulin, acrogranin, epithelin precursor, proepithelin and prostate cancer (PC) cell derived growth factor (He and Bateman, 2003). The protein is encoded by a single gene on chromosome 17q21, which produces a 593 amino acid, cysteine rich protein with a predicted molecular weight of 68.5 kDa. The full-length protein is subjected to proteolysis by elastase and this process is regulated by a secretory leukocyte protease inhibitor (SLPI) (Zhu et al., 2002). Progranulin and the various granulin peptides are implicated in a range of biological functions including development, wound repair and inflammation by activating signaling cascades that control cell cycle progression and cell motility (He and Bateman., 2003). Excess progranulin appears to promote tumour formation and hence can act as a cell survival signal. Despite the increasing literature on the function of progranulin, its role in neuronal function and survival remains unclear. In the human brain, *PGRN* is expressed in neurons but significantly is also highly expressed in activated microglia (Baker et al., 2006), with the result that *PGRN* expression is increased in many neurodegenerative diseases.

Since the original identification of null-mutations in FTLD in 2006, numerous novel mutations have been reported, spanning most exons, and to date more than 44 *PGRN* mutations have been described (Boeve et al., 2006; Gass et al., 2006; Masellis et al., 2006; Pickering-Brown et al., 2006; Snowden et al., 2006; Bronner et al., 2007; Mesulam et al., 2007; Spina et al., 2007; Benussi et al., in press).

Interestingly, all mutations identified create functional null alleles, with the majority causing premature termination of the *PGRN* coding sequence. This leads to the degradation of the mutant RNA by nonsense mediated decay, creating a null allele (Baker et al., 2006; Cruts et al., 2006). The presence of a null mutation causes a partial loss of functional progranulin protein, which in turn leads eventually to neurodegeneration (haploinsufficency mechanism), although how loss of *PGRN* causes neuronal cell death remains unclear. Estimates of the frequency of *PGRN* mutations in typical FTD patient populations suggests that they account for about 5-10% of all FTD cases, although numbers vary markedly depending on the nature of the populations considered (Cruts et al., 2006; Gass et al., 2006; Snowden et al., 2006).

While there is variability amongst cases, there are some common themes emerging regarding the age at disease onset. The clinical phenotypes of patients with *PGRN* mutations are mainly FTD, PA or CBD. The incidence of motor neuron disease appears to be low if not absent.

Neuropathology analysis revealed that ubiquitin immunoreactive neuronal cytoplasmatic and intranuclear inclusions were present in all cases with FTDP-17, where pathological findings were available (Mackenzie et al., 2006).

Furthermore, soon after the identification of mutations in *PGRN*, biochemical analyses demonstrated that truncated and hyperphosphorylated isoforms of the TAR-DNA binding protein (TDP-43) are major components of the ubiquitin-positive inclusions in families with *PGRN* mutations as well as in idiopathic FTD and a proportion of ALS cases (Neumann et al., 2006). TDP43 is a ubiquitously expressed and highly conserved nuclear protein that can act as a transcription repressor, an activator of exon skipping or a scaffold for nuclear bodies through interactions with survival motor neuron protein. Under pathological conditions, TDP-43 has been shown to relocate from the neuronal nucleus to the cytoplasm, a consequence of which may be the loss of TDP-43 nuclear functions (Neumann et al., 2006). The mechanism by which loss of progranulin leads to TDP-43 accumulation and whether this is necessary for neurodegeneration in this group of diseases is still to be clarified.

In conclusion, the function of progranulin in the brain is currently unclear and why loss of this protein leads to a neurodegenerative diseases in mid-life remains to be established, and its possible role as regulator of a repair activity in the central nervous system, as it is well known to happen in periphery, remains a challenge for science.

2.2. Chromosome 3

In 1995 Brown et al. reported linkage to the pericentromeric region of chromosome 3 in a large multigenerational family with FTLD from Denmark. Nevertheless, the aberrant gene in this family has only recently been identified (Skibinski et al., 2005). It consists in a mutation of the splice acceptor site of exon 6 of *CHMP2B* (charged multivescicular body protein 2B), which is part of the endosomal ESCRTIII-complex (Skibinski et al., 2005). The change from *G* to *C* results in an alteration of the splice acceptor site of exon 6, causing aberrant mRNA splicing of this transcript, which leads to the insertion of 201 base pairs of the intron between exons 5 and 6. In addition, a further transcript was identified, resulting from the use of a cryptic splice site consisting of 10 base pairs from the 5' end of exon 6. Anyway, mutations in *CHMP2B* appear as a rare genetic cause of FTLD mainly due to their rare frequency of occurrence, showing moreover that the *CHMP2B* locus does not increase the risk for FTLD (Rizzu et al., 2006).

2.3. Chromosome 9

The first evidence of linkage in families with Motor Neuron Disease (MND) and FTD was reported by Hosler et al. in 2000 and was addressed to the long arm of chromosome, 9q21-22. Despite the evidence of linkage to chr9q21-22 in several FTD-MND families, the gene responsible for the disease in this locus has yet to be identified and recently the validity of this linkage has been questioned (Hardy et al., 2006). More recently, two papers came up describing separate families with FTLD-MND linked to chromosome 9p (Morita et al., 2006; Vance et al., 2006). As Valosin Containing Protein (VCP) gene had been excluded as a cause of disease in these families, it appeared there are other genes that cause FTLD on the short arm of chromosome 9. The minimal disease region is defined by markers D9S2154 and D9S1791, which is approximately 10.3 Mb in physical size and contains 130 genes. The causal gene in this region has not been identified as well.

2.4. Chromosome 21

Recently, a novel *PSEN1* mutation (Gly183Val), associated with familial FTD neuropathologically characterized by Pick-type tauopathy, and absence of extracellular Aβ plaques was recently reported (Dermaut et al., 2004). Another mutation (M146L), which can also lead to the development of Pick bodies, has been identified by Halliday and colleagues (2005). However, in this particular case, amyloid pathology was also present (Halliday et al., 2005). Furthermore, an insertion at codon 352 of *PSEN-1* in a patient with a clinical diagnosis of FTD was reported (Tang-Wai et al., 2002). Cellular biological investigations into the functional consequences of this mutation demonstrated that it did not increase Aβ-42 levels as other *PSEN-1* mutations do. It was suggested that it could act in a dominant negative manner, decreasing Aβ production by inhibiting γ-secretase cleavage of the β-APP (Atmul et al., 2002).

Zekanowski and colleagues (2006) reported two additional novel *PSEN1* mutations (L226F and L424H) in two patients, one with a clinical diagnosis of FTD but with the typical AD neuropathology, and a second patient with AD but showing frontal lobe signs. Authors suggested that likely the two new *PSEN-1* mutations are indeed pathogenic, causing AD, with presumably an unidentified genetic modifier driving pathology to the frontal and temporal lobes (Zekanowski et al., 2006).

2.5. ApoE

The best well-known risk factor for late onset SAD, Apo E4, has also been considered as a risk factor for sporadic FTLD. A number of studies suggested an association between FTLD and APOE*4 allele (Farrer et al., 1995; Gustafson et al., 1997; Helisalmi et al., 1996; Stevens et al., 1997; Fabre et al., 2001; Bernardi et al., 2006). Other Authors however, did not replicate these data (Geschwind et al., 1998; Short et al., 2002; Riemenschneider et al., 2002). Recent findings demonstrated an association between the *APOE*4* allele and FTLD in males, but not females (Srinivasan et al., 2006), possibly explaining the discrepancies previously reported. An increased frequency of the *APOE*4* allele was described in patients with SD compared to those with FTD and PA (Short et al., 2002).

Concerning the *APOE*2* allele in the development of FTLD, heterogeneous data have been obtained in different populations. Bernardi et al. (2006) showed a protective effect of this allele towards FTLD, whereas other Authors failed to do so (Short et al., 2002; Riemenschneider et al., 2002; Engelborghs et al., 2003; Srinivasan et al., 2006). Despite these results, a recent meta-analysis comprising a total of 364 FTD patients and 2671 controls (CON) demonstrated an increased susceptibility to FTD in *APOE*2* carriers (Verpillat et al., 2002).

REFERENCES

Amtul Z, Lewis PA, Piper S, et al. A presenilin 1 mutation associated with familial frontotemporal dementia inhibits gamma-secretase cleavage of APP and Notch. *Neurobiol Dis* 2002; 9(2): 269–273.

Baker M, Litvan I, Houlden H, et al. Association of an extended haplotype in the tau gene with progressive supranuclear palsy. *Hum Mol Genet* 1999; 8(4): 711-715.

Baker M, Mackenzie IR, Pickering-Brown SM, et al. Mutations in progranulin cause tau-negative frontotemporal dementia linked to chromosome 17. *Nature* 2006; 442: 916–919.

Baki L, Shioi J, Wen P, et al. PS1 activates PI3K thus inhibiting GSK-3 activity and tau overphosphorylation: effects of FAD mutations. *EMBO J* 2004; 23: 2586–2596.

Bentahir M, Nyabi O, Verhamme J, et al. Presenilin clinical mutations can affect ɣ-secretase activity by different mechanisms. *J Neurochem* 2006; 96: 732–742.

Benussi L, Binetti G, Sina E, et al. A novel deletion in progranulin gene is associated with FTDP-17 and CBS. *Neurobiol Aging,* in press.

Bernardi L, Maletta RG, Tomaino C, et al. The effects of APOE and tau gene variability on risk of frontotemporal dementia. *Neurobiol Aging* 2006; 27(5): 702-709.

Bertram L, Tanzi RE. The genetic epidemiology of neurodegenerative disease. *J Clin Invest* 2005; 115(6): 1449-1157.

Blacker D, Wilcox MA, Laird NM, et al. Alpha-2 macroglobulin is genetically associated with Alzheimer disease. *Nat Genet* 1998; 19(4): 357-360.

Boeve BF, Baker M, Dickson DW, et al. Frontotemporal dementia and parkinsonism associated with the IVS1+1G→A mutation in progranulin: a clinicopathologic study. *Brain* 2006; 129: 3103–3114.

Bronner IF, Rizzu P, Seelaar H, et al. Progranulin mutations in Dutch familial frontotemporal lobar degeneration, *Eur J Hum Genet* 2007 15(3): 369–374.

Brown J, Ashworth A, Gydesen S, et al. Familial non-specific dementia maps to chromosome 3. *Hum Mol Genet* 1995; 4: 1625–1628.

Collins JS, Perry RT, Watson B Jr, et al. Association of a haplotype for tumor necrosis factor in siblings with late-onset Alzheimer disease: the NIMH Alzheimer Disease Genetics Initiative. *Am J Med Genet* 2000; 96(6): 823-830.

Combarros O, Infante J, Llorca J, Berciano J. No evidence for association of the monocyte chemoattractant protein-1 (-2518) gene polymorphism and Alzheimer's disease. *Neurosci Lett* 2004a; 360(1-2): 25-28.

Combarros O, Infante J, Llorca J, et al. The chemokine receptor CCR5-Delta32 gene mutation is not protective against Alzheimer's disease. *Neurosci Lett* 2004b; 366(3): 312-314.

Conrad C, Andreadis A, Trojanowski JQ, et al. Genetic evidence for the involvement of tau in progressive supranuclear palsy. *Ann Neurol* 1997; 41(2): 277-281.

Corder EH, Saunders AM, Strittmatter WJ, et al. Gene dose of apolipoprotein E type 4 allele and the risk of Alzheimer's disease in late onset families. *Science* 1993; 261(5123): 921-923.

Crawford F, Freeman M, Abdullah L, et al. No association between the NOS3 codon 298 polymorphism and Alzheimer's disease in a sample from the United States. *Ann Neurol* 2000; 47(5): 687.

Cruts M, Gijselinck I, van der Zee J, et al. Null mutations in progranulin cause ubiquitin-positive frontotemporal dementia linked to chromosome 17q21. *Nature* 2006; 442: 920–924.

Cruts M, Rademakers R, Gijselinck I, et al.Genomic architecture of human 17q21 linked to frontotemporal dementia uncovers a highly homologous family of low-copy repeats in the tau region. *Hum Mol Genet* 2005; 14: 1753–1762.

Dahiyat M, Cumming A, Harrington C, et al. Association between Alzheimer's disease and the NOS3 gene. *Ann Neurol* 1999; 46(4): 664-667.

Dermaut B, Kumar-Singh S, Engelborghs S, et al. A novel presenilin 1 mutation associated with Pick's disease but not beta-amyloid plaques. *Ann Neurol* 2004; 55(5): 617-626.

Di Maria E, Tabaton M, Vigo T, et al. Corticobasal degeneration shares a common genetic background with progressive supranuclear palsy. *Ann Neurol* 2000; 47(3): 374-377.

Du Y, Dodel RC, Eastwood BJ, et al. Association of an interleukin 1 alpha polymorphism with Alzheimer's disease. *Neurology* 2000; 55(4): 480-483.

Engelborghs S, Dermaut B, Goeman J, et al. Prospective Belgian study of neurodegenerative and vascular dementia: APOE genotype effects. *J Neurol Neurosurg Psychiatry* 2003; 74: 1148-1151.

Fabre SF, Forsell C, Viitanen M, et al. Clinic-based cases with frontotemporal dementia show increased cerebrospinal fluid tau and high apolipoprotein E epsilon4 frequency, but no tau gene mutations. *Exp Neurol* 2001; 168: 413–418.

Farrer LA, Abraham CR, Volicer L, et al. Allele epsilon 4 of apolipoprotein E shows a dose effect on age at onset of Pick disease. *Exp Neurol* 1995; 136: 162–170.

Fenoglio C, Galimberti D, Lovati C, et al. MCP-1 in Alzheimer's disease patients: A-2518G polymorphism and serum levels. *Neurobiol Aging* 2004; 25(9): 1169-1173.

Galimberti D, Fenoglio C, Lovati C, et al. CCR2-64I polymorphism and CCR5Delta32 deletion in patients with Alzheimer's disease. *J Neurol Sci* 2004; 225(1-2): 79-83.

Galimberti D, Venturelli E, Gatti A, et al. Association of neuronal nitric oxide synthase C276T polymorphism with Alzheimer's disease. *J Neurol* 2005; 252: 985-986.

Galimberti D, Scarpini E, Venturelli E, et al. Association of a NOS1 promoter repeat with Alzheimer's disease. *Neurobiol Aging,* in press.

Gass J, Cannon A, Mackenzie IR, et al. Mutations in progranulin are a major cause of ubiquitin-positive frontotemporal lobar degeneration. *Hum Mol Genet* 2006; 15(20): 2988–3001.

Geschwind D, Karrim J, Nelson SF, Miller B. The apolipoprotein E epsilon4 allele is not a significant risk factor for frontotemporal dementia. *Ann Neurol* 1998; 44: 134-138.

Goate A, Chartier-Harlin MC, Mullan M, et al. Segregation of a missense mutation in the amyloid precursor protein gene with familial Alzheimer's disease. *Nature* 1991; 349(6311): 704-706.

Goedert M, Jakes R. Mutations causing neurodegenerative tauopathies. *Biochim Biophys Acta* 2005; 1739: 240-250.

Griffin WS. Inflammation and neurodegenerative diseases. *Am J Clin Nutr* 2006; 83(suppl): 470S-474S.

Grimaldi LM, Casadei VM, Ferri C, et al. Association of early-onset Alzheimer's disease with an interleukin-1alpha gene polymorphism. *Ann Neurol* 2000; 47(3): 361-365.

Grupe A, Li Y, Rowland C, Nowotny P, et al. A scan of chromosome 10 identifies a novel locus showing strong association with late-onset Alzheimer disease. *Am J Hum Genet* 2006; 78(1): 78-88.

Guidi I, Galimberti D, Venturelli E, et al. Influence of the Glu298Asp polymorphism of *NOS3* on age at onset and homocysteine levels in AD patients. *Neurobiol Aging* 2005; 26(6): 789-794.

Gustafson L, Abrahamson M, Grubb A, et al. Apolipoprotein-E genotyping in Alzheimer's disease and frontotemporal dementia. *Dement Geriatr Cogn Disord* 1997; 8: 240–243.

Halliday GM, Song YJ, Lepar G, et al. Pick bodies in a family with presenilin-1 Alzheimer's disease. *Ann Neurol* 2005; 57: 139–143.

Hardy J, Momeni P, Traynor BJ. Frontal temporal dementia: dissecting the aetiology and pathogenesis. *Brain* 2006; 129: 830–831.

Hardy J, Selkoe DJ. The amyloid hypothesis of Alzheimer's disease: progress and problems on the road to therapeutics. *Science* 2002; 297(5580): 353-356.

He Z, Bateman A. Progranulin (granulin-epithelin precursor, PC-cell-derived growth factor, acrogranin) mediates tissue repair and tumorigenesis. *J Mol Med* 2003; 81: 600–612.

Helisalmi S, Linnaranta K, Lehtovirta M, et al. Apolipoprotein E polymorphism in patients with different neurodegenerative disorders. *Neurosci Lett* 1996; 205: 61–64.

Hosler BA, Siddique T, Sapp PC, et al. Linkage of familial amyotrophic lateral sclerosis with frontotemporal dementia to chromosome 9q21–q22. *JAMA* 2000; 284: 1664–1669.

Hou CE, Carlin D, Miller BL. Non-Alzheimer's disease dementias: anatomic, clinical, and molecular correlates. *Can J Psychiatry* 2004; 49(3): 164-171.

Huerta C, Alvarez V, Mata IF, et al. Chemokines (RANTES and MCP-1) and chemokine-receptors (CCR2 and CCR5) gene polymorphisms in Alzheimer's and Parkinson's disease. *Neurosci Lett* 2004; 370(2-3): 151-154.

Huppert SS, Ilagan MX, De Strooper B, Kopan R. Analysis of Notch function in presomitic mesoderm suggests a γ-secretase-independent role for presenilins in somite differentiation. *Dev Cell* 2005; 8: 677–688.

Hutton M, Lendon CL, Rizzu P, et al. Association of missense and 5′-splice-site mutations in tau with the inherited dementia FTDP-17. *Nature* 1998; 393: 702–705.

Lendon CL, Lynch T, Norton J, et al. Hereditary dysphasic disinhibition dementia: a frontotemporal dementia linked to 17q21–22. *Neurology* 1998; 50: 1546–1555.

Levy-Lahad E, Wasco W, Poorkaj P, et al. Candidate gene for the chromosome 1 familial Alzheimer's disease locus. *Science* 1995; 269(5226): 973-977.

Li Y, Grupe A, Rowland C, et al. DAPK1 variants are associated with Alzheimer's disease and allele-specific expression. *Hum Mol Genet* 2006; 15(17): 2560-2568.

Licastro F, Chiappelli M. Brain immune responses cognitive decline and dementia: relationship with phenotype expression and genetic background. *Mech Ageing Dev* 2003; 124: 539-548.

Liou YJ, Hong CJ, Liu HC, et al. No association between the neuronal nitric oxide synthase gene polymorphism and Alzheimer's disease. *Am J Med Gen* 2002; 114: 687-688.

Mackenzie IR, Baker M, West G, et al. A family with tau-negative frontotemporal dementia and neuronal intranuclear inclusions linked to chromosome 17. *Brain* 2006; 129: 853–867.

Masellis M, Momeni P, Meschino W, et al. Novel splicing mutation in the progranulin gene causing familial corticobasal syndrome. *Brain* 2006; 129: 3115–3123.

Mesulam M, Johnson N, Krefft TA, et al. Progranulin mutations in primary progressive aphasia: the PPA1 and PPA3 families. *Arch Neurol* 2007; 64: 43–47.

Monastero R, Cefalu AB, Camarda C, et al. No association between Glu298Asp endothelial nitric oxide synthase polymorphism and Italian sporadic Alzheimer's disease. *Neurosci Lett* 2003; 341: 229-232.

Morita M, Al-Chalabi A, Andersen PM, et al. A locus on chromosome 9p confers susceptibility to ALS and frontotemporal dementia. *Neurology* 2006; 66(6): 839–844.

Neary D, Snowden JS, Gustafson L, et al. Frontotemporal lobar degeneration: a consensus on clinical diagnostic criteria. *Neurology* 1998; 51: 1546–1554.

Neumann M, Sampathu DM, Kwong LK, et al. Ubiquitinated TDP-43 in frontotemporal lobar degeneration and amyotrophic lateral sclerosis. *Science* 2006; 314: 130–133.

Nicoll JA, Mrak RE, Graham DI, et al. Association of interleukin-1 gene polymorphisms with Alzheimer's disease. *Ann Neurol* 2000; 47(3): 365-368.

Papassotiropoulos A, Bagli M, Jessen F, et al. A genetic variation of the inflammatory cytokine interleukin-6 delays the initial onset and reduces the risk for sporadic Alzheimer's disease. *Ann Neurol* 1999; 45(5): 666-668.

Pericak-Vance MA, Bebout JL, Gaskell PC Jr, et al. Linkage studies in familial Alzheimer disease: evidence for chromosome 19 linkage. *Am J Hum Genet* 1991; 48(6): 1034-1050.

Pickering-Brown SM, Baker M, Gass J, et al. Mutations in progranulin explain atypical phenotypes with variants in MAPT. *Brain* 2006; 129: 3124–3126.

Poorkaj P, Bird TD, Wijsman E, et al. Tau is a candidate gene for chromosome 17 frontotemporal dementia. *Ann Neurol* 1998; 43: 815–825.

Raber J, Huang Y, Ashford JW. ApoE genotype accounts for the vast majority of AD risk and AD pathology. *Neurobiol Aging* 2004; 25(5): 641-650.

Rademakers R, Cruts M, Dermaut B, et al. Tau negative frontal lobe dementia at 17q21: significant finemapping of the candidate region to a 4.8 cM interval. *Mol Psychiatry* 2002; 7: 1064–1074.

Rademakers R, Cruts M, van Broeckhoven C. The role of tau (MAPT) in frontotemporal dementia and related tauopathies. *Hum Mutat* 2004; 24(4): 277-295.

Reif A, Herterich S, Strobel A, et al. A neuronal nitric oxide synthase (NOS-I) haplotype associated with schizophrenia modifies prefrontal cortex function. *Mol Psychiatry 2006*; 11(3): 286-300.

Riemenschneider M, Diehl J, Muller U, et al. Apolipoprotein E polymorphism in German patients with frontotemporal degeneration. *J Neurol Neurosurg Psychiatry* 2002; 72: 639–641.

Rizzu P, van Mil SE, Anar B, et al. CHMP2B mutations are not a cause of dementia in Dutch patients with familial and sporadic frontotemporal dementia. *Am J Med Genet B Neuropsychiatr Genet* 2006; 141: 944–946.

Rosen HJ, Hartikainen KM, Jagust W, et al. Utility of clinical criteria in differentiating frontotemporal lobar degeneration (FTLD) from AD. *Neurology* 2002; 58: 1608-1615.

Rosso SM, Kamphorst W, de Graaf B, et al. Familial frontotemporal dementia with ubiquitin-positive inclusions is linked to chromosome 17q21–22. *Brain* 2001; 124: 1948–1957.

Rovelet-Lecrux A, Hannequin D, Raux G, et al. APP locus duplication causes autosomal dominant early-onset Alzheimer disease with cerebral amyloid angiopathy. *Nat Genet* 2006; 38: 24–26.

Sánchez-Guerra M, Combarros O, Alvarez-Arcaya A, et al. The Glu298Asp polymorphism in the NOS3 gene is not associated with sporadic Alzheimer's disease. *J Neurol Neurosurg Psychiatry* 2001; 70: 566-567.

Saur D, Vanderwinden JM, Seidler B, et al. Single-nucleotide promoter polymorphism alters transcription of neuronal nitric oxide synthase exon 1c in infantile hypertrophic pyloric stenosis. *Proc Natl Acad Sci* 2004; 101(6): 1662-1667.

Scarpini E, Galimberti D, Guidi I, et al. Progressive, isolated language disturbance: its significance in a 65-year-old-man. A case report with implications for treatment and review of literature. *J Neurol Sci* 2006; 240(1-2): 45-51.

Seshadri S, Beiser A, Selhub J, et al. Plasma homocysteine as a risk factor for dementia and Alzheimer's disease. *New Engl J Med* 2002; 346: 476-483.

Sherrington R, Rogaev EI, Liang Y, et al. Cloning of a gene bearing missense mutations in early-onset familial Alzheimer's disease. *Nature* 1995; 375(6534): 754-760.

Short RA, Graff-Radford NR, Adamson J, et al. Differences in tau and apolipoprotein E polymorphism frequencies in sporadic frontotemporal lobar degeneration syndromes. *Arch Neurol* 2002; 59: 611–615.

Skibinski G, Parkinson NJ, Brown JM, et al. Mutations in the endosomal ESCRTIII-complex subunit CHMP2B in frontotemporal dementia. *Nat Genet* 2005; 37: 806–808.

Snowden JS, Neary D, Mann DM. Frontotemporal dementia. *Br J Psychiatry* 2002; 180: 140–143.

Snowden JS, Pickering-Brown SM, Mackenzie IR, et al. Progranulin gene mutations associated with frontotemporal dementia and progressive non-fluent aphasia. *Brain* 2006; 129: 3091–3102.

Spillantini MG, Murrell JR, Goedert M, et al. Mutation in the tau gene in familial multiple system tauopathy with presenile dementia. *Proc Natl Acad Sci USA* 1998; 95: 7737–7741.

Spina S, Murrell JR, Huey ED, et al., Clinicopathologic features of frontotemporal dementia with Progranulin sequence variation. *Neurology* 2007; 68(11): 820–827.

Srinivasan R, Davidson Y, Gibbons L, et al. The apolipoprotein E epsilon4 allele selectively increases the risk of frontotemporal lobar degeneration in males. *J Neurol Neurosurg Psychiatry* 2006; 77: 154-158.

Steiner H, Romig H, Grim MG, et al.The biological and pathological function of the presenilin-1 dExon 9 mutation is independent of its defect to undergo proteolytic processing. *J Biol Chem* 1999; 274: 7615–7618.

Stevens M , van Duijn CM, de Knijff P, et al. Apolipoprotein E gene and sporadic frontal lobe dementia. *Neurology* 1997; 48: 1526–1529.

Tang-Wai D, Lewis P, Boeve B, et al. Familial frontotemporal dementia associated with a novel presenilin-1 mutation. *Dement Geriatr Cogn Disord* 2002; 14: 13–21.

Tanzi RE, Gusella JF, et al. Amyloid beta protein gene: cDNA, mRNA distribution, and genetic linkage near the Alzheimer locus. *Science* 1987; 235(4791): 880-884.

Tedde A, Nacmias B, Cellini E, et al. Lack of association between NOS3 polymorphism and Italian sporadic and familial Alzheimer's disease. *J Neurol* 2002; 249: 110-111.

van der Zee J, Rademakers R, Engelborghs S, et al. A Belgian ancestral haplotype harbours a highly prevalent mutation for 17q21-linked tau-negative FTLD. *Brain* 2006; 129: 841–852.

Vance C, Al-Chalabi A, Ruddy D, et al. Familial amyotrophic lateral sclerosis with frontotemporal dementia is linked to a locus on chromosome 9p13.2–21.3. *Brain* 2006; 129: 868–876.

Venturelli E, Galimberti D, Fenoglio C, et al. Candidate gene analysis of IP-10 gene in patients with Alzheimer's disease. *Neurosci Lett* 2006; 404(1-2): 217-221.

Venturelli E, Galimberti D, Lovati C, et al. The T-786C NOS3 polymorphism in Alzheimer's disease: association and influence on gene expression. *Neurosci Lett* 2005; 382(3): 300-303.

Verpillat P, Camuzat A, Hannequin D, et al. Apolipoprotein E gene in frontotemporal dementia: an association study and meta-analysis. *Eur J Hum Genet* 2002; 10: 399–405.

Wang Y, Newton DC, Robb GB, et al. RNA diversity has profound effects on the translation of neuronal nitric oxide synthase. *Proc Natl Acad Sci USA* 1999; 96(21): 12150-12155.

Wilhelmsen KC, Forman MS, Rosen HJ, et al. 17q-linked frontotemporal dementia-amyotrophic lateral sclerosis without tau mutations with tau and alpha-synuclein inclusions. *Arch Neurol* 2004; 61: 398–406.

Wilhelmsen KC, Lynch T, Pavlou E, et al. Localization of disinhibition–dementia–parkinsonism–amyotrophy complex to 17q21–22. *Am J Hum Genet* 1994; 55: 1159–1165.

Zekanowski C, Golan MP, Krzysko KA, et al. Two novel presenilin 1 gene mutations connected with frontotemporal dementia-like clinical phenotype: genetic and bioinformatic assessment. *Exp Neurol* 2006; 200(1): 82-88.

Zhu J, Nathan C, Jin W, et al. Conversion of proepithelin to epithelins: roles of SLPI and elastase in host defense and wound repair. *Cell* 2002; 111: 867–878.

Chapter 16

EPIDEMIOLOGY OF DEMENTIA IN A FRENCH SPEAKING POPULATION: HIGH AGE-RELATED VARIABILITY OF SIMPLE BEDSIDE TESTS EFFICIENCIES

J.C. Bier [1]*, H. Slama [2], D. Van den Berge [2],
P. Fery [2] and M. Vokaer [1]

[1] Department of Neurology;
[2] Department of Neuropsychology – ERASME Hospital –
Université Libre de Bruxelles - Brussels – Belgium

ABSTRACT

We evaluated, from April 2001 to March 2007, the sensitivity and specificity of our French version of the Addenbrooke's Cognitive Examination (ACE), to detect dementia in the less than 66 year-old patient's population attending our outpatient's memory clinic. Validation of the French ACE has already been published but not assessed specifically on younger patients. The 149 included subjects had at least six months of follow-up. The diagnosis of a specific dementing illness was based on the consensus of the neurologist and neuropsychologists in the team. In this population of young patients, the sensitivity for diagnosing dementia with an MMSE score ≤ 24/30 was 59,5 %. The sensitivity of an MMSE score ≤ 27/30 was 83,8 % with a specificity of 88,6 %. The sensitivity of an ACE score ≤ 83/100 was 86,5 % with a specificity of 86 %, and the sensitivity of an ACE score ≤ 88/100 was 94,6 % with a specificity of 74,6 %. Three hundred thirty-nine patients older than 66 year-old were then selected identically. In this older population, the sensitivity for diagnosing dementia with an MMSE score ≤ 24/30 was 40,2 % while the sensitivity of an MMSE score ≤ 27/30 was 67,1 % with a specificity of 73,9 %. The sensitivity of an ACE score ≤ 83/100 was 84,6 % with a specificity of 73 %, and the sensitivity of an ACE score ≤ 88/100 was 94,4 % with a specificity of 47,8 %. We conclude that the French version of the ACE remains a very accurate test for the

---

* Jean-Christophe Bier, Hôpital Erasme, Service de Neurologie 3ème étage, 808 route de Lennik, 1070 Bruxelles, Belgium ;Email: Jean-Christophe.Bier@ulb.ac.be

detection of dementia in the youngest but that its benefit in comparison to MMSE is more intense in the older population.

INTRODUCTION

The Addenbrooke's Cognitive Examination (ACE)[1], has been proposed as a simple and effective instrument to detect dementia. It is used in Cambridge for a decade, and adopted in international sites from five continents[1-6].

The French ACE was validated on a general dementia population but its sensitivity and specificity to detect dementia in the youngest has not yet been investigated.

Age is however a crucial factor in development and prognosis of dementia. Indeed, younger subjects with MCI progressed to dementia at longer follow-up intervals than elderly subjects did. This is probably due to an earlier stage of the disease but it is also possible that the rate of progression of the neurodegenerative process is slower in younger subjects[7]. Symptoms of frontotemporal lobar degeneration (FTLD) classically begin at a lower age than Alzheimer's disease (AD)[8]. Moreover, epidemiologic studies have suggested that FTLD is the commonest cause of dementia in patients younger than 65, with a prevalence equivalent to that of AD[9]. Similar prevalence and increase of progression speed have been observed in the youngest in case of dementia associated with Lewy bodies (DLB)[10].

Education delays dementia diagnosis and argues this way for the cognitive reserve theory[11,12] confirming some prognosis variability of age onset.

METHODS

The Instrument

The French ACE has been previously validated and can be administered in 15 to 20 minutes[2,3].

Patients and Procedure

The ACE was administered to patients who were followed-up by one of the authors (J-C.B.) at the ERASME Hospital Memory Clinic every 3 to 12 months between April 2001 and March 2007. Patients were subjected to clinical, radiological (CT or MRI), and blood test investigations. All of them underwent standard neuropsychological test batteries, including the Raven progressive matrix (PM38), orientation in time and space, digit span, the Groeber and Buschke selective reminding task, an informal investigation of verbal expression and comprehension, a line-drawings naming task, verbal fluency tasks (P, R, animals, fruits), clock drawing, the Rey complex figure, the Trail Making test, the Stroop word-color interference test, the Tower of London and the Wisconsin Card Sorting test. The diagnosis of a specific dementing illness was based on the consensus of the neurologist and neuropsychologists in the team, who used evidence from all clinical and investigational results. Patients were retrospectively subdivided into two subgroups with 66 years old as cut-off value. Thereafter, in both groups (youngest and oldest) patients were classified in two categories, demented and non-demented according to Diagnostic and Statistical Manual of mental disorders, (DSM-III-R)[13]. The diagnosis of AD was based on National Institute of Neurological and Communicative Disorders and Stroke-AD and Related Disorders Association Criteria[14]. Patients who were diagnosed as FTLD fulfilled the clinical criteria of the Work Group on Frontotemporal Dementia and Pick's Disease[15] while the diagnosis of Dementia associated with Lewy Bodies (DLB) was based on the criteria published by McKeith et al[16]. Brain PET and/or SPECT scan were performed in all cases with a clinical diagnosis of FTLD and DLB

RESULTS

Four hundred and forty eight cases were included in the study. One hundred and forty nine were in the youngest group (33,3%). In this population younger than 66 years old, 112 subjects (75,2%) were found to be non-demented: 66 had a mood disorder with cognitive deterioration (58,9%), 8 had mild cognitive impairment (7,1%), 22 had no pathology (19,6%), 2 had primary progressive aphasia (1,8%), 3 had toxic cognitive impairments (2,7%), 5 had traumatic cognitive impairments (4,5%) and 6 had posttraumatic stress disorders (5,4%). Thirty-seven patients (24,8%) were diagnosed with a dementing illness: 16 with AD (43,2%), 5 with FTLD (13,6%), 2 with DLB (5,4%), 6 with vascular dementia (16,2%), 2 with mixed dementia (5,4%), 2 with toxic dementia (5,4%) and 4 with dementia from other causes (10,8%). Epidemiological data, MMSE and ACE scores of this youngest population are shown in table 1. In this population of young patients, the sensitivity for diagnosing dementia with an MMSE score ≤ 24/30 was 59,5 %. The sensitivity of an MMSE score ≤ 27/30 was 83,8 % with a specificity of 88,6 %. The sensitivity of an ACE score ≤ 83/100 was 86,5 % with a specificity of 86 %, and the sensitivity of an ACE score ≤ 88/100 was 94,6 % with a specificity of 74,6 %. Three hundred thirty-nine patients older than 66 years old were identically selected. In this population, 115 (33,9%) were found to be non-demented: 34 had a mood disorder with cognitive deterioration (29,6%), 37 had mild cognitive impairment (32,2%), 38 had no pathology (33%), 4 had primary progressive aphasia (3,5%), and 2 had hypothyroid cognitive disorder (1,7%). Two hundred and twenty-four patients (66,1%) were diagnosed with a dementing illness: 78 with AD (34,8%), 23 with FTLD (frontal form) (10,3%), 25 with DLB (11,2%), 41 with vascular dementia (18,3%), 39 with mixed dementia (17,4%), 2 with toxic dementia (0,9%) and 16 with dementia from other causes (7,1%). Epidemiological data, MMSE and ACE scores of this oldest group are shown in table 2. In this older population, the sensitivity for diagnosing dementia with an MMSE score ≤ 24/30 was 40,2 %. The sensitivity of an MMSE score ≤ 27/30 was 67,1 % with a specificity of 73,9 %. The sensitivity of an ACE score ≤ 83/100 was 84,6 % with a specificity of 73 %, and the sensitivity of an ACE score ≤ 88/100 was 94,4 % with a specificity of 47,8 %.

Table 1. Epidemiological data (younger than 65 years old)

		N	Gender	Age	MMSE			ACE		
			W	Year ; SD	Mean ; SD	> 24	≤ 24	Mean ; SD	> 83	≤ 83
Non-demented	Mood disorder	66	45	55,6 ; 7,1	29 ; 1,3	64	2	89,3 ; 6,9	58	8
	Normal	22	12	57,3 ; 4,5	28,7 ; 1,8	22	0	89,2 ; 8,9	22	0
	MCI	8	4	53,3 ; 7,6	28,1 ; 1,1	8	0	89,3 ; 6,9	6	2
	Toxic	3	3	52,3 ; 6,8	29,7 ; 0,6	3	0	93 ; 2	3	0
	Traumat	5	0	47,6 ; 6,9	28,2 ; 1,5	5	0	86,8 ; 9,8	3	2
	PTSD	6	5	38,5 ; 11,2	28,7 ; 1,8	6	0	89,2 ; 8,9	4	2
	PPA	2	0	60,5 ; 3,6	23,5 ; 4,9	1	1	64 ; 25,5	0	2
Demented	AD	16	11	57,4 ; 6	23,2 ; 3,2	6	10	68,4 ; 12	2	14
	FTLD	5	0	64 ; 18,9	22,2 ; 3,6	1	4	52 ; 9,3	1	4
	DLB	2	1	70,5 ; 2,1	22 ; 1,4	0	2	58,5 ; 2,1	0	2
	VaD	6	1	62,2 ; 19,9	25,3 ; 2,7	4	2	57,8 ; 5,5	0	6
	Mixed dementia	2	1	78 ; 19,8	24 ; 5,7	1	1	49 ; 18,4	1	1
	Toxic	2	0	72 ; 5,7	24 ; 5,7	1	1	60 ; 7,1	0	2
	Other	4	1	68,2 ; 16	24 ; 4,2	2	2	63,3 ; 3,5	1	3

N = number of patient; W = women; SD = standard deviation; MMSE = mini mental state examination; ACE = Addenbrooke's cognitive examination; MCI = mild cognitive impairment; PTSD: post traumatic stress disorder; PPA = pure progressive aphasia; AD = Alzheimer's disease; FTLD = frontotemporal lobar degeneration; DLB = dementia associated with Lewy bodies; VaD= vascular dementia

Table 2. Epidemiological data (older than 65 years old)

		N	Gender W	Age Year ; SD	MMSE Mean ; SD	>24	≤24	ACE Mean ; SD	>83	≤83
Non-demented	Mood disorder	34	20	73,8 ; 4,5	28,2 ; 1,7	32	2	73,8 ; 4,5	24	10
	Normal	38	23	76,2 ; 5	28,8 ; 1,9	36	2	90,1 ; 7,4	36	2
	MCI	37	15	77,2 ; 5,4	27,2 ; 2,3	33	4	83,5 ; 7,4	22	15
	Hypothyroid	2	2	68,5 ; 2,1	27 ; 0,0	2	0	88,5 ; 7,8	1	1
	PPA	4	2	77 ; 6,7	27 ; 1,4	4	0	82,3 ; 5,4	1	3
Demented	AD	78	58	77,7 ; 5,9	24,6 ; 2,6	47	31	70,6 ; 1,1	9	69
	FTLD	23	8	74,7 ; 4	25,7 ; 2,5	15	8	73,1 ; 12,2	5	18
	DLB	25	17	72,2 ; 11,1	24,8 ; 2,6	13	12	76 ; 5,6	4	21
	VaD	41	20	78,3 ; 5,5	25,9 ; 2,8	30	11	73,4 ; 13,5	12	29
	Mixed dementia	39	22	77,9 ; 5,5	24,2 ; 2,9	17	22	67,8 ; 13,2	4	35
	Toxic	2	0	71 ; 2,8	27 ; 2,8	2	0	83 ; 0,0	0	2
	Other	16	6	76,4 ; 5,8	25,2 ; 2,6	10	6	72,6 ; 12,6	2	14

N = number of patient; W = women; SD = standard deviation; MMSE = mini mental state examination; ACE = Addenbrooke's cognitive examination; MCI = mild cognitive impairment; PPA = pure progressive aphasia; AD = Alzheimer's disease; FTLD = frontotemporal lobar degeneration; DLB = dementia associated with Lewy bodies; VaD= vascular dementia.

DISCUSSION

Our results are concordant with other observations[1-6]. We confirm the good sensitivity of an ACE score $\leq 83/100$ to detect dementia in the youngest (86,5%) and the oldest (84,6%). Specificity was especially good at 86%, in the youngest for 79% in patients older than 66-years old. Similarly, our sensitivity to detect dementia with an MMSE score $\leq 27/30$ was better than previously reported in our youngest subgroup (83,8%) but not in the oldest (67,1%) one. However in our youngest population, an MMSE score $\leq 27/30$ was highly specific (88,6%) to dementia syndromes with a much lower specificity in the oldest (73,9%). This is in part due to the possible bias of selection induced by the specialization of our memory clinic. Furthermore, this specialization explains the weak proportion of AD in our oldest demented population. Additionally, there could be an impact of the inclusion of depressed patients in ours series. Indeed, depression could have more impact on cognitive functions in older patients. In clinical practice, depression is often associated with, and may precede degenerative dementia[17] and the acuity of a single test to detect dementia has thus, in our opinion, to be confronted to cases of depression. Noteworthy, the youngest consults more easily psychiatrist than the oldest. We could therefore observe more mood disorders in our oldest population than in the youngest one. In the ACE, despite the absence of consideration of the age, education and ethnicity of the evaluated patients, the sensitivity and specificity of the test was good but clearly unequal, at least, in front of age. This could also be due to a ceiling effect in the oldest population or to a floor one in the youngest. In conclusion, the French version of the ACE remains a very accurate test for the detection of dementia in the youngest but its benefit in comparison to MMSE is more intense in the older population.

REFERENCES

[1]   Mathuranath PS, Nestor PJ, Berrios GE, Rakowicz W and Hodges JR. A brief cognitive test battery to differentiate Alzheimer's disease and frontotemporal dementia. *Neurology* 2000; 55: 1613-20.

[2]   Bier JC, Ventura M, Donckels V, Van Eyll E, Claes T, Slama H, Fery P, Vokaer M, Pandolfo M. "Is the Addenbrooke's Cognitive Examination effective to detect frontotemporal dementia?" *Journal of Neurology* 2004, 251: 428-431.

[3]   Bier JC, Donckels V, Van Eyll E, Claes T, Slama H, Fery P, Vokaer M. The French Addenbrooke's Cognitive Examination is effective to detect dementia in French speaking population. *Dementia and Geriatric Cognitive Disorders* 2005, 19(1): 15-17.

[4]   Diego Sarasola; María De Luján Calcagno; Liliana Sabe; Lucia Crivelli; T. Torralva; M. Roca; Alejandro García Caballero; Facundo Manes. El Addenbrooke's Cognitive Examination en español para el diagnóstico de demencia y para la diferenciación entre enfermedad de Alzheimer y demencia frontotemporal. *Revista de Neurologia* 2005; 41(12): 717.

[5]   H Bak, T T Rogers, L M Crawford, V C Hearn, P S Mathuranath, J R Hodges. Cognitive bedside assessment in atypical parkinsonian syndromes. *Journal of Neurology Neurosurgery and Psychiatry* 2005; 76: 420-422

[6]   Garcia-Caballero A, Garcia-Lado I, Gonzalez-Hermida J, Recimil M, Area R, Manes F, Lamas S, Berrios G. Validation of the Spanish version of the Addenbrooke's Cognitive Examination in a rural community in Spain. *Int. J. Geriatr. Psychiatry* 2006 Mar; 21(3): 239-45.

[7]   Pieter Jelle Visser, Arnold Kester, Jellemer Jolles, and Frans Verhey. Ten-year risk of dementia in subjects with mild cognitive impairment. *Neurology.* 2006; 67: 1201-1207

[8]   E.D. Roberson, J.H. Hesse, K.D. Rose, H. Slama, J.K. Johnson, K. Yaffe, M.S. Forman, C.A. Miller, J.Q. Trojanowski, J.H. Kramer, and B.L. Miller. Frontotemporal dementia progresses to death faster than Alzheimer disease. *Neurology.* 2005; 65: 719–725.

[9]   J.R. Hodges, R. Davies, J. Xuereb, J. Kril, and G. Halliday. Survival in frontotemporal dementia. *Neurology* 2003; 61: 349–354.

[10]   Monique M. Williams, Chengjie Xiong, John C. Morris and James E. Galvin. Survival and mortality differences between dementia with Lewy bodies vs Alzheimer disease. *Neurology.* 2006; 67: 1935-1941.

[11]   Soininen and M. Kivipelto T. Ngandu, E. von Strauss, E. -L. Helkala, B. Winblad, A. Nissinen, J. Tuomilehto, H. Education and dementia: What lies behind the association? *Neurology.* 2007; 69: 1442-1450.

[12]   D. S. Knopman, J. A. Lucas, T. J. Ferman, N. Graff-Radford and R. J. I G. E. Smith, V. S. Pankratz, S. Negash, M. M. Machulda, R. C. Petersen, B. F. Boeve.A plateau in pre-Alzheimer memory decline: Evidence for compensatory mechanisms? *Neurology.* 2007; 69: 133-139.

[13]   American Psychiatric Association. Diagnostic and Statistical Manual of Mental Disorders. 3. Washington DC: American Psychiatric Association; 1980.

[14]   Mc Kahnn G, Drachman D, Folstein M, Katzman R, Price D, Stadlan EM. Clinical diagnosis of Alzheimer's disease: report of the NINCDS-ADRDA Work Group under the auspices of Department of Health and Human Services Task Force on Alzheimer's Disease. *Neurology.* 1984; 34: 939-944.

[15]   Mc Kahnn G, Albert M, Grossman M, Miller B, Dickson D, Trojanowski JQ; Work Group on Frontotemporal Dementia and Pick's Disease. Clinical and Pathological Diagnosis of Frontotemporal Dementia: report of the Work Group on Frontotemporal Dementia and Pick's Disease. *Arch. Neurol.* 2001; 58: 1803-1809.

[16]   McKeith IG, Galasko D, Kosaka K, Perry EK, Dickson DW, Hansen LA, Salmon DP, Lowe J, Mirra SS, Byrne EJ, Lennox G, Quinn NP, Edwardson JA, Ince PG, Bergeron C, Burns A, Miller BL, Lovestone S, Collerton D, Jansen EN, Ballard C, de Vos RA, Wilcock GK, Jellinger KA, Perry RH. Consensus guidelines for the clinical and pathological diagnosis of dementia with Lewy bodies (DLB): report of the consortium on DLB international workshop. *Neurology.* 1996; 47: 1113-1124.

[17]   Bier JC, Fery P, Ellincx S, Claes T, Ventura M, Goldman S. Depression may mimic the clinical and metabolic patterns of degenerative diseases. *Alzheimer's report,* 2002; 5: 41-44.

INDEX

B

C

E

H

N

S

X

W

Y